Errors of Omission

Errors

of

Omission

HOW MISSED NURSING CARE IMPERILS PATIENTS

Beatrice J. Kalisch, PhD, RN, FAAN

American Nurses Association
Silver Spring, Maryland
2015

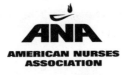

The American Nurses Association is the only full-service professional organization representing the interests of the nation's 3.4 million registered nurses through its constituent/state nurses associations and its organizational affiliates. The ANA advances the nursing profession by fostering high standards of nursing practice, promoting the rights of nurses in the workplace, projecting a positive and realistic view of nursing, and by lobbying the Congress and regulatory agencies on healthcare issues affecting nurses and the public.

American Nurses Association
8515 Georgia Avenue, Suite 400
Silver Spring, MD 20910-3492
1-800-274-4ANA
http://www.Nursingworld.org

Library of Congress Cataloging-in-Publication Data
Kalisch, Beatrice J., 1943- , author.
 Errors of omission : how missed nursing care imperils patients / by Beatrice J. Kalisch.
      p. ; cm.
 Includes bibliographical references and index.
 ISBN 978-1-55810-631-4
 I. American Nurses Association, issuing body. II. Title.
 [DNLM: 1. Nursing Care—standards. 2. Medical Errors—nursing. 3. Nurse's Role. 4. Nursing Staff, Hospital—organization & administration. 5. Patient Harm. WY 100.1]
 R729.8
 610.289—dc23
                                    2015029770

The research reported in this book was largely supported by the Blue Cross Blue Shield Foundation of Michigan.

ISBN-13: 978-1-55810-631-4 SAN: 851-3481 1.0K   11/2015R
Second printing: November 2015

This book is dedicated to staff nurses everywhere, my heroes

Contents

PART 2: STRATEGIES TO DECREASE MISSED NURSING CARE

Acknowledgments

The research completed for this book would not have been possible without many people and several organizations. The ideas for the research reported in this book came from staff nurses and managers in many hospitals where it was my privilege to serve as a consultant. In particular, the vice president for nursing, Millie Curley, RN, MS, of Parrish Medical Center in Titusville, Florida, who supported the work wholeheartedly and stuck in there when the going got rough. Not too many nurse leaders have shown the vision that she exhibited. I feel honored to have worked beside her. Also very instrumental in the success of this work were the contributions of her direct reports— Susan Stefanov, Kathy Myer, Joann Chapman, Donna Shearer, Pat Hurley, Deb Landers, Deb Lindemuth, and the nursing staff throughout the hospital. All of these dedicated and talented people were absolutely instrumental in identifying the problem of missed nursing care and developing solutions to decrease missed nursing care. It was my privilege to conduct numerous interviews and focus groups with the staff and managers, to observe them while they worked, to facilitate workshops for strategic planning, to provide managers with leadership training, and to participate in committee work with the staff and managers.

Second, funding for many of the studies reported in this book was provided by the Blue Cross Blue Shield Foundation of Michigan. Nora Maloy, PhD, program officer, gave vital support and facilitation for this work. Without this Foundation's support, this work would not have been completed.

Third, I want to thank the three organizations and their leaders that selected me to be the 2013–2014 distinguished nurse scholar in residence at the Institute of Medicine, Washington, D.C.: The American Academy of Nursing (Cheryl Sullivan), the American Nurses Foundation (Kate Judge), and the American Nurses Association (Marla Weston). All three of these individuals went out of their way to help me. Part of the requirements for the fellowship includes a project and this book was the result of my project. The year in Washington, D.C., was a tremendous opportunity for me to bring the research on missed nursing care and teamwork together in one volume and to develop strategies to move missed nursing care onto the policy agenda.

Fourth, my faculty colleagues at the University of Michigan who worked with me on various aspects of this research over the past 10 years were absolutely critical. Dana Tschannen, RN, PhD, collaborated with me in the early years to conceptualize the research, collect and analyze the data, and publish the results. Ada Sue Hinshaw, RN, PhD, former dean, participated in the development of a concept analysis of missed nursing care. Reg Williams, RN, PhD, was essential in the development and psychometric testing of the *MISSCARE Survey*. Chris Friese, RN, PhD, offered advice throughout the projects and coauthored several publications. AkkeNeel Talsma, RN, PhD, conducted research on missed nursing care in the perioperative area and contributed a chapter to this book on the subject. Michelle Aebersold also collaborated on several studies.

Another person who made a substantial contribution to this research was Gay Landstrom, RN, PhD, who was the chief nurse for Trinity Health in Livonia, Michigan and is now chief nurse at Dartmouth Hitchcock Medical Center in New Hampshire. She gathered the data for the first study of three hospitals and participated in the concept analysis, tool development, and data analysis. PhD students Suzanne Begeny Miyamoto, Christine Anderson, Henna Lee, Seung Hee Choi, Monica Rochman, Kyung Hee Lee, Ronald Piscotty, Beverly Dabney, Rhonda Schoville, Peg Mclaughlin, Sung Hee Choi, and Boqin Xie served as data collectors and analysts applying their outstanding analytics skills and knowledge to this research as well as to the writing of results. Ron Piscotty studied the use of electronic health record reminders on the incidence of missed nursing care for his dissertation and authored the chapter in this book on technological solutions. All of these students, most of whom have graduated, are truly awesome nurse researchers who will undoubtedly continue to make significant and important contributions to nursing science in the years to come. A number of master's degree students in the Nursing Business and Health Systems program at the University of Michigan participated in data collection and analysis including Laura Shakarjian, RN, MS; Susan Wright, RN, MS; Julie Juno, RN, MS; Kate Gosselin, RN, DNP, MS; Aimee Elizabeth Labelle, RN, MS; and Katherine Russell, RN, MS. Without their contributions, this research would not have been possible. I am very indebted to them. A special thanks to Sarah Lane, RN, MS, nurse manager, who opened her unit to the testing of interventions and to all of the managers in the over 130 patient care units in my studies for their willingness to participate and for their facilitation of the research. I am also grateful to Eduardo Salas, PhD, Professor & Trustee Chair, University of Central Florida, the author of the theory upon which my teamwork studies are built, for his ongoing assistance and support. His student, Sallie J. Weaver, PhD, was also very helpful.

In addition, a number of international colleagues were outstanding to work with and made the countries comparison possible. These include:

University of Iceland, Reykjavik, Iceland: Helga Bragadottir RN, PhD; Sigridur Briet Smaradottir, Cand. Psych.; and Heiður Hrund Jonsdottir MS

Hacettepe University, Ankara, Turkey: Fusun Terzioglu, RN, PhD; Sergul Duygulu, RN, PhD; and Cigdem Yucel, RN, PhD

Lebanese American University, Beirut, Lebanon: Myrna Doumit, RN, PhD, and Joanna El Zein, RN, MSN

University of São Paulo, Ribeirão Preto, Brazil: Maria Helena Larcher Caliri, RN, PhD; Lillian Dias Castilho Siqueira, RN, MS; and Rosana Aparecida Spadoti Dantas

Princess Alexandra Hospital, Brisbane, Australia: Kerri Holzhauser, RN, MS, and Liz Burmeister, RN, MS, PhD

Kyngpook National University, Daegu, South Korea: Eunjoo Lee, RN, PhD

Azienda Ospedaliera Policlinico di Modena, the Italian Missed Care Study Group, Modena, Italy: Annamaria Ferraresi, Luisa Sist, Anna Bandini, Stefania Bandini, Carla Cortini, Massa Licia Massa, and Roberta Zanin.

I have many wonderful memories of my visits to their countries and feel very fortunate to have had them as collaborators. The quality of their participation was superb.

Last, but definitely not least, I want to give a special thanks to Betsy Hetrick, RN, MS, who painstakingly reviewed every word in every chapter, correcting errors and ensuring appropriate style. I am also thankful to Erin Walpole, the American Nurses Association editor assigned to this book, for also reading every word many times and substantially improving it. And, Joe Vallina, CAE, publisher for the American Nurses Association. Finally, thanks to Philip and Melanie, my son and daughter, whose love and affection continuously sustain me.

Introduction

The content of this book addresses the problem of missed nursing care (standard, required care that is not provided), ramifications of missed nursing care, and strategies to decrease missed nursing care. The research underlying this book was the result of listening to nursing staff members and observing them at work over several years. Thanks to all of you for your contributions to this research. Addressing missed nursing care is a part of the overall patient safety movement which began to receive attention when the Institute of Medicine (IOM) published *To Err is Human* in 1999. This ground-breaking study reported that there were close to 100,000 unnecessary and preventable deaths each year due to errors made in the delivery of health care. Up to this point, there was a tendency to ignore errors or even to cover them up. Patients and families were not always told that something had gone wrong.

The IOM report recommended creating an environment where it is safe to report errors, meaning that errors would not lead to punishment as in the past. Only by openly reporting errors can the causes be identified and solutions developed to avoid them in the future. The report strongly recommended that the culture of blame present in most healthcare organizations be replaced with a culture of safety and teamwork where providers feel safe to disclose their mistakes, challenge authority, and ask questions of others. This report also underlined the importance of teamwork in achieving patient safety.

This early work in patient safety focused primarily on errors of commission (e.g., amputating the wrong leg, giving too high a dosage of a medication or one the patient is allergic to, etc.). But there are also **errors of omission**, such as omitting surveillance, not administering ordered medications, not preparing the patient and family for discharge, not ambulating, not teaching patients and families, and so forth. In fact, the Agency for Healthcare Research and Quality (AHRQ) states that there are likely more errors of omission than commission. A study of the parenteral drug administration for 1,328 patients in 113 intensive care units (ICUs) in 27 countries, 861 errors affecting 441 patients were identified. Three-quarters of those errors were classified as errors of omission (Valentin et al., 2009). In a study conducted in U.S. Department of Veterans Affairs Hospitals, errors averaged 4.7 per case, of which 95.7% represented problems of underuse (for example, inadequate diagnostic testing and the failure to obtain sufficient data from histories and physical examinations). Of the 2,917 errors uncovered in this study, 27 (97%) were rated as highly serious and 26 of these (96%) were errors of omission (Hayward et al., 2005).

The "omission bias" where nurses and other providers would rather do nothing than do something that causes harm contributes to errors of omission. Both of these actions—providing or not providing care—potentially cause harm, but not giving care is considered more acceptable. For example, a nurse may feel that it would be better to not ambulate a patient than to have the patient fall in the process.

Like healthcare providers in general, nurses have been reluctant to report their own and coworkers' errors. Somehow nurses, at least when they first start to practice, believe they should be able to practice for 40 or 50 years and almost never make a mistake. I vividly remember the first mistake I made, and I was fully convinced I could not be a nurse because of it.

Nurses carry a heavy sense of guilt and experience moral distress when their patients do not receive all the care they need. In fact, the more nursing care that is missed, the higher the rate of job dissatisfaction and intent to leave their current position or occupation. Nurses want to do a good job! Because of these feelings and the culture of blame that still exists in many healthcare organizations, nurses do not readily discuss the nursing care they miss or other mistakes they make. But just like any error, unless it is acknowledged and the causes examined, the problem will not be fixed. At my presentations of this research, nurses often come up afterward and thank me for bringing this issue out in the open. They refer to it as a hidden secret. Regret and self-blame are palpable.

One of the key strategies for addressing the problem of missed nursing care is teamwork. Building a safety culture requires teamwork. Basic human behaviors lead to the normal competitiveness and pride among members of work groups and often result in defensive statements about how someone else is the problem. Nurses and other healthcare providers need to believe that if anyone fails, the whole organization or patient care unit fails. Leaders need to emphasize the word "we" instead of "they." For example one RN says: "Why do you have 4 patients and I have 5?" This comment demonstrates that the most important concern of this nurse is probably herself and her workload, not the team and the patients who need care. If collective orientation is present, the response would be "We have 9 patients to take care of. How can we work together to get the work done?"

Hand washing is another opportunity for team accountability. Many staff members believe if they wash their own hands, that is the end of their responsibility. But they are also accountable for hand washing by everyone else on the team (if they witness it). If a teammate (e.g., nurse, physical therapist, physician, etc.) does not wash their hands and no one brings it to that person's attention, the teammates are not fulfilling their responsibilities. Everyone makes mistakes and it takes a team to catch each other's errors. The patient care unit staff needs to see themselves as a team which must work together and help each other to yield safe and successful outcomes. Teamwork is essential to decreasing errors including missed nursing care.

The book is divided into two sections. Part one presents the findings of the research conducted on how much nursing care is missed in the United States and in seven other countries. It also reports the reasons for missing nursing care and the impact of not completing care on patients, nursing staff, and organizations. Finally, it reports on several studies of nursing teamwork. Part two contains strategies for decreasing missed care including culture change, leadership, teamwork, patient and family engagement, and technology. Taken all together they offer the reader an in-depth view of errors of omission in nursing care and ways to diminish their frequency.

Who Should Read This Book?

This book will be worthwhile to a wide range of audiences including staff nurses, nurse executives and managers in acute and long-term care, nursing faculty and students in nurse preparation programs, healthcare administrators and chief executives of acute and long-term care facilities, researchers, physicians and other healthcare providers (e.g., pharmacy, respiratory, physical and occupational therapy, etc.), and policy makers.

Staff nurses and managers will find this book very valuable in their work of providing safe, quality nursing care. It identifies areas of missed nursing care, the consequences of not providing care, methods of monitoring and studying it, and the importance and the role of management and leadership in addressing the issue of missed nursing care. Staff nurses and managers will find the strategies outlined in the book helpful in decreasing missed nursing care in their team or organization.

The basic nurse preparation program curricula in most schools of nursing does not include content and practice in what to do when a mistake is made. Students in nursing schools, physicians, pharmacists, physical therapists, and other providers who read this book will be exposed to the high value and impact of nursing care and the problems associated with not providing it. They will gain an understanding of the science behind nursing care. Researchers will be able to identify topics in need of additional study. For example, there is a large gap in research on the impact of basic nursing care and on interventions to decrease missed nursing care. They will also learn the language of explaining the value of nursing to others, such as hospital administrators, financial officers, legislators, and congressmen, to name a few.

Administrators who read this book will gain an appreciation of the work of nurses and the difference it makes for patient and staff outcomes, thus providing a basis for resource allocation decisions. This book will give them insight into how to balance the costs and benefits. Nurse leaders, lobbyists, professional association executives, and others will also find this book useful in documenting the importance and impact of nursing care or the lack of it as they advocate for resources and policy.

There is a tendency to diminish the importance of nursing ("So what if the patient isn't ambulated or doesn't eat for a day? What's the big deal?"). This book contains evidence that nursing care is a big deal. It also provides a strong reminder of the value of nursing care. Even nurses often lose sight of the importance of their work, given the stereotypes of nursing as the "lower half of medicine," the poor media portrayals of nursing, and other factors which diminish the true importance and contributions of nurses and nursing care. What if all the nurses in the world took a day off? What would be the consequences? The impact would be far greater, and more detrimental than if all the members of other occupations took a day off. A day without lawyers, a day without accountants, a day without professors for example, would not result in the same level of harm and suffering as a day without nurses. There are three nurses for every physician, thus a day without physicians, while disastrous, would probably not be as detrimental as a day without nurses. Nurses are an indispensable and exceedingly valuable contributor to the health and well-being of society. What nurses do and the difference they make must be recognized and supported to ensure that this essential resource is available in future years and for decades to come.

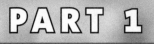

PART 1

THE PROBLEM

Patient Safety: Errors of Omission

A Patient Experience

The U.S. healthcare delivery system does not consistently provide high-quality nursing care to all citizens who need it. The public should be able to count on receiving at least the standard required nursing care that meets their needs and is based on evidence—yet, research shows us that this is not the case. Nursing care routinely fails to deliver its potential benefits. Indeed, between the nursing care that we now experience and the nursing care that we could have, there exists not just a gap, but what the Institute of Medicine has called a chasm.

How different the view of the hospital is from the bed of a patient. Suddenly, the paradigm is flipped, and the insights revealed about hospital care can be quite astounding. It is toward this end that I am sharing my experience as an inpatient for seven days in an acute care hospital. I was hospitalized out of town. The following does not describe everything that happened, but includes some of the major gaps in my care.

First Impressions: The Emergency Department (ED)

Arriving at the Emergency Department as most patients do, I was triaged. Not knowing what was wrong with me, just that I was in intense pain, I immediately suggested an EKG to the triage nurse. I was placed on a stretcher in the hall (no room was available) for the EKG and remained there for over two and half hours during which the only contact with staff was when my friend asked for an emesis basin which was handed to her; this staff member, who I assume was an RN, didn't even look my way. This nurse was assigned to me but she never presented herself, despite my obvious and intense pain. My friend noted that during this time, several staff members were laughing and talking at the desk.

Finally, I was moved into an ED room. I mentioned to the nurse that she must be really busy. She replied rather briskly, giving me the impression that I was off-base: "You're lucky; yesterday it was a six-hour wait." The care I received once in the room in the ED was good. They started a morphine IV, sent me for a CT scan, and diagnosed my problem as pancreatitis.

Then, I was told that I was to be transferred to an inpatient unit. My pain was coming back; the morphine was wearing off. I asked the nurse if I could have pain medication before being transferred to the unit, knowing that once on the unit, an assessment would need to be made by the nurse and physician orders would need to be obtained before I could receive pain medication. She said "Honey, you will get it when you get to the unit." Thirty minutes later, my pain was getting worse and the transporter had not shown up to take me to the unit. I asked again for pain medication and the nurse repeated that I would receive medication on the unit. Another half hour passed and no one came to take me to the unit; I asked for pain medication and again met with the same response from the ED staff. At that point, I asked when I was going to be transferred and wondered out loud if one of the ED techs could take me. Apparently, they realized at that point that I had waited a very long time for transportation (I wonder when it would have dawned on them if I had not asked the question). They decided to give up on the transporter and finally had a tech take me up 45 minutes later. As my ED room was across from the nurses' station, I noted during my two or more hour wait that the staff were gathered at the desk, laughing and talking. So much for my first impressions!

Second Impression: On the Unit
On the unit, in my room, I waited for what seemed like an intermi-
nable time and I was in very intense pain. A nursing assistant finally
came in and I asked for pain medication once again. She apparently
let the nurse know because the nurse came in with the computer to
do my assessment. Her first comment was "No one let us know you
were here!" I again asked for pain medication, and she predictably
said she couldn't give me anything until she finished her assessment.
I said, "Well, can we hurry?" She was pleasant and moved through the
process quickly. After another period of time, a nurse came in with
pain medication. She said, "I have overridden the Pyxis to get this
and I can only do it one time." I am not sure why she said this but my
internal response was, "Shame on me; I am getting special favors that
are a great inconvenience to the staff. And don't ask again! I hope this
kills my pain!"

The Hospitalists
Since I was out of town, the hospitalists were my sole physicians,
except for one referral to a gastroenterologist. Over the course of the
hospital stay, I estimated that I had five different hospitalists. The first
one came into my room after I was admitted to the unit and said,
"Your pain is not exactly in the right place." I was miserable and far
from the problem-solving mode. I wondered what he wanted to do.
Then he said that I would be on IVs, and I could have a catheter if I
wanted it so I wouldn't have to get up to go to the bathroom. I rose out
of the bed and said, "NO!" That would be all I needed—a urinary tract
infection and more immobility. That was my last glimpse of a hospitalist for another three days. I asked the nurse why no one had come
in to see me and she said, "Oh, he was here. Maybe you were sleeping."
    Several days into the hospitalization, a referral was made to a
gastroenterologist and he ordered an upper GI for the next morning.
When I arrived in the diagnostic area, the nurse questioned me several
times about my pain location and finally said that I didn't have to have
the procedure if I didn't want to. What if it was a pulmonary embolism (PE)? Not being fully capable of decision-making, to say the least,
this was alarming, and I was not sure what to do. She was trying to
tell me something. My oxygen saturation rate was low at 85. She was
obviously coaching me. When the physician came back in, I asked
him what the implications of me having a possible PE with the procedure he was about to do. He said, "I shouldn't put you under anesthesia for two hours if that is the case." Instead he ordered a CT scan

where they found pneumonia. He mentioned that it was probably hospital-acquired. I never had the procedure.

Nursing Care

In order to describe the nursing care on the medical unit I was on for seven days, I have presented it in the following categories of basic care, psychosocial care, and discharge planning. Since I was too sick to evaluate medication doses or accuracy of IVs, I assume that everything was correct and on time, but given the other nursing care I received, I was anxious that there could be errors.

Basic care. As far as hygiene care, there was practically none. Being on nothing by mouth (NPO), my mouth was extremely dry and my lips were crusted (worse than I had ever experienced). I asked for ice chips but was told I couldn't have them. I asked for mineral oil and received one small tube to apply myself. When I asked for more, they gave me a disposable mouth care packet with two swabs to stick into a cup of water which sat there for 36 hours until I asked for fresh water. I knew I should not use the same swabs over and over, but no one offered additional ones and I was too sick to ask. It seemed low on the priority list at that point.

I had only two baths (showers) during the seven days, and the second one I insisted upon (the day I was discharged). When I rang to go to the bathroom, the staff came in a reasonable time but they repeatedly scolded me that I was making "a mess" of my tubes, which took them time to straighten out. After about the fifth time, I said, practically in tears, "I am not doing it on purpose." Shortly afterwards, the nurse came in with a Velcro cord she had taken off of the computers to tie the tubes together. I felt heard at that point.

Ambulation was also totally absent throughout the hospitalization. I turned myself and got up into the chair on my own whenever I could, but no one came to get me out of bed, much less ambulate me, through the entire hospital stay. After several days, I felt good enough to think about the need to walk, and I started out down the hall but the staff said, "No, you have to have your oxygen," and chased me back to my room. So, I went back to my room, thinking they would come and assist me to ambulate but they never did, and I felt too sick to do anything about it. There was no physical therapy ordered either. Consequently, it took seven weeks after discharge in costly physical therapy for me to become conditioned again.

The issue of hand washing was revelatory. I searched the room for Purell and finally found it over in front of my roommate's bed that was closest to the window (an odd place). I wondered why it was located so far out of the way. The staff would have had to walk in front of me to use it, and I saw only one staff member do that. I wondered if there was a sink outside my room and assumed there was because the thought that my caretakers were not washing their hands was too frightening to contemplate. Later, when I was moved to another room, I saw that there was no such sink and wondered what infections I might have acquired.

Intake and output documentation was scant at best. I often told the staff that I had used the toilet, but I didn't see anyone measure it. I was concerned because I was aware that my output was extremely low. When I told them, they did not seem concerned. I also had received too much fluid, which was inhibiting my breathing (along with the pneumonia).

Emotional support. In terms of what I will call psychological support, staff did not listen to me on repeated occasions. In the midst of all of this missed nursing care, I had one excellent nurse intervention. I was hallucinating and asked the nurse if I could talk with her. She sat down by my bed, and I told her I was seeing things. She said: "You are exhausted. Your roommate is going to be out of the room for two hours, and we will put a sign on the door to not disturb you and you can get two hours of sleep." After that I had no more mental disturbances.

Discharge planning/teaching. Through all of the hospital days, no one mentioned anything about post-discharge arrangements until the day before I finally did leave. On the sixth day, a hospitalist I had never seen before came into the room and stood by the door (as far away from me as she could get), and said, "You are being discharged today." I looked at the clock, saw that it was 10:30 a.m., and asked when that would be. She said by noon. I felt panicked. The best way to describe my discomfort was an extreme bloating sensation in my chest and stomach (from over-hydration). I had also gained 15 pounds without eating or drinking much of anything. My Sat rate without oxygen was still 85%, and I had pitting edema on my ankles. I had been on oxygen 24 hours a day.

Since I was out of town and felt absolutely horrible, I was very confused as to what to do. I very much wanted to get back home, but I couldn't imagine how I would make it. I expressed my concern to the nurse who said, "Well, you can't stay here just because you don't feel good. Most people want to go home for Christmas." My thoughts were "Not me, I want to spend Christmas right here in this wonderful environment!" I also thought "If I am discharged, I know I will have to come back to the ED and go through that terrible experience again. I am not sure I can make it."

Then, I received a phone call from the social worker with whom I had never had contact before this point in time. She said she lived an hour away and didn't want to come in. She stated, "You need to leave the hospital today." Somehow I felt I had been labeled a deadbeat of some kind. Her first question was "Where did you come from?" I answered a hotel. I said I had to get a plane reservation—frankly I was confused and anxious as to what to do. She said, "Can you go back there (hotel)?" I said they didn't have a restaurant. She quickly, without listening and without giving me a chance to say what I was worried about, levied several more questions. Since they knew I was in town to get my mother into assisted living, she asked "Can you go to your mother's home?" "Can you go to assisted living?" "Maybe you can go to the assisted living your mother is going to go to. You have to leave the hospital. We have several places you can go but you can't stay in the hospital." At that point, my anxiety was skyrocketing. I was also angry (why did they wait until now to discuss this with me?). I was so frustrated that this social worker was not giving me a chance to say anything and that she would not even listen to me. I just hung up, which is something I never do.

About 30 minutes later, the nurse came in again and said, "Just because you hung up doesn't mean you can stay here. The doctor wants me to tell you that you can't stay in the hospital just because you don't feel well. You haven't been getting out of bed and walking." Now it was my fault that I was deconditioned, not the fact that ambulation had been entirely omitted in my care.

At that point the respiratory therapist appeared and saw my distress. She subsequently walked me down the hall and stayed with me for over an hour, recognizing my frustration and trying to help me deal with my anxiety. I told her I had a friend that I could stay with for a short time but her husband was very sick, and I was afraid that if I went there feeling the way I did, she would need to bring me back to the ED. It appeared that she was helpless to keep me in the hospital but she arranged for oxygen to be delivered to my friend's house and for oxygen to take on the airplane.

My friend came to the hospital and she was clearly worried about taking me home in the condition I was in. She asked the staff why I had gained 15 pounds—she knew something was wrong with me. At this point, I had reached my wit's end and asked to see the administrator in charge. They sent the house supervisor who came in and said, "You don't have to leave until midnight" as if that was going to solve my problem of being barely able to get out of bed. My friend asked her about the weight gain and she looked puzzled. My friend talked to the supervisor for about a half hour, pleading for help with this situation.

I asked the nurse if I should have Lasix for what I felt was excess fluid. She said, "We are afraid of the side effects." I asked "Is there anything I can take?" basically pleading for help. She answered, "You are a nurse; you know the answer to that." I thought, "What do I not remember. Everyone, except my friend, seems to think there is no problem."

At 7 p.m., this same nurse (going off-duty, I presume) came in and said they decided to keep me another day and I would receive Lasix . She said the night nurse would administer it, which occurred three hours later. I was thinking, "I wish she would have given it to me earlier," since I imagined I would not be able to sleep getting up to the bathroom all night. I voided more than 1,500 ccs in the next several hours (although the staff did not measure my output and did not ask me about it). I felt like a new person and was able to be discharged (without oxygen).[1]

There were major gaps in my care including lack of surveillance, missed nursing care, shaming and blaming, not being listened to, lack of discharge planning, and poor practices. To begin, there were gaps in surveillance. In the ED, I was ignored until I was placed in a room. No one checked on me for over two hours as I lay there waiting in pain. Then, when I was to be transported to the unit for admission, I waited unattended another few hours in pain while they repeatedly said, "You will get pain medication when you get to the unit." The transport to the unit occurred 45 minutes after I suggested that a tech in the ED could take me (the ordinary patient would not have the information to know what was causing the delay—unavailable transporters). How long I would have been there had I not intervened is unknown. Once I got to the unit, my nurse was not notified of my presence and didn't come into my room for another hour. Meanwhile, my pain was escalating. This gave me little confidence that my nursing staff were observing me. Just the opposite; I seemed invisible wherever I went!

Care was missed repeatedly. Missed nursing care, defined as any aspect of required patient care that is omitted (either in part or in whole) or delayed, is the subject of this book and was the area of research I had been working on for some time before this incident. Basic care was virtually nonexistent—ambulating, turning, monitoring intake and output, bathing, mouth care, and so forth. These were important to my well-being and are truly patient safety issues—acts of omission.

Another element of missed care was emotional support. It was not just the lack of support; the staff seemed to have a strong need to control their patients. Not being listened to by the staff proved to be a prevailing theme. Repeatedly, the staff communicated that they knew what was best and it didn't matter what I said. It was not until I asked to see an administrator on the sixth day that someone (the house supervisor) looked at the situation from my point of view and arranged for me to receive Lasix and stay in the hospital another day. There were many instances of blaming me for problems, such as not ambulating, and telling me I should know, since "after all you are a nurse." (I kept it a secret as long as I could but somehow the dean of the local school of nursing found out I was hospitalized and came to visit me. Much later she told me she talked to them about the lack of care I was receiving.) The lack of preparation for discharge was remarkable. This experience underlined the critical importance of planning for discharge early in the hospital stay.

It took me weeks, even months, to process and recover from the entire experience. I could not even write about it for a year. Although there were instances of excellent nursing care, on the whole, it was severely lacking. If nursing care had been up to standard, my illness would still have been trying, but perhaps I would not have contracted pneumonia (from poor mouth care practices, no ambulation, etc.), become debilitated, experienced feelings of shame, and run the risk of infection; I could have avoided the associated stress and anxiety. Although this could, conceivably, be a rare occurrence, I am afraid it is not. These gaps in care, or errors of omission, are not only unsafe but are also costly to the healthcare system.

The Patient Safety Movement

In 1999, *To Err is Human* was published by the Institute of Medicine (IOM). This study, which reported that tens of thousands of patients die each year as a result of preventable mistakes in their care, launched a national, and later worldwide, movement to increase patient safety and decrease errors. Following this study, the IOM published *Crossing the Quality Chasm: A New Health System for the 21st Century* (2001). This study called for a total revamping of the current healthcare system, and the need for innovative approaches for caring for patients. It called for major changes to the healthcare system's processes to improve the level of quality and safety. It also explored potential ways in which the required changes could be implemented. These two documents were instrumental in raising patient safety to be viewed as a major concern in health care and among policymakers.

In addition, a large number of reports, in what is referred to as the Quality Chasm Series, were issued that addressed leadership, systems issues, the health workforce, medication errors, priorities, academic health centers, health literacy, partnership with engineering, and others.

One of these reports was devoted to nursing: *Keeping Patients Safe: Transforming the Work Environment of Nurses* (2004). The report is significant for three reasons:

1. It documents the key role that nurses play in patient safety and makes specific recommendations for changing their work environments to improve patient safety.

2. It highlights the role that an organization's governing boards, executive leadership, other management personnel, and practices play in patient safety by shaping organizational work environments.

3. It identifies generic workplace processes and characteristics that threaten or protect patient safety, not just with respect to nurses' actions, but by affecting the actions of all healthcare practitioners.

Keeping Patients Safe identifies eight overarching safeguards to protect patient safety that need to be in place within all healthcare organizations: (1) organizational governing boards that focus on safety; (2) the practice of evidence-based management and leadership; (3) effective nursing leadership; (4) adequate staffing; (5) provision of ongoing learning and clinical decision-making support to nursing staff; (6) mechanisms that promote interdisciplinary collaboration; (7) work design practices that defend against fatigue and unsafe work; and (8) a fair and just error reporting, analysis, and feedback system with training and rewards for patient safety (Table 1.1).

Patient Errors

Errors are classified in a number of ways. One way that they are classified is to view them as underuse, overuse, or misuse. Overuse refers to providing care that potentially could harm the patient more than the expected benefit. Giving antibiotics for a viral infection like a cold, for which antibiotics are ineffective, constitutes overuse. Adverse reactions and the development of increases in antibiotic resistance

TABLE 1.1.   Necessary patient safeguards in the work environment of nurses.

Governing Boards That Focus on Safety
• Are knowledgeable about the link between management practices and patient safety.
• Emphasize patient safety to the same extent as financial and productivity goals.

Leadership and Evidence-Based Management Structures and Processes
• Provide ongoing vigilance in balancing efficiency and patient safety.
• Demonstrate and promote trust in nursing staff.
• Actively manage the process of change.
• Engage nursing staff in nonhierarchical decision-making and work design.
• Establish the organization as a "learning organization."

Effective Nursing Leadership
• Participates in executive decision-making.
• Represents nursing staff to management.
• Achieves effective communication between nurses and other clinical leadership.
• Facilitates input from direct-care nursing staff into decision-making.
• Commands organizational resources for nursing knowledge acquisition and clinical decision-making.

Adequate Staffing
• Is established by sound methodologies as determined by nursing staff.
• Provides mechanisms to accommodate unplanned variations in patient care workload.
• Enables nursing staff to regulate nursing unit workflow.
• Is consistent with best available evidence on safe staffing thresholds.

Organizational Support for Ongoing Learning and Decision Support
• Uses preceptors for novice nurses.
• Provides ongoing educational support and resources to nursing staff.
• Provides training in new technology.
• Provides decision support at the point of care.

Mechanisms That Promote Interdisciplinary Collaboration
• Use interdisciplinary practice mechanisms, such as interdisciplinary patient care rounds.
• Provide formal education and training in interdisciplinary collaboration for all healthcare providers.

Work Design That Promotes Safety
• Defends against fatigue and unsafe and inefficient work design.
• Tackles medication administration, hand washing, documentation, and other high-priority practices.

Organizational Culture That Continuously Strengthens Patient Safety
• Regularly reviews organizational success in achieving formally specified safety objectives.
• Fosters a fair and just error-reporting, analysis, and feedback system.
• Trains and rewards workers for safety.

Source: Reprinted with permission from *Committee on the Work Environment for Nurses and Patient Safety, 2004*, pages 16–17, by the National Academy of Sciences, Courtesy of the National Academies Press, Washington, D.C.

are potential harms. Misuse occurs when an appropriate process of care has been selected but a preventable complication occurs and the patient does not receive the full potential benefit of the care. Avoidable complications of surgery or medication use are misuse problems. A patient who suffers a rash after receiving penicillin for strepthroat, despite having a known allergy to that antibiotic, is an example of misuse. A patient who develops a pneumothorax after an inexperienced operator attempts to insert a subclavian line would represent another example of misuse. Underuse refers to the failure to provide a healthcare service or nursing intervention when it would have produced a favorable outcome for a patient. Missed nursing care is an error of underuse.

Another way to classify errors is as active and latent. Active errors occur at the point of contact between a human and some aspect of a larger system (e.g., a human–machine interface). They are generally readily apparent (e.g., ignoring an alarm). Active failures are sometimes referred to as errors at the sharp end, figuratively referring to a scalpel. Errors at the sharp end are made by frontline staff or providers closest to the patient. This person may figuratively or literally be holding a scalpel (e.g., a nurse administering the wrong dose of a medication or a surgeon operating on the wrong eye). Latent errors (or latent conditions), on the other hand, refer to fewer apparent failures of the system that contributed to the errors that occur. Latent errors are those at the other end of the scalpel—the blunt end—referring to the policies, management practices, design of medical devices, and other people and forces, which, despite being removed in time and space from direct patient care, nonetheless affect how care is delivered. For example, when a nurse fails to give a medication because it has not been made available by the pharmacy, or when the wrong amount of IV fluid is administered because of a manufacturer's mistake in programming the IV pump.

Errors can also be dichotomized as either slips or mistakes. Slips refer to failures of schematic behaviors or lapses in concentration (e.g., overlooking a step in a routine task such as urinary catheterization because of a lapse in memory). Slips occur when there are competing sensory or emotional distractions, fatigue, and stress. Reducing the risk of slips requires paying attention to the designs of procedures, medical devices, and work environments—using checklists so key steps are not omitted, not allowing high-risk work by staff who are fatigued, eliminating interruptions and other distractions—in areas where work requires intense concentration (e.g., medication administration).

Slips can be contrasted with mistakes, which are failures that occur in attentional behavior such as active problem-solving. Rather than lapses in concentration (as with slips), mistakes typically involve insufficient knowledge or the failure to correctly interpret available information, such as a nurse who gives the wrong dose of a medication. Mistakes often reflect lack of experience or insufficient training. Unfortunately, health care has typically responded to all errors as if they were mistakes, with remedial education or added layers of management. Most errors are actually slips, which are failures that occur because of distractions, fatigue, stress, or emotional states.

Errors of Commission versus Errors of Omission

Errors are also classified as errors of commission and errors of omission. Acts of commission (doing something wrong) or omission (failing to do the right thing) can both lead to undesirable outcomes. For a nurse, administering a medication to a patient with a documented allergy to that medication would be an act of commission, while not giving the medication at all is an act of omission. Acts of omission are believed to be greater in number than acts of commission (Hayward, Asch, Hogan, Hofer, & Kerr, 2005).

In a study conducted in 12 U.S. Department of Veterans Affairs Hospitals, errors averaged 4.7 per case, of which 95.7% represented problems of underuse (for example, inadequate diagnostic testing and the failure to obtain sufficient data from histories and physical examinations). Of the 2,917 errors uncovered in this study, 27 were rated as highly serious and 26 were errors of omission (Hayward et al., 2005). In a 2009 report regarding the administration of parenteral drugs to 1,328 patients in 113 intensive care units (ICUs) in 27 countries, 861 errors affecting 441 patients were identified, and three quarters of the errors were classified as errors of omission (Valentin et al., 2009).

The Missed Nursing Care Model

Nursing quality care and patient safety are major challenges facing nurses and nurse leader today. Although the relationship between the level and type of nurse staffing and patient outcomes is well-established, it is unclear what other variables shape the quality of nursing care, and ultimately, patient outcomes (Needleman et al., 2011; Cho, Ketefian, Barkauskas, & Smith, 2003; Kane, Shamliyan, Mueller, Duval, & Wilt, 2007; Mark & Harless, 2007). Missed nursing care has been developed and studied to determine what happens in the process of nursing care or the black box of nursing care.

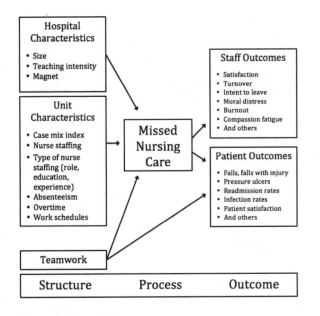

FIGURE 1.1   **The Missed Nursing Care Model.**

The Missed Nursing Care Model serves as a conceptual framework for this book (Figure 1.1). This framework is based on Donabedian's structure, process, and outcome framework (Donabedian, 1988). This model hypothesizes that hospital, unit, and staff characteristics (structure variables) lead to missed nursing care (process variable), which in turn affects outcomes.

Structure variables include hospital, patient unit, and individual characteristics. Nursing staff characteristics include gender, age, education, experience levels, job title, and work schedules. The unit characteristics are the type of unit (i.e., medical–surgical, rehabilitation, intermediate, intensive care unit, etc.), staffing levels and type, case mix index, and teamwork. Hospital variables include size, ownership, teaching intensity, and Magnet status.

The process variable is missed nursing care. Quality measures of the process of nursing care in acute care hospitals are lacking. We can access input variables (the process of nursing care) such as staffing levels, type of hospital, and staff characteristics, and we can evaluate certain output variables such as patient falls, pressure ulcers, and infection rates. What we struggle to measure is the process, or black box, of nursing care. If we cannot systematically evaluate the process of nursing care, we will not be able to develop interventions to improve it.

The two outcomes of this Model are separated as relating to patient outcomes (e.g., falls, pressure ulcers, infection rates, readmission rates, etc.) and staff outcomes (i.e., job satisfaction, occupation satisfaction, intent to leave, and turnover).

The Missed Nursing Care Model postulates a number of relationships: missed nursing care predicts job and occupation satisfaction, intent to leave, and turnover; missed nursing care predicts patient outcomes; staffing levels and type predict missed nursing care; teamwork predicts missed nursing care; Magnet status predicts missed nursing care; size of hospital predicts teamwork; type of patient unit predicts missed nursing care; and so forth. These relationships will be the subject of this book.

Summary

In this chapter, an illustration with a personal experience is used to introduce types of errors, including errors of omission and commission. The history of the patient safety movement, initiated by the first book in the chasm series, *To Err is Human*, is traced. Finally, the Missed Care Nursing Model, used to test the contributors and results of missed nursing care, is presented.

References

Cho, S. H., Ketefian, S., Barkauskas, V. H., & Smith, D. G. (2003). The effects of nurse staffing on adverse events, morbidity, mortality, and medical costs. *Nursing Research, 52*(2), 71–79.

Committee on Engineering and the Health Care System, Institute of Medicine, & National Academy of Engineering. (2005). *Building a better delivery system: A new engineering/health care partnership*. Washington, DC: National Academies Press.

Donabedian, A. (1988). The quality of care. How can it be assessed? *Journal of the American Medical Association, 260*(12), 1743–1748.

Hayward, R. A., Asch, S. M., Hogan, M. M., Hofer, T. P., & Kerr, E. A. (2005). Sins of omission: Getting too little medical care may be the greatest threat to patient safety. *Journal of General Internal Medicine, 20*(8), 686–691.

Institute of Medicine. (1999). *To err is human: Building a safer health system*. Washington, DC: National Academies Press.

Institute of Medicine. (2001). *Crossing the quality chasm: A new health system for the 21st Century*. Washington, DC: National Academies Press.

Institute of Medicine. (2002). *Leadership by example: Coordinating government roles in improving health care quality*. Washington, DC: National Academies Press.

Institute of Medicine. (2003). *Fostering rapid advances in health care: Learning from system demonstrations.* Washington, DC: National Academies Press.

Institute of Medicine. (2003). *Health professions education: A bridge to quality.* Washington, DC: National Academies Press.

Institute of Medicine. (2003). *Priority areas for national action: Transforming health care quality.* Washington, DC: National Academies Press.

Institute of Medicine. (2004). *Academic health centers: Leading change in the 21st century.* Washington, DC: National Academies Press.

Institute of Medicine. (2004). *Patient safety: Achieving a new standard of care.* Washington, DC: National Academies Press.

Institute of Medicine. (2004). *The 1st annual Crossing the Quality Chasm summit: A focus on communities.* Washington, DC: National Academies Press.

Institute of Medicine. (2006). *Performance measurement: Accelerating improvement.* Washington, DC: National Academies Press.

Institute of Medicine. (2007). *Preventing medication errors.* Washington, DC: National Academies Press.

Institute of Medicine. (2007). *The learning healthcare system. Workshop summary.* Washington, DC: National Academies Press.

Institute of Medicine. (2007). *The state of quality improvement and implementation research: Expert views. Workshop summary.* Washington, DC: National Academies Press.

Institute of Medicine. (2008). *Knowing what works in health care: A roadmap for the nation.* Washington, DC: National Academies Press.

Institute of Medicine. (2008). *Training the workforce in quality improvement and quality improvement research.* Paper presented at the Forum on the Science of Health Care Quality Improvement and Implementation, Washington, DC.

Institute of Medicine. (2009). *Leadership commitments to improve value in health care: Finding common ground. Workshop summary.* Washington, DC: National Academies Press.

Institute of Medicine. (2010). *Redesigning continuing education in the health professions.* Washington, DC: National Academies Press.

Institute of Medicine. (2011). *Clinical guidelines we can trust.* Washington, DC: National Academies Press.

Institute of Medicine. (2011). *Crossing the quality chasm: The IOM health care quality initiative. Announcement.* Washington, DC: National Academies Press.

Institute of Medicine. (2011). *Finding what works in health care: Standards for systematic reviews.* Washington, DC: National Academies Press.

Institute of Medicine. (2011). *Leading health indicators for Healthy People 2020. Letter report.* Washington, DC: National Academies Press.

Institute of Medicine. (2011). *The common rule and continuous improvement in health care: A learning health system perspective. Discussion paper.* Washington, DC: National Academies Press.

Institute of Medicine. (2011). *The future of nursing: Leading change, advancing health.* Washington, DC: National Academies Press.

Institute of Medicine, & National Academy of Engineering. (2011). *Engineering a learning healthcare system: A look at the future: Workshop summary.* Washington, DC: National Academies Press.

Institute of Medicine. (2004). *Keeping patients safe: Transforming the work environment of nurses.* A. Page (Ed.). Washington, DC: National Academies Press.

Kalisch, B. J. (2010). Missed nursing care: View from the hospital bed. *Reflections on Nursing Leadership, 36*(3), 4.

Kane, R. L., Shamliyan, T., Mueller, C., Duval, S., & Wilt, T. (2007). *Nursing staffing and quality of patient care. Evidence report/technology assessment no. 151.* AHRQ Publication No. 07-E005. Rockville, MD: Agency for Healthcare Research and Quality.

Mark, B. A., & Harless, D. W. (2007). Nurse staffing, mortality, and length of stay in for-profit and not-for-profit hospitals. *Inquiry, 44*(2), 167–186.

Needleman, J., Buerhaus, P., Pantratz, V. S., Leibson, C. L., Stevens, S. R., & Harris, M. (2011). Nurse staffing and inpatient hospital mortality. *The New England Journal of Medicine, 364*(11), 1037–1045.

Nielsen-Bohlman, L., Panzer, A. M., & Kindig, D. A. (Eds.). (2004). *Health literacy: A prescription to end confusion.* Washington, DC: National Academies Press.

Swain, A. D., & Guttman, H. E. (1983). *Handbook of human reliability analysis with emphasis on nuclear power plant applications*

Valentin, A., Capuzzo, M., Guidet, B., Moreno, R., Metnitz, B., Bauer, P., & Metnitz, P. (2009). Errors in administration of parenteral drugs in intensive care units: Multinational prospective study. *BMJ, 338.* http://dx.doi.org/10.1136/bmj.b814

Wilson, R. M., Runciman, W. B., Gibberd, R. W., Harrison, B. T., Newby, L., & Hamilton, J. D. (1995). The quality in Australian health care study. *The Medical Journal of Australia, 163*(9), 458–471.

Endnote

1   Parts of this personal story have been published previously in Kalisch, B. J. (2010). Missed nursing care: View from the hospital bed (part one and part two). *Reflections on Nursing Leadership, 36*(3). Reproduced here with permission from *Reflections on Nursing Leadership, Sigma Theta Tau.*

— 2 —

Missed Nursing Care

Missed nursing care is defined as any aspect of standard, required nursing care that is not provided. These are errors of omission. A large number of studies have established the fact that nurse staffing levels and types impact patient outcomes: the better the staffing, the fewer the adverse outcomes (e.g., falls, infections, pressure ulcers, etc.). But we don't know a lot about what characterizes the process of nursing care that makes a difference. I call it the black box of nursing care. In other words, what happens in the process of giving care that results in poorer outcomes.

In this chapter, we will summarize the study findings, which demonstrate the extent of missed nursing care and the specific elements of nursing care that were not completed. In other words, what is the problem and how extensive is it? We will also report on how missed care varies across hospitals.

Studies of Specific Elements of Nursing Care
Selected aspects of missed nursing care have been investigated, including the impact of failure to complete the following: ambulation, turning and positioning, medication administration, hand washing

and other infection control procedures, mouth care, emotional support, promoting sleep, discharge planning, patient teaching, nourishment, bathing and skin care, and interdisciplinary conferences and rounds. These studies are reviewed below.

Ambulation

Several researchers have examined the frequency of patient ambulation that occurs in acute care hospitals. Callen, Mahoney, Grieves, Wells, and Enloe studied the frequency of hallway walking by adults hospitalized on a medical unit and found that 73% of patients did not walk at all, only 19% walked once, 5% twice, and 3% more than twice (2004). Brown, Friedkin, and Inouye also uncovered inadequacies in inpatient mobilization. Observation of 45 hospitalized medical patients indicated that, on average, 83% of the hospital stay was spent lying in bed. The amount of time spent standing or walking ranged from 0.2% to 21% (Brown et al., 2004).

Turning and Positioning Patients

Although an accepted standard of care is turning immobilized patients every two hours, Krishnagopalan, Johnson, Low, and Kaufman (2002) found in an observational study of 74 intensive care patients for 566 hours of patient care (7.7 hours per patient) that 97% of patients did not receive the minimum standard of body repositioning every two hours. Of the patients observed, 49.3% were not repositioned for more than two hours. Only 2.7% of patients had a demonstrated change in body position every two hours. A total of 80% to 90% of respondents to the survey agreed that turning every two hours was the accepted standard and that it prevented complications, but only 57% believed it was being achieved in their intensive care units.

Medication Administration

There have also been studies which point to missed medications (Anselmi, Peduzzi, & Dos Santos, 2007; Holley, 2006). In fact, omission of ordered medications has been found to be the most common medication error (Anselmi et al., 2007; Holley, 2006). One investigator discovered that 6% of all medication doses were omitted (Barker, Flynn, Pepper, Bates, & Mikeal, 2002). Greene, Du-Pre, Elahi, Dunckley, and McIntyre (2009) found 20% of prescriptions affecting 17% of patients did not reach patients. Other studies revealed 14% to 69% of all medication errors were errors of omission (Anselmi et al., 2007; Holley, 2006; Rinke, Shore, Morlock, Hicks, & Miller, 2007). In

England at the National Health Service (NHS), the National Patient Safety Agency received reports of 27 deaths, 68 severe harms, and 21,383 other patient safety incidents relating to omitted or delayed medicines from 2006 and 2009. They point out that "wider evidence suggests that the true rate of harm may be much higher, as events such as these are often not reported" (National Patient Safety Agency, 2010). A prevalence survey of 162 medical and surgical patients across four sites in England revealed that the number of patients who missed at least one medication was 80% with a total of 1,077 doses omitted. The most commonly missed medications were analgesia and anti-inflammatory drugs, which were missed 28% of the time (Warne et al., 2010). Another research team in England extracted data on drug administration during 2010 and found that 60,763 (12.4%) of the 491,894 doses were omitted (National Patient Safety Agency, 2010). In addition, time spent by the nurses tracking missed doses takes away from time available for direct patient care (Committee on Drugs and Committee on Hospital Care, 1998).

Hand Washing

Hand washing is essential to the prevention of healthcare-associated infections and improving hand hygiene compliance is a major goal for the World Health Organization Patient Safety Challenge and is one of The Joint Commission's National Patient Safety Goals (The Joint Commission, 2014; World Health Organization, 2014). Compliance of healthcare workers with recommended hand washing practices remains unacceptably low, often in the range of 30% to 50% (Boyce, 1999). Erasmus and colleagues (2010), in a systematic review of existing studies, found an overall median compliance rate of 40%. Compliance rates were lower in intensive care units (30% to 40%) than in other settings (50% to 60%), lower among physicians (32%) than among nurses (48%), and lower before (21%) rather than after (47%) patient contact.

Another potential source of infection arises with the use of intravenous catheters. Deficient routines in use, care, handling, and documentation of peripheral intravenous vein cannulae (PIV) have been reported, and complications have been noted in 50% to 75% of the patients (Lundgren & Wahren, 1999). Urinary catheters that are not handled appropriately and not removed in a timely manner are also a source of infection.

Mouth Care

A series of studies by Kalisch and colleagues (2011, 2012, 2013), reviewing the current state of mouth care practices, have demonstrated that for many hospitalized patients, mouth care is not being completed. In 2011, nursing staff reported that mouth care was the third most frequent element of nursing care to be missed after ambulation and attendance at interdisciplinary care rounds. Of the nurses surveyed, 39% reported missing mouth care occasionally, 25.5% reported frequently missing it, and 2% reported always missing mouth care (Kalisch, Tschannen, Lee, & Friese, 2011). In 2012, Kalisch surveyed patients' perceptions of missed care and found that patients uniformly reported not receiving assistance with mouth care (Kalisch, McLaughlin, & Dabney, 2012). Patients identified mouth care as the most missed aspect of nursing care, with 50.3% reporting not receiving any mouth care (Kalisch, Xie, & Dabney, 2013). It is worth noting that the patients surveyed indicated that mouth care was very important to them (Kalisch, McLaughlin, & Dabney, 2012).

When Kalisch and colleagues (2011) compared intensive care units (ICUs) and medical–surgical units, the researchers found that intensive care nurses report missing less mouth care (14%) than medical–surgical nurses (29.2%). However, based on the potential impact of missed mouth care in ICUs, the percentage of patients who do not receive the care is of significant concern. Feider, Mitchell, and Bridges (2010) sought to describe the oral care practices of critical care nurses with a high-risk population of orally intubated, critically ill patients and concluded that although 47% of nurses report oral care to be a high priority, many are not aware of published oral care guidelines for their patients. A discrepancy was found between national oral care standards and nurse-reported oral care practices when the care was completed.

Pettit, McCann, Schneiderman, Farren, and Campbell (2012) found a similar deficit in knowledge when conducting a study of certain dimensions of oral care in Texas hospitals. The results of this study suggested that 78.6% of nurses did assess the oral cavity of their patients, yet after taking a follow-up, knowledge-based mouth care written test, the mean grade of the nurses surveyed was 51%. Combined, the above studies demonstrate a deficit in mouth care being performed among hospitalized patients as well as a lack of uniform knowledge among nurses as to how to properly provide the care.

Emotional Support
In their book, Adler and Page (2008) note the lack of emotional support for inpatients is a problem. The authors state that the advances in biomedical care for cancer patients have not been matched by achievements in providing high-quality care for the psychological and social effects of the disease. Numerous cancer survivors and their caregivers report that cancer care providers did not understand their psychosocial needs, failed to recognize and adequately address depression and other symptoms of stress, were unaware of or did not refer them to available resources, and generally did not consider psychosocial support to be an integral part of quality cancer care (Adler & Page, 2008; Hupcey, 2000).

Promoting Sleep
Poor sleep is an undiagnosed problem of hospitalized patients. Despite use of hypnotic agents, people in hospitals often do not get enough sleep (Resnick et al., 2011). Sleep disturbances are caused by noise, light, interruptions, pain, alterations to the patients' diurnal rhythm (wake and sleep times), and not allowing patients to maintain their routines at bedtime (Hilton, 1976). A study of 280 patients aged 65 or older admitted to the hospital who reported sleep problems (37%) on the third day of hospitalization found that patients with sleep problems scored significantly worse on the cumulative index rating scale severity index (a measure of multi-morbidity) and on the activities of daily living scale (Isaia et al., 2011).

Discharge Planning
A number of studies have pointed to inadequacies with discharge planning from acute care hospitals. In one study using a mixed methods approach, Ubbink and colleagues (2014) found that one-third of the adult patients and nearly half of the children (or their parents) felt their personal situation and assistance needed at home was insufficiently taken into account before discharge. Patients were least satisfied with the information given about what they were allowed to do or what they should avoid after discharge and their involvement in the planning of their discharge (Ubbink et al., 2014).

Patient Teaching
Teaching has a wide range of definitions and meanings from handing the patient pamphlets or showing them a video to completing a thorough review, including return demonstrations and evaluation where

appropriate. The failure to adequately teach patients has also been investigated. In a survey of patients discharged from medical–surgical units, almost half stated they needed additional information or specific directions concerning their self-care (Lee, Wasson, Anderson, Stone, & Gittings, 1998).

Nourishment
Malnutrition is common in hospitalized patients, particularly the elderly. A number of studies have investigated the nutritional status of inpatients. In a study by Covinsky and colleagues (1999), 59.3% of inpatients were well nourished, 24.4% were moderately malnourished, and 16.3% were severely malnourished. Mudge, Ross, Young, Isenring, and Banks (2011) studied 134 inpatients and found that only 41% met estimated resting energy requirements. Mean energy intake was 1,220 kcal/day. Other studies have found malnutrition in 30% to 50% of hospital patients. Rasmussen and colleagues (2004) found that out of 590 patients, 39.9% were nutritionally at risk, with the highest prevalence in departments of gastrosurgery (57%). BMI was less than 18.5 in 10.9%, and between 18.5 and 20.5 in 16.7% of the patients.

Lack of knowledge of the extent of malnutrition of hospitalized patients is due to a lack of reliable and valid assessments tools. No nutritional screening tool is considered the gold standard for identifying nutritional risk. Using four different tools, Velasco and colleagues found that the prevalence of nutritional risk in hospitalized patients was high with all of them (Velasco et al., 2011).

Studies of Missed Nursing Care
While there have been these focused studies of omitted nursing care, they do not address the global issue of missed nursing care. They also do not describe the variation in care across settings, nor do they identify factors associated with missed nursing care.

The term "missed nursing care" was coined in 2006 and further defined in 2009 (Kalisch, 2006; Kalisch, Landstrom, & Hinshaw, 2009). Recognition of this concept was based on the experience of conducting over 400 focus groups and interviews with staff nurses, and engaging in an estimated 350 hours of observations of nurses at work in my role as a consultant to hospitals. I asked the question "What don't you get done?" This question elicited a large amount of information about what nursing care is not completed and also how nurses feel about it. This turned out to be a highly emotionally laden subject. Nurses have said to me that having the opportunity to verbalize this issue in a safe environment was psychologically very therapeutic for them and they were grateful that the hidden secret was out in the open. It was very clear that nurses want to do a good job caring for patients and are distressed when they cannot or do not do so.

Qualitative Study

Based on these experiences, I decided to conduct a systematic qualitative study to determine the extent of missed nursing care and the specific elements of nursing care that are missed. A total of 107 registered nurses (RNs), 15 licensed practical nurses (LPNs), and 51 nursing assistants (NAs) providing nursing care in medical–surgical and intensive care patient care units were interviewed in 25 focus groups in two hospitals. The staff members were segregated by job title in the focus groups to maximize honesty in the sharing of issues that they might have been reluctant to verbalize if other members of the team were present (e.g., nurses discussing problems with nursing assistants, etc.). The focus group interviews, which lasted 90 to 120 minutes, used a semi-structured design. Participants were asked to commit to confidentiality (not to quote the others outside the focus group). They were assured of the confidentiality of their comments by the investigator and encouraged to be as open and honest as possible. Ethics approval was obtained from each hospital to conduct the study.

All interviews were tape-recorded, fully transcribed, and analyzed by a research associate and myself independently, using NVivo 2.0 by QRS International, a qualitative analysis software. The themes from the first and second analyses, although differently grouped, extracted the same issues from the transcribed focus groups. To be included as a theme, supporting data had to be contained in all the focus groups from both hospitals (Kalisch, 2006).

Findings revealed the following nine areas of missed care:

- **Ambulation:** "Sometimes a nurse will come and ask, 'Can you walk this patient if you get time?' If we get time, we can do it. But if we don't, we can't do it. We don't do it." (NA)

- **Turning:** Instead of turns every two hours, they often turned the patient every four, six, eight hours, or even longer.

- **Delayed or missed feedings:** "You would really be surprised to find out how many trays get returned to dietary untouched because no one got around to feeding the patients."

- **Patient teaching:** "I never have time for diabetic teaching."

  "If you want to get out on time, do you think you do as much teaching as you really should, or do you turn around and run for the computer to get your charting done?"

- **Discharge planning:** "I really rarely know much about where the patient is going after hospitalization and whether there have been adequate preparations made."

- **Emotional support:** "I know the patient needs to talk with me, but I am afraid of getting in a situation where I can't easily get away."

  "There's many times when I've been in the room listening to somebody and my beeper goes off with two or three rings. I feel like, great, now I have to tell this person, I'm sorry, can you hold that statement so I can go check on these two or three other people? That to me is saying that this person isn't important and that's what they're feeling. I'm not important because she has to go to another room."

- **Hygiene:** "We have patients that haven't had a bath in two to three days."

  "One day I came to work, I had three patients 'on strike.' One refused to get back into her bed until the sheets were changed."

- **Intake and output documentation:** Tray being picked up before the staff recorded what was eaten, patients going to the bathroom when the staff members were not present, a lack of a systematic way to record the filling of water pitchers, etc.

- **Surveillance:** "I hold my breath as I leave one wing and round the corner to the other wing. I think it has been an hour since I was in his room. Will he be alright?"

  "Sometimes you have to remind yourself to go in a room to a patient who is pretty much taking care of himself. You say 'Oh my God! I've been so busy with these other ones, I haven't been in his room.'"

The *MISSCARE Survey*

Based on this study, it was evident that missed nursing care deserved further study on a wider basis using a quantitative methodology in order to determine the extent and specific nature of the problem. To do this, we developed and tested the *MISSCARE Survey* designed to measure the phenomenon empirically (Kalisch & Williams, 2009).

The *MISSCARE Survey* has two parts: (Part A) aspects of nursing care that are missed and (Part B) the reasons for missing care. In Part A, respondents are asked how often specifics elements of nursing care are missed on their unit by all of the staff, including themselves using the scale "rarely," "occasionally," "frequently," "always," or "non-applicable." In Part B of the *MISSCARE Survey*, the respondents were asked to rate each item using the scale significant factor," "moderate factor," "minor factor," or "not a reason for missing nursing care" (see Chapter 3). In addition, a demographic and background data section contained questions about the characteristics of the respondents, their satisfaction with their job and occupation, intent to leave, number of patients cared for on the last shift they worked, and assessment of the adequacy of staffing (from 0% to 100 % of the time).

The initial generation of items for the survey was based on the findings from the qualitative study described above, along with 95 interviews with staff nurses in four settings including an academic healthcare setting, a Veteran's Administration hospital, and two community hospitals.

The psychometric testing of the *MISSCARE Survey* involved measures of acceptability, validity, and reliability. The results of the testing revealed that acceptability was high for the *MISSCARE Survey*, with 85% of the respondents answering all items on the survey. The validity, or the extent to which it actually measures what it claims to measure, was assessed with content, construct, and contrasting group validity. Content validity was established by having the survey reviewed and rated on clarity and relevance by three panels of staff nurse experts (Lynn, 1985). The content validity index was 0.89, indicating a clear and relevant tool.

The further evaluation of the missed nursing care tool, the *MISSCARE Survey,* involved two studies in four hospitals: Study 1 (n = 459) and Study 2 (n = 639). The sample in study 1 was made up of staff nurses working on 35 inpatient units including maternity, intensive care, intermediate care, cardiac, surgical, medical, renal, oncology, and rehabilitation. The study 2 sample consisted of nurses and nursing assistants working on 18 patient care units including surgical, renal, and intermediate care.

Factor and confirmatory analyses, while not appropriate for Part A of the survey because it contains a list of independent nursing actions (not necessarily related to one another), were applied to Part B, reasons for missing care. A three-factor solution (i.e., communication and teamwork, labor resources, and material resources) emerged with Cronbach values ranged from 0.64 to 0.86. Confirmatory factor analysis demonstrated a good fit for the data.

For contrasting group validity, a comparison of nursing staff perceptions of missed care on intensive care units versus rehabilitation units was completed and resulted, as hypothesized, in a significantly lower amount of missed care on intensive care units.

In this study, reliability was evaluated by assessing the internal consistency of the items representing the factors in Part B and the test–retest coefficients (which determines the likelihood that a given measure will yield the same description of a given phenomenon if that measure is repeated). In this study, identical forms of the instrument were administered to the same nurses, two weeks apart. Pearson correlation coefficient on a test–retest of the same subjects yielded a value of 0.87 on Part A and 0.86 on Part B.

Quantitative Studies

Using the *MISSCARE Survey*, we have conducted studies in 14 acute care hospitals and 138 patient care units. The *MISSCARE Survey* was administered to nursing staff (n = 5134) who provided direct patient care (RNs, n = 4010, 78.1%; LPNs, n = 105, 2%; and NAs, n = 1019, 19.8%). The return rate for the surveys was 60%.

Of the 5,134 respondents, 91% were female, and 51% held a baccalaureate degree or higher. The majority of respondents (77%) were RNs, and the remaining 23% were NAs. Since the percentage of LPNs was so low, these were eliminated from the data set. Day shift was the most frequently reported work schedule (50%), followed by nights (32%), then evenings or rotating shifts (18%); most participants (74%) worked 12-hour shifts. Work experience was widely distributed; 34% reported more than ten years, 27% reported less than two years, and the remainders was distributed across two to ten years of experience. Of all the participants, 32% reported missing one shift in the last three months and 27% reported missing two or more shifts (Table 2.1). The majority of participants worked in medical–surgical units (52%), followed by intensive care (24%), intermediate care (19%), and rehabilitation (4%).

Amount and Type of Missed Care

The mean score of missed care was 1.57 (SD = .42) on a four-point scale from 1 = rarely missed to 4 = always missed. Figure 2.1 shows the elements of the least and most missed care across the 14 hospitals.

The six most frequently missed care activities were ambulation (75.7%), attending interdisciplinary care rounds/conferences (65.8%), mouth care (64.1%), timely medication administration (60.4%), turning (59.8%), and feeding patients (57.9%). Conversely, completing shift patient assessments (10%), glucose monitoring (14.5%), checking vital signs (26.3%), discharge planning (27%), reassessments (26.7%), and hand washing (27.1%) were the six least frequently missed nursing care. Analysis of the data retrieved for vital signs, discharge planning, reassessment, and hand washing illustrate that one out of four patients misses this care.

TABLE 2.1.   **Demographic characteristics of sample (n = 5134).**

		Frequency (n)	Percentage (%)*
Education	Diploma	393	9.5
	Associate degree of nursing	1651	39.9
	Baccalaureate degree of nursing or greater	2099	50.7
Gender	Female	447	8.9
	Male	4571	91.1
Age	<25 years	674	14.5
	26–34 years	1448	31.1
	35–44 years	1158	24.9
	45–54 years	940	20.2
	>55 years	437	9.4
Job titles	RNs	4010	78.1
	LPNs	105	2
	NAs	1019	19.8
Full-time equivalency	Full time	4147	81.1
	Part time	968	18.9
Shifts	Days	2549	49.9
	Evenings	588	11.5
	Nights	1638	32.1
	Rotations	332	6.5
Experience in role	<2 years	1243	26.7
	2–5 years	948	20.4
	5–10 years	871	18.8
	>10 years	1580	34
Experience on current unit	<2 years	1764	38.1
	2–5 years	1128	24.3
	5–10 years	884	19.1
	>10 years	859	18.5
Overtime	None	1419	30.5
	1–12 hours	2006	43.1
	>12 hours	1229	26.4
Absenteeism	None	2040	44
	1 day or shift	1489	32.1
	>1 day or shift	1109	26.9

Note: * valid percentage

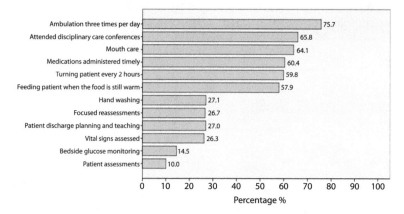

FIGURE 2.1. **The six most missed and the six least missed elements of nursing care.**
Note: The solid bars represent the means across all 14 hospitals, and the range lines indicate the standard deviations.

Table 2.2 shows the distribution of responses for how frequently each element of care was reported as missed (always missed, frequently missed, occasionally missed, or rarely missed). Table 2.3 demonstrates the percentages of each element of missed care (occasionally, frequently, and always missed) from most to least.

In addition to our studies of missed nursing care, other researchers have studied similar phenomena, namely unfinished care, rationed care, and care left undone. Sochalski (2004) found that the quality of nursing care was significantly related to nurse-reported rates of unfinished care. A Swiss team has investigated what they term "rationed nursing care," or care that does not take place when nurses lack sufficient time to provide the care. Although these researchers

TABLE 2.2. **Missed nursing care, 14 hospitals (n = 5134).**

Items of the MISSCARE Survey	Rarely Missed (n %)	Occasionally Missed (n %)	Frequently Missed (n %)	Always Missed (n %)
1. Ambulation 3 times per day or as ordered	1133(24.3)	2009(43.1)	1408(30.2)	107(2.3)
2. Turning patient every 2 hours	2003(40.2)	2179(43.7)	768(15.4)	38(0.8)
3. Feeding patient when the food is still warm	1918(42.1)	1843(40.4)	755(16.6)	44(1.0)
4. Setting up meals for patients who feed themselves	2919(64.4)	1238(27.3)	332(7.3)	47(1.0)

Items of the MISSCARE Survey	Rarely Missed (n %)	Occasionally Missed (n %)	Frequently Missed (n %)	Always Missed (n %)
5. Medications administered within 30 minutes before or after scheduled time	1879(39.6)	2023(42.7)	789(16.6)	48(1.0)
6. Vital signs assessed as ordered	3726(73.7)	1097(21.7)	194(3.8)	39(0.8)
7. Monitoring intake/output	2619(51.5)	1622(31.9)	785(15.4)	61(1.2)
8. Full documentation of all necessary data	2203(43.8)	2106(41.9)	667(13.3)	55(1.1)
9. Patient teaching about procedures, tests, and other diagnostic studies	2057(42.7)	1973(41.0)	742(15.4)	41(0.9)
10. Emotional support to patient and/or family	2824(55.9)	1610(31.9)	580(11.5)	36(0.7)
11. Patient bathing/skin care	2679(53.5)	1909(38.1)	386(7.7)	34(0.7)
12. Mouth care	1793(35.9)	1922(38.5)	1187(23.8)	94(1.9)
13. Hand washing	3711(72.9)	1092(21.5)	240(4.7)	46(0.9)
14. Patient discharge planning and teaching	3356(73.0)	972(21.1)	239(5.2)	32(0.7)
15. Bedside glucose monitoring as ordered	4273(85.5)	598(12.0)	76(1.5)	53(1.1)
16. Patient assessments according to patient condition	4374(90.0)	368(7.6)	69(1.4)	51(1.0)
17. IV/central line site care and assessments according to hospital policy	3013(63.6)	1401(29.6)	302(6.4)	19(0.4)
18. Response to call light is initiated within 5 minutes	2474(49.3)	1822(36.3)	688(13.7)	39(0.8)
19. PRN medication requests acted on within 5 minutes	2573(54.2)	1710(36.0)	443(9.3)	22(0.5)
20. Assess effectiveness of medications	2238(47.2)	1961(41.4)	518(10.9)	20(0.4)
21. Attend interdisciplinary care rounds whenever held	1492(34.2)	1475(33.8)	1108(25.4)	293(6.7)
22. Assist with toileting needs within 5 minutes request	2503(50.0)	1982(39.6)	493(9.8)	32(0.6)
23. Skin/wound care	3037(68.0)	1281(28.7)	126(2.8)	19(0.4)

TABLE 2.3.   **Elements of missed care from most to least frequency (n = 5134).**

Elements of nursing care	%*
Ambulation 3 times per day or as ordered	75.7
Attend interdisciplinary care rounds whenever held	65.8
Mouth care	64.1
Medications administered within 30 minutes before or after scheduled time	60.4
Turning patient every 2 hours	59.8
Feeding patient when the food is still warm	57.9
Patient teaching about procedures, tests, and other diagnostic studies	57.3
Full documentation of all necessary data	56.2
Assess effectiveness of medications	52.8
Response to call light is initiated within 5 minutes	50.7
Assist with toileting needs within 5 minutes request	50.0
Monitoring intake/output	48.5
Patient bathing/skin care	46.5
PRN medication requests acted on within 5 minutes	45.8
Emotional support to patient and/or family	44.1
IV/central line site care and assessments according to hospital policy	36.4
Setting up meals for patients who feed themselves	35.6
Skin/wound care	32.0
Hand washing	27.1
Focused reassessments according to patient condition	26.7
Patient discharge planning and teaching	27.0
Vital signs assessed as ordered	26.3
Bedside glucose monitoring as ordered	14.5
Patient assessments performed each shift	10.0

Note: *In this table, the percentages of occasionally, frequently, and always missed were categorized as "missed" care

reported a low rate of rationed care, the occurrence of rationed care (i.e., missed care) was associated with poor patient outcomes (e.g., medication errors, patient falls, infections, pressure ulcers, etc.; Schubert et al., 2008). In another study they found that patients who were cared for in the hospital with the highest rationing level were 51% more likely to die than those in peer institutions (Schubert,

Clarke, Aiken, & DeGeest, 2012). In Cypress, a study of the rationing of nursing care, which included a sample of 393 nurses from medical and surgical units, discovered that the highest level of rationing was reported for the "reviewing of patient documentation," followed by "oral and dental hygiene," and "coping with the delayed response of physicians" (Papastavrou, Andreou, Tsangari, Schuber, & DeGeest, 2014).

The prevalence and patterns of incomplete nursing care have been investigated by Ausserhofer and colleagues (2014). They studied 33,659 nurses in 488 hospitals across 12 European countries and found that the most frequent nursing care activities left undone were comforting and talking with patients (53%), developing or updating nursing care plans or care pathways (42%), and educating patients and families (41%). Ball and colleagues (2014) conducted a survey of 2,917 RNs working in 401 general medical/surgical wards in 4 general acute care hospitals in the National Health Service in England. A total of 86% of the nurses reported that one or more elements of care had been omitted due to lack of time on their last shift. Specific elements of nursing care which were not completed include comforting or talking with patients (66%), educating patients (52%), and developing/ updating nursing care plans (47%). The larger number of patients per registered nurse was significantly associated with the incidence of missed care ($p < 0.001$). A mean of 7.8 activities per shift were left undone on patient care units which were rated as 'failing' on patient safety, compared with 2.4 where patient safety was rated as 'excellent' ($p < 0.001$). More information about international missed nursing care will be presented in Chapter 5.

Staff and Unit Characteristics and Missed Nursing Care

Using the overall sample, a series of bivariate regression analyses using robust cluster estimation were conducted to find significant variations reported in missed care by unit staff characteristics, work schedules, and staffing. It was found that eight variables were significantly associated with missed nursing care: sex, age, job title, shift worked, years of experience, absenteeism, number of patients cared for, and perceived adequacy of staffing. When nursing staff members were female ($\beta = 0.84$; robust standard error [SE] = 0.02; $p < .001$), older ($\beta = 0.03$; robust SE = 0.01; $p < .001$), RNs (versus NAs; $\beta = 0.19$; robust SE = 0.03; $p < .001$), working on a day shift (compared with those on night shifts; $\beta = 0.05$; robust SE = 0.02; $p < .05$), or more experienced ($\beta = 0.04$; robust SE = 0.01; $p < .001$), they reported more missed nursing care.

Higher levels of missed care correlated with nursing staff who missed more shifts in the past three months (compared with those who did not miss any shifts; $\beta = 0.08$; robust SE = 0.02; $p < .001$), higher numbers of staff reporting staffing levels as inadequate ($\beta = 0.11$; robust SE = 0.01; $p < .001$), or staff who had a greater number of patients assigned to them ($\beta = 0.01$; robust SE = 0.00; $p < .05$). Education level, weekly work hours, and type of unit were not significantly associated with missed care. Significant independent variables were then entered into the following multivariable analysis to determine the significant predictors of missed care.

Predictors of Missed Nursing Care

A multiple regression model that includes significant variables from the bivariate analyses is shown in Table 2.3. The model significantly predicted the missed care score ($R^2 = 0.16$; $F[19, 109] = 28.0$; $p < .001$). NAs (versus RNs) and staff with fewer years of experience reported significantly less missed care ($p < .001$). Night-shift workers reported less missed care than day-shift workers ($p < .01$). Nursing staff who missed two or more shifts in the past three months reported missed care more often than those who did not miss any shifts ($p < .01$). Those who cared for more patients on the previous shift reported more missed care ($p < .001$), whereas nursing staff who perceived their staffing as adequate were more likely to report fewer instances of missed nursing care ($p < .001$). Age and gender were not significantly associated with missed nursing care.

Variations Across Hospitals

The next aim was to determine the extent to which nursing care varied by hospital. We found differences in the elements of missed nursing care across hospitals but generally they were similar (F = 55.49, $p < .001$). Figure 2.2 contains a description of the amount of missed nursing care by hospital.

Figure 2.3 shows the six most missed elements of nursing care by hospital and Figure 2.4 shows the six least missed elements of nursing care by hospital. Although the percentages differed slightly, the least and the most missed care items were the same across all hospitals. Bedside glucose monitoring and shift assessments were reported as being missed the least frequently. Conversely, ambulation was among the top six elements of missed nursing care reported

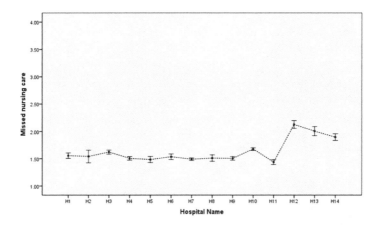

FIGURE 2.2. **The amount of missed nursing care across hospitals (n = 5134).**
Note: The bar line indicates the 95% confidence interval.

across all 14 hospitals. Although some pairs of hospitals were significantly different in the amount of missed care (e.g., Hospital 2 had significantly higher rates of not turning patients than Hospital 7), the most missed and least missed elements of care were similar across the hospitals.

Summary

In this chapter, the concept of missed nursing care and studies that show the prevalence and type of nursing care that is left undone were reviewed. From this research, it can be concluded that the problem of missed nursing care is extensive and widespread. Particular areas of care tend to be missed more often than others (i.e., ambulation, interdisciplinary rounds, mouth care, timely medication administration, turning, and feeding patient). On the other hand, completing shift patient assessments, glucose monitoring, vital signs, discharge planning, reassessments, and hand washing were the six least frequently missed aspects of nursing care. Although some pairs of hospitals were significantly different in the amount of missed care (e.g., Hospital 2 had significantly higher rates of not turning patients than Hospital 7), the most missed and least missed elements of care were similar across the hospitals. In the next chapter, reasons for missing nursing care will be described.

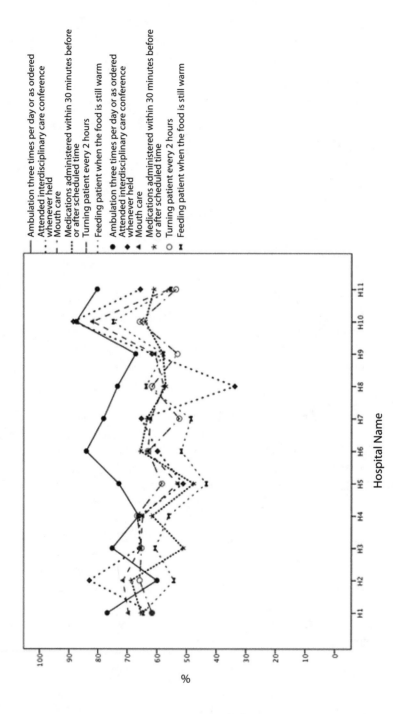

Ambulation three times per day or as ordered
Attended interdisciplinary care conference whenever held
Mouth care
Medications administered within 30 minutes before or after scheduled time
Turning patient every 2 hours
Feeding patient when the food is still warm

Ambulation three times per day or as ordered
Attended interdisciplinary care conference whenever held
Mouth care
Medications administered within 30 minutes before or after scheduled time
Turning patient every 2 hours
Feeding patient when the food is still warm

Hospital Name

%

FIGURE 2.3.   The six most frequently missed elements of nursing care across hospitals.

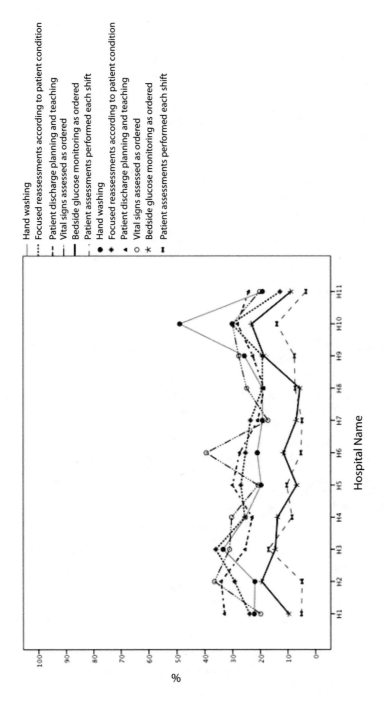

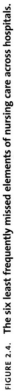

FIGURE 2.4. **The six least frequently missed elements of nursing care across hospitals.**

References

Adler, N. E., & Page, A. E. K. (Eds.). (2008). *Cancer care for the whole patient. Meeting psychosocial needs.* Washington, DC: National Academies Press.

Aiken, L. H., Clarke, S. P., Sloane, D. M., Sochalski, J. A., Busse, R., Clarke, H., ... Shamian, J. (2001). Nurses' reports on hospital care in five countries. *Health Affairs, 20*(3), 43–53.

Anselmi, M. L., Peduzzi, M., & Dos Santos, C. B. (2007). Errors in the administration of intravenous medication in Brazilian hospitals. *Journal of Clinical Nursing, 16*(10), 1839–1847.

Ausserhofer, D., Zander, B., Busse, R., Schubert, M., De Geest, S., Rafferty, A. M., ... Schwendimann, R. (2014). Prevalence, patterns and predictors of nursing care left undone in European hospitals: Results from the multicountry cross-sectional RN4CAST study. *BMJ Quality & Safety, 23*(2), 126–135.

Ball, J. E., Murrells, T., Rafferty, A. M., Morrow, E., & Griffiths, P. (2014). 'Care left undone' during nursing shifts: Associations with workload and perceived quality of care. *BMJ Quality & Safety, 23*(2), 116–125.

Barker, K. N., Flynn, E. N., Pepper, G. A., Bates, D. W., & Mikeal, R. L. (2002). Medication errors observed in 36 health care facilities. *Archives of Internal Medicine, 162*(16), 1897–1903.

Boyce, J. M. (1999). It is time for action: Improving hand hygiene in hospitals. *Annals of Internal Medicine, 130*(2), 153–155.

Brown, C. J., Friedkin, R. J., & Inouye, S. K. (2004). Prevalence and outcomes of low mobility in hospitalized older patients. *Journal of the American Geriatrics Society, 52(8), 1263–1270.*

Callen, B. L., Mahoney, J. E., Grieves, C. B., Wells, T. J., & Enloe, M. (2004). Frequency of hallway ambulation by hospitalized older adults on medical units of an academic hospital. *Geriatric Nursing, 25*(4), 212–217.

Committee on Drugs and Committee on Hospital Care. (1998). Prevention of medication errors in the pediatric inpatient setting. *Pediatrics, 102*(2), 428–430.

Covinsky, K. E., Martin, G. E., Beyth, R. J., Justice, A. C., Sehgal, A. R., & Landefeld, C. S. (1999). The relationship between clinical assessments of nutritional status. *Journal of the American Geriatrics Society, 47*(5),532–8.

Erasmus, V., Daha, T. J., Brug, H., Richardus, J. H., Behrendt, M. D., Vos, M. C., & van Beeck, E. F. (2010). Systematic review of studies on compliance with hand hygiene guidelines in hospital care. *Infect Control and Hospital Epidemiology, 31*(3), 283–294.

Feider, L. L., Mitchell, P., & Bridges, E. (2010). Oral care practices for orally intubated critically ill adults. *American Journal of Critical Care, 19*(2), 175–183.

Greene, C. J., Du-Pre, P., Elahi, N., Dunckley, P., & McIntyre, A. S. (2009). Omission after admission: Failure in prescribed medications being given to inpatients. *Clinical Medicine, 9*(6), 515–518.

Holley, J. L. (2006). A descriptive report of errors and adverse events in chronic hemodialysis units. *Nephrology News & Issues, 20*(12), 57–58, 60–61, 63.

Isaia, G., Corsinovi, L., Bo, M., Santos-Pereira, P., Michelis, G., Aimonino, N., & Zanocchi, M. (2011). Insomnia among hospitalized elderly patients: Prevalence, clinical characteristics and risk factors. *Archives of Gerontology and Geriatrics, 52*(2), 133–137.

Hupcey, J. E. (2000). Feeling safe: The psychosocial needs of ICU patients. *Journal of Nursing Scholarship, 32*(4), 361–367.

The Joint Commission. (2014). Hospital national patient safety goals. Retrieved from http://www.visimobile.com/wp-content/uploads/2014/05/2014-National-Patient-Safety-Goals.pdf

Kalisch, B. J. (2006). Missed nursing care: A qualitative study. *Journal of Nursing Care Quality, 21*(4), 306–313.

Kalisch, B. J., Landstrom, G., & Hinshaw, A. (2009). Missed nursing care: A concept analysis. *Journal of Advanced Nursing, 65*(7), 1509–1517.

Kalisch, B. J., McLaughlin, M., & Dabney, B. W. (2012). Patient perceptions of missed nursing care. *The Joint Commission Journal on Quality and Patient Safety, 38*(4), 161–167.

Kalisch, B. J., Tschannen, D., Lee, H., & Friese, C. R. (2011). Hospital variation in missed nursing care. *American Journal of Medical Quality, 26*(4), 291–299.

Kalisch B. J., & Williams R. A. (2009). Development and psychometric testing of a tool to measure missed nursing care (MISSCARE Survey). *The Journal of Nursing Administration, 39*(5), 211–219.

Kalisch, B. J., Xie, B., & Dabney, B. W. (2013). Patient-reported missed nursing care correlated with adverse events. *American Journal of Medical Quality.* Advance online publication. doi: 10.1177/1062860613501715

Krishnagopalan, S., Johnson, E. W., Low, L. L., & Kaufman, L. J. (2002). Body positioning of intensive care patients: Clinical practice versus standards. *Critical Care Medicine, 30*(11), 2588–2592.

Lee, N. C., Wasson, D. R., Anderson, M. A., Stone, S., & Gittings, J. A. (1998). A survey of patient education postdischarge. *Journal of Nursing Care Quality, 13*(1), 63–70.

Lundgren, A., & Wahren, L. K. (2011). Effect of education on evidence-based care and handling of peripheral intravenous lines. *Journal of Clinical Nursing, 8*(5), 577–585.

National Patient Safety Agency. (2010, February). Reducing harm from omitted and delayed medicines in hospital. Rapid Response Report. Retrieved from http://www.nrls.npsa.nhs.uk/alerts/?entryid45=66720

NVivo 2.0 is the current version of QSR's NVivo product. QSR International Pty Ltd, 2nd Floor, 651 Doncaster Road, Doncaster, Victoria 3108, Australia. Available at: http://www.qsrinternational.com/products_nvivo.aspx

Papastavrou, E., Andreou, P., Tsangari, H., Schubert, M., & De Geest, S. (2014). Rationing of nursing care within professional environmental constraints: A correlational study. *Clinical Nursing Research, 23*(3), 314–335.

Pettit, S. L., McCann, A. L., Schneiderman, E. D., Farren, E. A., & Campbell, P. R. (2012). Dimensions of oral care practices in Texas hospitals. *Journal of Dental Hygiene, 86*(2), 91–103.

Rasmussen, H. H., Kondrup, J., Staun, M., Ladefoged, K., Kristensen, H., & Wengler, A. (2004). Prevalence of patients at nutritional risk in Danish hospitals. *Clinical Nutrition, 23*(5), 1009–1015.

Rinke, M. L., Shore, A. D., Morlock, L., Hicks, R. W., & Miller, M. R. (2007). Characteristics of pediatric chemotherapy medication errors in a national error reporting database. *Cancer, 110*(1), 186–195.

Resnick, H., Perla, R., Ilagan, P., Kaylor, M., Mehling, D., & Alwan, M. (2012). TEAhM—technologies for enhancing access to health management: A pilot study of community-based telehealth. *Telemedicine and e-Health. 18*(3): 166–174. doi:10.1089/tmj.2011.0122

Schubert, M., Clarke, S. P., Aiken, L. H., & De Geest, S. (2012). Associations between rationing of nursing care and inpatient mortality in Swiss hospitals. *International Journal for Quality in Health Care, 24*(3), 230–238.

Schubert, M., Glass, T. R., Clarke, S. P., Aiken, L. H., Schaffert-Witvliet, B., Sloane, D. M., & De Geest, S. (2008). Rationing of nursing care and its relationship to patient outcomes: The Swiss extension of the International Hospital Outcomes Study. *International Journal for Quality in Health Care, 20*(4), 227–237.

Sochalski, J. (2004). Is more better?: The relationship between nurse staffing and the quality of nursing care in hospitals. *Medical Care, 42*(2 suppl), 1167–1173.

Ubbink, D. T., Tump, E., Koenders, J. A., Kleiterp, S., Goslings, J. C., & Brolmann, F. E. (2014). Which reasons do doctors, nurses, and patients have for hospital discharge? A mixed-methods study. *PLOS ONE, 13*(9), e91333.

Velasco, C., García, E., Rodríguez, V., Frias, L., Garriga, R., Álvarez, J., García-Peris, P., & León, M. (2011) Comparison of four nutritional screening tools to detect nutritional risk in hospitalized patients: A multicentre study. *European Journal of Clinical Nutrition* (65), 269–274.

Warne, S., Endacott, R., Ryan, H., Chamberlain, W., Hendry, J., Boulanger, C., & Donlin, N. (2010). Non-therapeutic omission of medications in acutely ill patients. *Nursing in Critical Care, 15*(3), 112–117.

World Health Organization. (2014). About save lives: Clean your hands. Retrieved from http://www.who.int/gpsc/5may/background/en/

3

Reasons for Missed Nursing Care

In order to determine strategies to decrease missed nursing care, we need to understand why it occurs. We conducted several studies addressing this question.

Qualitative Study

The first was the focus group study reported in Chapter 2 where we explored the reasons for missed nursing care (Kalisch, 2006). The following reasons were identified:

- Too few staff members:

    An inadequate staff-to-patient ratio; shifts in which the full complement of budgeted staff are not present (e.g., sickness, absence, unfilled positions); unexpected heavy work demands (e.g., declining health of a patient, a large number of discharges and admissions).

- Poor use of existing staff resources:

    Too few of a particular category of staff, usually nursing assistants (NAs); too many inexperienced staff members on a given shift; patient assignments based solely on numbers; inconsistent patient assignments from day to day.

- Time required for the nursing intervention:

  If a nursing action takes a lot of time, it is less likely to be done.

- It's-not-my-job syndrome:

  RNs believed that the work delegated to the NAs is not their responsibility (e.g., not answering patient call light because it's the NA's job.)

- Ineffective delegation:

  Failure of the nurse to obtain the buy-in of the NA; no reports between NAs and RNs; RNs not retaining accountability; inability to deal with conflict management and give effective feedback.

- Habit:

  "To be honest, when you skip ambulation one day because you don't have time, and nothing happens, even though we know the patient goes home debilitated, I think it is easier to skip it the next day, and the next, and the next." [RN]

- Denial:

  Nurses reported engaging in denial about the care that was not completed, particularly care they delegated to NAs; they "do not want to know that care is being missed."

  "We don't let ourselves think about it. It is the way we cope. Underneath, we don't feel good about it."

Quantitative Studies

As explained in Chapter 2, after conducting this qualitative study, we developed the *MISSCARE Survey* with two parts: Part A, which includes elements of missed nursing care, and Part B, the reasons for missed nursing care (Kalisch & Williams, 2009). The psychometric studies of the *MISSCARE Survey* are described in Chapter 2. As noted there, we have conducted studies in 14 acute care hospitals and 138 patient care units with 5,134 staff members (RNs, 78.1%; LPNs, 2%; and NAs, 19.8%; Kalisch, Landstrom, & Williams, 2009; Kalisch, Tschannen, Lee, & Friese, 2011).

Reasons for missing nursing care were treated dichotomously, with the item being considered as a reason if "significant reason" or "moderate reason" was marked but not a reason if "minor reason" or " not a reason." Figure 3.1 shows the three subscales that emerged from the Part B component of the *MISSCARE Survey*: 1. labor

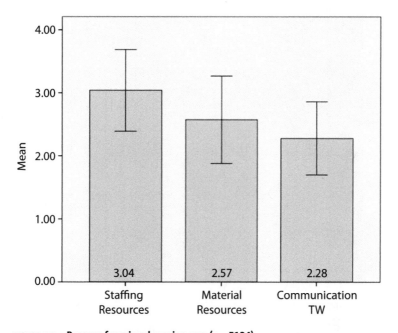

FIGURE 3.1. **Reasons for missed nursing care (n = 5134).**
Note: The solid bars represent the means of each reason for missed nursing care, and range lines indicate one standard deviation.

resources; 2. material resources; and 3. communication and team-work. Inadequate labor resources was the most often cited reason for missed nursing care (73.9% across the 14 hospitals), followed by material resources (50.6%), and then communication and teamwork (36.5%). Overall, these three reasons were observed consistently in the studies conducted in the United States and most other countries. The reasons are quite similar across organizations; the variation across the 14 hospitals is illustrated in Figure 3.2. Staffing was 3.5 with little varia-tion. Material resources ranged between 3.0 and 3.5. Hospital 1 had the fewest problems in this area (scoring 2.29) while Hospital 12 had the highest scores (scoring 2.94). This suggests that individual hospitals vary in the availability of medications and equipment, which impacts the ability of nursing staff to complete their work. Communication and teamwork varied from the lowest, 2.18, to the highest, 2.36, which shows that this is a consistent problem across hospitals.

Labor Resources
As noted in Table 3.1, the specific items under labor resources ranged from an inadequate number or type of staff to emergencies and other

TABLE 3.1. Reasons for missed nursing care across 14 hospitals (%) (n = 5134).

	Total (n=5134)	H1 (n=241)	H2 (n=47)	H3 (n=734)	H4 (n=506)	H5 (n=234)	H6 (n=218)	H7 (n=912)	H8 (n=199)	H9 (n=577)	H10 (n=754)	H11 (n=253)	H12 (n=164)	H13 (n=119)	H14 (n=176)
Staffing Resources															
Inadequate number of staff	70.1	79.8	63	62.7	57.1	77.7	69.4	72.9	74.9	68.2	71.8	64.6	84	87.2	79.2
Urgent patient situation	73.3	75.1	71.7	70.7	67.5	66.1	68.8	73.1	75.9	69.4	77.7	75.9	84	84.7	83.7
Unexpected rise in patient volume and/or acuity on the unit	82.1	84.9	84.4	70.4	76	83.3	86.1	83.5	79.5	82.4	85.8	85.1	93.9	94.9	90.8
Inadequate number of assistive and/or clerical personnel	74.9	78.6	71.7	66.8	69.9	72.2	72.9	74.8	77.5	74.5	81.6	76.3	82.8	84.7	77.6
Heavy admission and discharge activity	69	70.3	82.6	68.7	69.5	68.7	82.2	75.3	66.2	74.7	73.4	82.2	22.6	29.1	32.4
Material resources															
Medications were not available when needed	70.1	42.9	67.4	67.3	71.7	62.2	75.9	70.9	81.3	80.7	73	71	70.7	68.6	53.2
Supplies/equipment not available when needed	46.7	38	47.8	45.6	35.8	51.1	47.7	42.8	59.8	46.9	49.3	46.1	78	54.7	46.8
Supplies/equipment not functioning properly when needed	34.9	25.8	41.3	36.6	22.8	37.1	34.8	31.9	44.1	34.2	35.9	43.2	65.2	34.7	34.3

Communication/ Teamwork

Unbalanced patient assignments	56.9	66.5	41.3	56.4	57.8	58.7	62.9	60	49	59.6	57.9	69.8	37.9	47.5	23.6
Inadequate handoff from previous shift or sending unit	37.3	33	51.1	38.9	39.8	37.5	46.5	31.7	35.4	34.5	43.3	37.3	36.6	31.4	33.7
Other departments did not provide the care needed	34.7	21.9	30.4	42.7	32.7	39.4	34.4	32	41.1	29.6	36.8	36.5	38.4	33.9	27.9
Lack of back-up support from team members	36	36.1	37	37.2	31.3	38.3	43.3	32.8	36.7	30.1	41.4	35.5	44.8	34.7	36.2
Tension or communication breakdowns with other ancillary/support departments	31.5	29.3	26.1	31.4	22.6	33.2	30.7	24.1	29	31.4	43.5	25.7	55.8	36.8	32.2
Tension or communication breakdowns within the nursing team	29.8	31.5	33.3	31.6	24.7	33.9	31	23.7	25.9	25.5	36.9	28.5	46	30.5	31
Tension or communication breakdowns with the medical staff	36.2	29.3	48.9	35.7	29.8	39	38.2	27.7	29	34.3	47.1	31.6	69.8	40.7	39.2
Nursing assistant did not communicate that care was not done	43	38.5	29.5	45.1	43.2	40.4	49.3	44	38.5	36.6	48	37.8	42.3	48.3	43
Caregiver off unit or unavailable	22.8	22.6	13.6	26.8	16.9	23	26	20.8	22.3	21.6	24.7	22.8	27.4	28	19.3

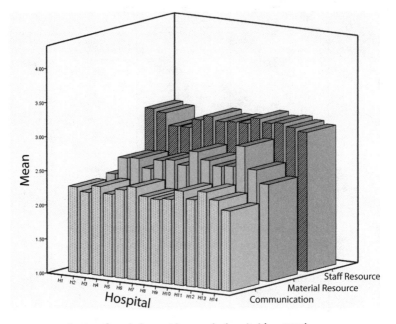

FIGURE 3.2. **Reasons for missing nursing care by hospital (n = 5134).**

increases in volume. Specifically, within this subscale, an unexpected rise in patient volume, acuity, or both was consistently identified as the top reason for missed care (82.1% for all respondents), with a range in frequency from 70.4% to 94.9% across hospitals. Below are some examples of nursing staff explaining how staffing levels and type leads to missed nursing care:

- "Labor resources, to me, is the biggest reason for missed care as far as I can see. You are always short-staffed of a tech (NA) and/or an assistant charge nurse. When we're short-staffed, it is not that people are not willing to help you, it is just that they do not have the time themselves." (RN)

- "Patient acuity defines what nursing care is required and when you don't have the adequate number of staff to give that required care, things get missed. We have seen that time and time again throughout the years. Unfortunately, things like oral care and ambulation get missed. Those things that have that effect downstream. You don't think they matter currently, but then you see the problems downstream. Things like pressure ulcers are directly related to inadequate staffing numbers." (RN)

- "Today, we are supposed to have ten nurses on day shift, but someone called off and we have nine. We can still staff the full unit with nine nurses, but it is just a heavier workload for everybody so maybe not everyone gets ambulated the number of times that they should be." (RN)

Material Resources

The most common item reported in the material resources subscale was the lack of availability of medications when needed (70.1% overall, range across hospitals 42.9% to 81.3%). Nursing staff give examples as follows:

- "Ever since we moved to [a new hospital building], the pharmacy has been a nightmare. And we have been here for what? Two years now? And meds are still always missing, you still have fights with the pharmacy about chemo orders and them not sending things when you ask them to. I called pharmacy this morning for hydrocortisone pre-med and 45 minutes later I didn't have it so I called the pharmacy again, 'Hey, is it en route?' And they are shuffling through meds and said, 'Oh, its sitting right here; we will tube it.' Well, why is it sitting right there?" (RN)

- "It has gotten to the point with me that I will check all my medications for the day the second I get to work so that I call pharmacy to remind them to bring some of my 9 o'clock medications. I knew if I did not do it in advance, I would not have it in time." (RN)

- "So we had a nurse, she has been a nurse here for a very long time. She is an exceptional nurse, she does not make mistakes. She spent so much time messing with that [new IV] pump that she forgot to have someone come in and check her chemo rate and it was the wrong rate. So she accidently made it run too slow for about an hour. It wasn't a huge error, but she was beside herself. She had to spend so much time dealing with that pump, figuring out the pump." (RN)

- "I had a nurse the day before come in to talk to the NA and I could hear the conversation. She was just frustrated because during a twelve-hour day, nine hours into her shift all the IVs she had administered so far required her to override the settings on the IV pump. That's not safe or efficient." (RN)

Communication

The level of communication/teamwork was less similar across hospitals; however, the most frequently reported item in this scale was unbalanced patient assignments (56.9% overall, range across hospitals 37.9% to 66.5%). Nursing staff give examples of communication and teamwork issues as follows (more details contained in Chapter 12):

- "Sometimes the things you delegate are not done. They are not done when they are asked to be done and it is not often communicated that it hasn't been done so then you do not know that it has been missed." (RN)

- "There is about 60 nurses, how many of those 60 will be helpful? 20. It seems like once one nurse doesn't want to help, neither will two or three other nurses that same day." (RN)

- "Personally, on the floor that I worked on, the techs were a tight-knit group. They were tight in the sense that all together they kind of weren't going to do all the little details of the work. Personally, I was outside of that group because I was always doing something. I was never sitting down. Literally, I don't understand how they could sit down in 12 hours having all that stuff to do. And, so I guess, I don't know. I don't know if it's a culture that develops on a floor." (Former NA, Current RN)

- "The nurses won't answer the call lights no matter what. The response when you are down a tech, you get another nurse. That doesn't help at all. They should do aid work, but they don't." (NA)

Several other studies have investigated the causes of missed nursing care (or similar concepts). Papastavrou, Andreou, Tsangari, Schubert, and De Geest (2013) studied the relationship between nurses' perceptions of their professional practice environment and care rationing (missed nursing care). Using regression analyses, teamwork, leadership and autonomy, and communication about patients accounted for 18.4% of the variance in rationing. Ausserhofer and colleagues (2014) found that in hospitals with more favorable work environments, lower patient to nurse ratios, and lower proportions of nurses carrying out non-nursing tasks frequently, had less nursing care left undone. Schubert, Clarke, Aiken, and De Geest (2012) found that patients treated in the hospitals with higher work-environment quality ratings from nurses had a significantly lower likelihood of death. Comparatively, those treated in the hospital with the highest measured patient-to-nurse ratio (10:1) had a 37% higher risk of death.

Other Reasons for Missed Nursing Care

In our analysis of the data from the 14 hospitals, we found that the reasons for missed care (derived from Part B of the Survey), explained only 9.4% of variance in missed nursing care (Part A of the Survey), indicating that the *MISSCARE Survey* does not capture all of the reasons why nursing staff are missing care. Based on this finding, we conducted a qualitative study where we interviewed over 50 staff nurses as to other reasons for missed nursing care. The findings from this study uncovered additional reasons (to the three described above):

1. interruptions, multitasking, and task switching;
2. fatigue and physical exhaustion;

3. cognitive biases;
4. lack of patient and family engagement;
5. lack of physician resources;
6. leadership issues;
7. moral distress and compassion fatigue;
8. documentation load;
9. large proportion of new nurses on unit; and
10. complacency.

Interruptions, Multitasking, and Task Switching
Interruptions

The interviewees pointed to interruptions and multitasking as reasons for missed nursing care. They indicated that they were often interrupted and this caused them to forget about aspects of care they needed to do. Similarly, frequent multitasking led to missed nursing care because they would forget what they hadn't finished on a previous task while completing something else. They often remembered they had not completed an aspect of nursing care after they had already left the unit, sometimes waking up in the middle of the night and remembering it.

- "I totally missed charting my patient assessment on one of my four patients last week and I was reminded by the next shift nurse. So, I charted it four days later. I was just very busy with the discharges, admits, etc., and it just skipped my mind." (RN)

- "I asked one of the techs to get blood vitals for me because I was in the middle of something and then she totally forgot, and then I came back and asked, 'So what were those vitals?' And I looked them up and asked 'Did you just not put it in the computer?' And she was like 'No, I totally forgot!'" (RN)

- "I will wake up in the middle of my sleep and remember I didn't do x or y." (RN)

- "When I do two or more tasks at a time, it is easy to forget everything." (RN)

An interruption is a signal indicating there is an event that needs attention (American Psychological Association, 2006). Nurses use various strategies to handle interruptions, including task switching and multitasking. For example, a nurse may be asked a question by a physician and she can respond by stopping the current activity and answering the question (task switching) or by continuing the task while concurrently answering the physician's question, which is multitasking.

Nurses' work is characterized by this interruptive, multitask-driven, fast-paced, and unpredictable environment. Consequently, nurses' cognitive load is exceptionally heavy (Ebright, Patterson, Chalko, & Render, 2003; Simmons, Lanuza, Fonteyn, Hicks, & Holm, 2003). The environment in which nurses work is complex and fragmented, with many competing demands on nurses' time and cognitive processes (Simmons et al., 2003; Biron, Lavoie-Tremblay, & Loiselle, 2009). A study showed that nurses, balancing multiple patients and their families with changing needs and problems, engage in a recursive cognitive process that uses inductive and deductive cognitive skills (Ebright et al., 2003).

Interruptions, multitasking, and task switching are felt to predispose people to make errors (Coiera, Jayasuriya, Hardy, Bannan, & Thorpe, 2002; Laxmisan, et al., 2007). In other high-risk industries, such as nuclear power plant operations and aviation, interruptions, multitasking, and task switching are known human factors that contribute to errors and even catastrophic events (Dismukes, Young, & Sumwalt, 1998; Reason, 1990). They are seen as particular sources of concern in that they negatively affect an individual's working memory, which is limited in its capacity and is transient in nature. The working memory is the system that actively holds multiple pieces of transitory information in the mind. People may be able to remember a massive number of facts, but only a handful are held in the working memory, able to be accessed at any given moment.

In recent years, there has been evidence that the limitation of working memory is somewhere between one and four information chunks (Cowan, 2001; Izawa & Ohta, 2005). Information chunks refers to concepts split into small pieces or "chunks" of information to make reading and understanding faster and easier. This is why it is not unusual to forget items at the grocery store when relying on a mental shopping list. Some researchers are suggesting that it may only be possible to remember one fact. In a study by Brian Mcelree (2001), participants underwent a test of working memory called "n-back" (Verhaeghen & Basak, 2005). In the task, the participants read a series of numbers that were presented one at a time on a computer screen. In the easiest version of the task, the computer presents a new digit, then prompts participants to recall what number immediately preceded the current one. More difficult versions might ask participants to recall what number appeared two, three, or four digits previously. Mcelree found that participants recalled the immediately preceding numbers in a fraction of the time it took them to recall numbers presented more than one number ago.

The problem with working memory is that when items are stored temporarily (short-term store), they can easily be bumped out by more information coming in (Woloshynowych, Davis, Brown, & Vincent, 2007). Working memory has been referred to as the Post-It notes of the brain (Woloshynowych et al., 2007). Task switching involves several parts of the brain. Brain scans during task switching show activity in four major areas. The pre frontal cortex (PFC) is involved in shifting and focusing attention, and selecting which task to do when. The posterior parietal lobe activates rules for each task, the anterior cingulate gyrus monitors errors, and the pre motor cortex prepares the body for movement.

Juggling tasks can be very stressful. In the short term, stress makes you feel bad. In the long run, it can become a serious threat to health— and that's not even counting the dangers such as talking on the phone while driving or taking care of a patient while talking on the phone. Working memory is also impaired by stress. This phenomenon was first discovered in animal studies by Arnsten (1998), who demonstrated that stress-induced catecholamine release in the PFC rapidly decreases PFC neuronal firing and impairs working memory performance. This research was extended to humans, and confirms that stress leads to reduced working memory capacity. The more stress, the lower the efficiency of working memory in performing simple thinking tasks.

Individual differences among nurses can have various influences on their working memory. People vary in their ability to ignore sensory input, and this is closely linked to their working memory capacity. The greater a person's working memory capacity, the greater their ability to resist sensory capture (Fukuda & Vogel, 2009). The limited ability to override attentional capture is likely to result in the unnecessary storage of information in working memory, suggesting not only that having a poor working memory affects attention but that it can also limit the capacity of working memory even further (Fukuda & Vogel, 2009). Also, working memory is sensitive to age. Research shows that its capacity tends to decline with age.

Multitasking
Multitasking involves actively thinking about more than one thing at a time, which can overload the brain's working memory. Dividing

attention across multiple activities is taxing on the brain, and as a result, productivity often suffers. There are some cases where it may be possible to do what is called 'perfect time-sharing,' but this typically happens when each of the two tasks are pretty routine (Schumacher et al., 2001).

Humans are typically good at balancing tasks that use unrelated mental and physical resources. For instance, most people are able to sweep the floor and listen to music without too much trouble. However, when tasks become more complicated, such as determining the rate of flow of an IV and talking to a patient about their illness, there's going to be interference with one or more of the tasks. The person has two alternatives—either slow down on one of the tasks (e.g., talking to a patient) or risk making a mistake (with the IV rate).

The brain is designed to handle multitasking when actions or activities are so familiar they have become habits. This is why, when a child is learning how to ride a tricycle, each movement requires intense concentration, but adults generally have no trouble riding a bike while talking. If a task becomes a habit, such as how a person drives to work every day, it can be done without thinking. In fact, people sometimes drive to work when they want to go to the dentist's office. Yet some activities, no matter how many times they have been performed, require too much engagement and active thinking to become truly habitual (e.g., determining correct flow of fluid, assessing a patient's condition, preparing medications, etc.). Even though some nurses may be better than others in completing more than one task at a time, if the task is complicated and involves the same part of the brain, it will not be possible to do more than one thing at a time.

Task switching

Research has shown that task switching takes more time to get tasks completed than if they were performed one at a time. It has been shown that people make more errors when they switch than if they do one task at a time. The more complicated the task, the more likely errors will occur. If there is a lot of task switching during a shift, it can add up to as much as 40% loss in productivity (Verhaeghen & Hoyer 2007). Task switching in health care has been studied less than interruptions and multitasking. Walter, Li, Dunsmuir, and Westbrook (2014) compared multitasking and task switching of physicians and nurses in an emergency department and general units. They found that task switching rates-per-hour were higher in the ED than on the general medical–surgical units, while multitasking occurred more on the general units than the ED. Nurses were more apt to multitask, while physicians were more prone to switch tasks.

For decades, research in psychology has shown that people can only attend to one cognitive task or mental activity at a time. For example, a person can be reading or typing, or listening or reading. Because humans are pretty good at switching back and forth quickly, they think they are actually multitasking, but in reality they are not. The only exception that the research has uncovered is that if a person is doing a physical task that they have done very, very often and are good at, then they can do that physical task while doing a mental task. For example, adults can and walk and talk at the same time. Even this doesn't work as well as we think. In a study by Hyman, Boss, Wise, McKenzie, and Caggiano in 2009, people talking on their cell phones while walking ran into people more often than those who weren't and didn't notice what was going on around them. The researchers had someone in a clown suit ride a unicycle. The people talking on a cell phone were much less likely to notice or remember the clown. Clifford Nass's (2013) study found that when people are asked to deal with multiple streams of information, they can't pay attention to them, can't remember as well, and don't switch as well as they thought they would.

Westbrook, Duffield, Li, and Creswick (2011) found in a study of emergency departments, physicians were interrupted 6.6 times per hour and 3.3% more than once. Physicians multitasked 12.8% of the time. Interruptions were associated with a significant increase in time spent on a task. However, when length-biased sampling was accounted for, interrupted tasks were unexpectedly completed in a shorter time than uninterrupted tasks. Physicians failed to return to 18.5% of interrupted tasks (Westbrook et al., 2011; Westbrook, Woods, Rob, Dunsmuir, & Day, 2010).

Studies have shown the extent to which nurses in acute care settings (medical–surgical, intensive care units) are interrupted (Rivera-Rodriguez & Karsh, 2010). In one study, nurses were interrupted 10 times per hour, or 1 interruption per 6 minutes (Kalisch & Aebersold, 2010). Ebright and colleagues (2003) found that RNs were interrupted 6.3 times per hour, while Potter and colleagues (2005), using both an RN and a human factors engineer (HFE) as observers, uncovered 5.9 per hour (HFE) and 3.4 per hour (RN). A third study conducted reported 14 interruptions per hour (McGillis Hall et al., 2010). Kosits and Jones (2011) found 3.3 interruptions per hour for nurses in the emergency department. Biron, Lavoie-Tremblay, and

Loiselle (2009) found that interruptions during medication administration were 6.3 per hour.

In the Kalisch and Aebersold study, nurses were most frequently interrupted by patients (28%), other nurses (25%), assistive personnel (10%), and physicians (9%). Task switching, where the nurse had to suspend an activity for greater than 10 seconds, occurred in 38% of the interruptions. After being interrupted during a task and switching to a different one, personnel were often interrupted again, even multiple times. Nurses engaged in multitasking 30% of the time in Hospital 1 and 40% in Hospital 2. The events associated with multitasking were communication (38%), nursing interventions (15%), medication administration (13%), documentation (13%), and assessment (10%) (Kalisch & Aebersold, 2010).

Tucker and Spear (2006) conducted an observational study of 11 nurses and found that there was an average of 8.4 work system failures per 8-hour shift. The five most frequent types of failures, accounting for 6.4 of these obstacles, involved medications, orders, supplies, staffing, and equipment. Survey questions asking nurses how frequently they experienced these five categories of obstacles yielded similar frequencies. For an average 8-hour shift, the average task time was only 3.1 minutes, and in spite of this, nurses were interrupted mid-task an average of eight times per shift.

Another recent phenomenon, which leads to greater amounts of interruptions and multitasking, is staff members talking on cell phones, checking personal email, and using social media sites, such as Facebook and Twitter.

- "Another problem is just a change in society where you are not able to be disconnected from anything. And I think that that also can lead... to missed care because you're not focused on being there, you're focused on being somewhere else." (RN)

- "Now our [personal] cell phones chirp 100 times a day. And you look at your cell phone 100 times a day." (RN)

- "I can picture the people on our unit consistently on something [Pinterest or Facebook]." (RN)

Multiple alarms also interrupt the work of nurses.

- "So literally, there are days [the telemetry monitor] is going off every minute, just with normal alarms. So what happens is that you miss the real things. Some days up here it is awful. Especially when you are trying to make a phone call [to a doctor] and it is alarming in your ear and you are like, 'Oh sorry what was that?'" (RN)

Studies on the impact of interruptions, multitasking, and task switching on actual errors have produced mixed results. Westbrook and colleagues (2010) found that procedural failures proportionally increased from 70% with no interruptions to 92% with four interruptions. They also reported a statistically significant relationship (coefficient of 0.18, SE ¼ 0.05, $p < .001$) between interruptions and clinical errors. Kalisch and Aebersold (2010), who observed 200 errors and 1,354 interruptions in two hospitals, found that errors were no more common when nurses were interrupted or when they multitasked than when the nurses were focused on a single task without interruption. Potter et al. (2005) reported that 24% of the interruptions experienced by nurses on medical–surgical units occurred prior to a cognitive shift, defined as a shift in attention; the authors did not find an association with errors.

Other investigators explored relationships between interruptions and the time it takes to resume the interrupted activity (Grundgeiger & Sanderson, 2009). Grundgeiger, Sanderson, MacDougall, and Venkatesh (2010) provided evidence that interruptions affected cognitive activity for nurses working in intensive-care settings. The duration of the interruption as well as a change in the nurses' physical location increased the time before the nurse resumed the initial task. Additionally, it was noted that nurses employed strategies such as "holding items in their hands" or "placing items in conspicuous locations" as reminders to resume the initial task (Grundgeiger, Sanderson, MacDougall, and Venkatesh, 2010). Brixey and colleagues (2008) also noted that interruptions caused delays in resuming the initial task. Disruption of workflow has also been associated with interruptions. For example, in a study of physicians, workflow interruptions were significantly related to physicians' workload (Weigl, Muller, Vincent, Angerer, & Sevdalis, 2012). Kowinsky and colleagues (2012) noted that frequent interruptions in work flow led to a lack of reliable completion of routine, predictable patient care tasks (e.g., ambulating, turning, repositioning, feeding, routine bedside procedures), and a lack of timely attention to non-routine, unpredictable patient care tasks (e.g., answering call bells, taking patients to the bathroom, blood draws, transporting patients on and off the unit for tests or therapy, admissions, discharges, and transfers).

Fatigue and Exhaustion
The third reason uncovered in this study was that fatigue due to long work hours or shifts (12 hours or more), rotating shifts, mandated

overtime, not having breaks, and working more than one job leads to missed nursing care. Nurse interviewees said that sometimes they were just tired and exhausted and found themselves skipping care. They pointed to such occurrences as not getting breaks and working long shifts. Being mandated to stay after their shift was particularly difficult. Older nurses especially said the 12-hour shift is increasingly difficult for them to work.

Long work hours

Sleep loss and fatigue have been shown to have a negative effect on cognitive performance (Alhola & Polo-Kantola, 2007; Cohen et al., 2010; Harrison & Horne, 2000; Killgore, 2010). Dembe, Erickson, Delbos, and Banks (2005) found that working in jobs with over-time schedules was associated with a 61% higher injury hazard rate compared to jobs without overtime. Working at least 12 hours per day was associated with a 37% increased hazard rate. Impairments in higher-level domains of executive function and decision-making have been noted in physicians who work during long, and especially night-time, shifts (Rothschild et al., 2009; Scott et al., 2007).

In a review paper, Caruso (2006) summarizes research linking long work hours to a wide range of risks. The risks are theorized to stem from less time to recover from work, longer exposure to workplace hazards, and less time to attend to non-work responsibilities. Risks to workers include sleep deprivation, poor recovery from work, decre-ments in neuro-cognitive and physiological functioning, illnesses, adverse reproductive outcomes, and injuries. Risks to employers include reduced productivity and increases in workers' errors. One study also found that longer shifts led to higher nurse burnout and less patient satisfaction (Stimpfel, Sloan, & Aiken, 2012).

As indicated above, there are several practices which may contribute to fatigue in nursing. Twelve-hour shifts are everywhere in nursing. Although some nurses, especially those over 50 years of age, do not like working twelve-hour shifts, the majority of nurses prefer them, because they gain an extra day off. They typically work three twelve-hour shifts, but sometimes they work longer on overtime in order to complete their work.

Rogers and colleagues (2004) conducted a study of 393 hospital staff nurses who kept logbooks of their work hours and errors made at work. The results showed that nurses usually worked longer than scheduled and that approximately 40% of the 5,317 work shifts they logged exceeded twelve hours. The risks of making an error were significantly increased when work shifts were longer than twelve hours, when nurses worked overtime, or when they worked more than forty hours per week.

In a study of critical care nurses, 502 subjects completed logbooks about their work hours, overtime, days off, and sleep–wake patterns. During work days, the respondents completed all work-related questions and questions about difficulties in remaining awake while on duty. Space was provided for descriptions of any errors or near errors that might have occurred. On their days off, the nurses completed only those questions about sleep–wake patterns, mood, and caffeine intake. The respondents consistently worked longer than scheduled and for extended periods. Longer work duration increased the risk of errors and near errors and decreased nurses' vigilance (Scott, Rogers, Hwang, & Zhang, 2006).

Dean, Scott, and Rogers (2006) used a case study method to determine the relationship between fatigue and error in caring for neonatal patients. They conclude that employing good sleep habits, minimizing shift rotations and excessive work hours, and using strategic naps can reduce the adverse effects of fatigue that put patients at risk.

These case studies reinforce the concept that neonatal intensive care (NICU) nurses need to be alert enough to provide safe care for their patients, as well as alert enough to detect and correct the errors made by others. Investigations indicate that long shifts worked by hospital staff nurses are associated with higher risk of errors, especially when coupled with insufficient sleep and fatigue. Scott, Hofmeister, Rogness, and Rogers (2010) reported that most of the nurses in a study they conducted experienced poor sleep quality, severe daytime sleepiness, and decreased alertness at work and while operating a motor vehicle.

Trinkoff and colleagues (2011) found that work schedules were related significantly to patient mortality when staffing levels and hospital characteristics were controlled. Pneumonia deaths were significantly more likely to occur in hospitals where nurses reported schedules with long work hours (odds ratio [OR] = 1.42, 95% confidence interval [CI] = 1.17–1.73, $p < .01$) and lack of time away from work (OR = 1.24, 95% CI = 1.03–1.50, $p < .05$). Abdominal aortic aneurysm was also associated significantly with the lack of time away from work (OR = 1.39, 95% CI = 1.11–1.73, $p < .01$). For patients with congestive heart failure, mortality was associated with nurses working while sick (OR = 1.39, 95% CI = 1.13–1.72, $p < .01$), whereas acute myocardial infarction was associated significantly with weekly burden (hours per week; days in a row) for nurses (OR = 1.33, 95% CI = 1.09–1.63, $p < .01$).

In another study, 546 nurses responded to a survey containing several instruments measuring sleep quality and quantity, and sleepiness, as well as clinical decision self-efficacy. Decision regret was reported by 157 of 546 (29%) nurses. Nurses with decision regret reported more fatigue, more daytime sleepiness, less inter-shift recovery, and worse sleep quality than did nurses without decision regret (Scott, Arslanian-Engoren, & Engoren, 2014).

Rotating shifts

Circadian rhythm misalignment, inadequate and poor-quality sleep, and sleep disorders, such as sleep apnea, insomnia, and shift work disorder (excessive sleepiness, insomnia, or both temporally associated with work schedules), contribute to these problems. Falling asleep at work at least once a week occurs in 32% to 36% of shift workers. Risk of occupational accidents is at least 60% higher for non-day shift workers. Shift workers also have higher rates of cardiometabolic diseases and mood disturbances. Road and workplace accidents attributable to excessive sleepiness, to which shift work is a significant contributor, are estimated to cost $71 to $93 billion per annum in the United States (Rajaratnam, Howard, & Grustein, 2013).

Rotating shifts are still scheduled, although they have been reduced in number in recent years. Sometimes a shift even changes within a week, causing a nurse to work both days and nights. In a review of studies on the impact of rotating shifts in nursing, it was concluded that rotating night shifts resulted in adverse psychological and physiological effects when compared with their permanent night duty peers, particularly for those over 40 years of age. Evidence also suggests that the effects of fatigue on nurse performance may negatively affect the quality of patient care (Muecke, 2005).

Mandated overtime

When it is not possible to find a replacement for a nurse or the demands on the unit increase, some hospitals mandate the staff to stay for either all or part of the next shift. This means that a nurse could be working 16 or more hours in a row. There is an increase in missed nursing care at the end of this long time period. This nurse explains:

> *There are also issues when you have to mandate people to stay. So say you just worked a 12-hour shift and we're short and you're the next person on the list to be mandated, you have to be mandated. You may be working for 16 hours. At the end of a 16-hour shift you*

*are more likely to miss things and have errors. And then you have
to be back the next day at 7:00 am. (RN)*

Lack of breaks
Breaks are also a problem in nursing. In one study, nurses reported
having a break or meal period free of patient care responsibilities in
less than half of the shifts they worked. There were no differences in
the risk of errors, however, reported by nurses who had a break free of
patient care responsibilities compared with those who were unable to
take a break (Rogers, Hwang, Scott, Aiken, & Dinges, 2004).

Multiple jobs
Another issue that has been reported is nurses "stacking" working
days so that they work six days in a row and can have a week off. This
occurs most often when the nurse works more than one job.

Cognitive Biases
Cognitive biases are glitches in thinking that cause people to make
questionable decisions and reach erroneous conclusions. A cognitive
bias is a deficiency or limitation in thinking—a flaw in judgment that
arises from errors of memory, social attribution, and miscalculations.
Psychologists say that cognitive biases help people process information more efficiently, especially in stressful situations (where nursing
staff spend a great deal of their time). Still, they can also lead people
to make serious miscalculations. Heuristic thinking is associated with
cognitive biases. Heuristic thinking refers to experience-based techniques for problem-solving, learning, and discovery that give a solution that may not be optimal (Gigerenzer & Gaissmaier, 2011). When
a thorough examination of all of the factors is not possible, heuristic
methods are used to speed up the process of finding a satisfactory
solution via mental shortcuts to ease the cognitive load of making
a decision. Examples of this method include using a rule of thumb,
an educated guess, an intuitive judgment, a stereotype, or common
sense. This works well under most circumstances, but in certain cases
leads to systematic errors or cognitive biases.

Cognitive dissonance
Cognitive dissonance is one of the most well-known types of cognitive
biases. It is the feeling of tension or anxiety that is caused by holding
two opposing beliefs or thoughts at the same time. A common example
of this type of bias is when a person holds a certain belief about him

or herself. An individual may believe he or she is honest but proceed to act in a dishonest way. A nurse may hold the belief that he or she is an excellent nurse, yet does not complete standard, required nursing care.

Status-quo bias

People tend to be apprehensive about change, which often leads them to make choices that guarantee that things remain the same, or change as little as possible. Needless to say, this has ramifications in everything from politics to economics. People like to stick to their routines, political parties, and favorite meals at restaurants. Part of the perniciousness of this bias is the unwarranted assumption that another choice will be inferior or make things worse. The status-quo bias can be summed up with the saying "If it ain't broke, don't fix it"—an adage that fuels our conservative tendencies. And in fact, some commentators say this is why the United States. has not been able to enact true universal health care, despite the fact that most individuals support the idea of reform. Even the market-driven Affordable Care Act (ACA) has been unpopular with many Americans.

Bandwagon effect

Although often unconscious of it, people love to go with the flow of the crowd. When the masses start to pick a winner or a favorite, that's when our individualized brains start to shut down and enter into a kind of groupthink or hive-mind mentality. It has also been referred to as herding (Raafat, Chater, & Frith 2009). But it doesn't have to be a large crowd or the whims of an entire nation; it can include small groups, like a family or even a small group of coworkers. The bandwagon effect is what often causes behaviors, social norms, and memes to propagate among groups of individuals, regardless of the evidence or motives in support. This is why opinion polls are often maligned, as they can steer the perspectives of individuals according to the goals of those giving the surveys. Much of this bias has to do with our built-in desire to fit in and conform, as demonstrated by the famous Asch Conformity Experiments, a series of experiments in the 1950s that demonstrated the degree to which an individual's own opinions and perceptions are influenced by those of a majority group. Two related concepts are groupthink and herd behavior. Groupthink is when a poor decision emerges because a group of people have a desire for harmony. In fact, the more harmonious the group, the more the danger of lacking independent critical thinking increases. Herd behavior occurs when people are influenced by their peers to act in certain ways (Asch, 1955, 1956).

Omission bias

Omission bias—the tendency to judge harmful actions as worse or less moral than equally harmful omissions (inactions)—may contribute to nurses' decisions as to what care to complete and what to leave undone. This is due to the fact that actions are more visible and tangible than inactions, and because actions tend to be seen as more causative in nature than omissions (Spranca, Minsk, & Baron, 1991). For example, people perceive a death resulting from a vaccine as much worse than a death resulting from not getting a vaccine (Kahneman & Tversky, 1979). Likewise, a nurse giving a medication that results in a bad outcome may be considered worse than a nurse not giving a medication at all, which also results in a bad outcome. In other words, when a decision leads to a bad outcome relative to what might have been, people think that the decision is worse if the outcome results from action than if it results from inaction (Baron & Ritov, 1994; Kahneman & Tversky, 1982; Miller & Taylor, 1995; Ritov & Baron, 1990; Spranca et al., 1991). Further, self-blame and regret depends on perception of causality (Fincham & Jaspers, 1980).

The bias toward omission is also prevalent where the outcome of the option not chosen is unknown. For example, the outcome of many nursing actions such as ambulation, mouth care, teaching, etc. will not be evident until after discharge from the acute care hospital. Even though this information might be difficult to obtain, nurses could theoretically investigate the outcomes for their patients after discharge. However, they may not do so because they want to avoid regret in regard to their care decisions.

Regret aversion

Such anticipated regret might be especially conspicuous when the decision-maker knows the outcome of the choice not to do something, because learning that the outcome was bad and could have been avoided often leads to regretful feelings. Interestingly, and somewhat ironically, avoiding (outcome) regret in the short-run could lead to greater self-blame and outcome regret in the long run, as they have not sought nor received feedback for their actions which could have led to better decisions in the future. However, it is not common for nursing staff in acute care settings to seek out information about their patients' status after discharge. It is possible that they are avoiding potential regret, although if they did obtain this information, they would likely make different decisions in the future (Josephs, Larrick, Steele, & Nisbett, 1992; Kahneman, 2011).

Scientific studies show that people tend to overestimate the level of regret associated with a decision, and that the majority of people regret inaction above all else (Connolly & Zeelenberg, 2002). When faced with a hypothetical decision, study participants believe that they are much more likely to regret things they do than things they don't do. When asked about real-life experiences, however, an overwhelming majority regretted the things they hadn't done much more than the things they had.

Regret is a painful cognitive emotion. Recent research suggests it has two major components, outcome regret and self-blame regret (Connolly & Zeelenberg, 2002). Outcome regret results from an unfavorable comparison of the consequences of one's decisions with a better outcome such as what could have been had one chosen differently (Zeelenberg, 1999). Self-blame regret results from the feeling that one's decision was not sufficiently justified (Reb & Connolly, 2005). Regret is the second most mentioned emotion in day-to-day conversations (Shimanoff, 1984). Regret aversion might keep nurses from seeking feedback out of fear. Feedback avoidance due to regret aversion seems quite innocent and perhaps even reasonable. After all, regret is painful, and nothing useful could be learned by getting feedback on the outcomes for specific patients since they are no longer under their care.

The importance of feedback is heightened when the same kind of decision is faced repeatedly, which is certainly the case in nursing. Feedback avoidance in such repeated decision-making results in reduced information gain. As a consequence, the nurse decision-maker will be less prepared to choose the best available options in the future. This has been labeled myopic regret aversion. Feedback avoidance results in decreased learning and subsequently reduced quality.

Lack of Patient or Family Engagement

Another reason some nursing care is missed is that patients and families are not fully engaged in the patient's care. Nursing staff often said that nursing care is missed because the patient or family refuses the care such as ambulation.

- "There are patients that do not want to ambulate, so for the rest of your shift you just stop trying." (RN)

- "We had this young girl a while ago. Her boyfriend [the patient] didn't want to go to therapy and she kept saying we were bothering him, but we only wanted to motivate him to go to therapy. She wasn't making it any better, so our supervisor made it that she couldn't come up here anymore." (RN)

- "[Family resistance] is a big problem. It's hard when the family does not support the nurse." (RN)

Lack of Physician Resources

In addition to a lack of material resources, focus group participants pointed to not having the human resources they need to do their jobs. For example, they might have needed a physician's order for something, could not read their writing, or the orders did not make sense and they could not contact the physician. This kept them from providing aspects of nursing care.

- "So, it could be a lack of communication in the sense that you never know... who's rounding for the attending, and you don't know if they have resident coverage and then you don't know if they've consulted a different team to work on it, and then you don't know if the consulting team is handling it and I will literally page six wrong people before I figure out the one person who can give me an answer. So I feel like a lot of times I'm chasing down pain meds; I'm chasing down testing times; I'm chasing down all of these other things instead of being at the bedside and doing care. That's why I think I miss things." (RN)

- "Now we have 15 different services on our floor at one time. It's insane. I don't know who to contact; I don't know these people. I've never met them; they don't know me." (RN)

- "The paging list is never up-to-date." (RN)

- "Half of the time doctors are ordering things and you can't find a reason as to why they would order that, so I am constantly paging them and asking, 'Did you mean to put this on for this person?' Half of the time they didn't mean to put the order in for that patient and the other half, yes, they did mean to. If you had just let me know that this is what you are ordering and why, I wouldn't have to ask you about it or clarify or say, 'What are we doing this for?'" (RN)

- "I think where I work, the biggest reason or complaint that I would have, or feeling like I miss certain care, is because I'm spending too much of my time fulfilling things that aren't really my job. Things that the doctor should be doing. I'm hunting people down to get really simple things, or I'm making five phone calls that should be one phone call, or doctors are missing orders because they are just assuming that the nurse will put in orders for them, or they assume that we know the bowel prep they want, and then I'm spending all this time investigating things. So I feel like my time was better spent making sure I had all the right information and knowing what I needed to do related to something different, than if I didn't get to the patient's IV. I'm thinking, 'Well that was like the least important thing on the list today.' So I feel like my hospital is just lacking policies and procedures, and it's also lacking follow-through from physicians and that there's just a lot of responsibility on the nurses that we're going to follow-up with everything. So a lot of the time I'm at the computer looking up information, I'm spending a lot of time paging physicians, and chasing things down instead of them just being there." (RN)

Leadership Gaps

Leadership and management issues were noted by the interviewees as another common factor that leads to missed nursing care, especially exemplified by leaders not dealing with performance issues and not recognizing good performers. The most frequent area of concern is inadequate performance management of unproductive staff members: Staff members who do not perform well are not counseled or dealt with. They are allowed to continue to work in the same manner as they have been, even though they are missing essential elements of nursing care.

- "I never get it! Are they walking their patients? Are they bathing their patients? Because I always see them in the break room and I don't understand it. It's always the same people. And I just want to follow them, and look at their charting and see what they chart." (RN)

- "If you see other people who get to be lazy and they get paid the same as you and the repercussions are exactly the same, then why would you want to do anything extra? Why are you working so hard?" (RN)

- "Some of them are lazy, there is a lazy component. I've been doing this 33 years, all on this unit, some of it is definitely a lazy component." (Unit Supervisor)

- "The nurses won't answer the call lights no matter what. The response when you are down a tech, you get another nurse. That doesn't help at all. They should do aid work, but they don't." (NA)

Another leadership issue is not recognizing and valuing the work of the staff who are good performers. They feel they are not valued by their leaders and worry about getting blamed for things that go wrong.

- "I think that there's not really any incentive to be a subpar nurse, a great nurse, or just an ok nurse." (RN)

- "You can be the worst or the best and it doesn't matter." (RN)

Staff also feel that managers are not visible on the unit and would like them to help when they are overwhelmed and serve as role models for the staff.

- "If management was out on the floor though, if management got up from their desk and helped with anything, your lights wouldn't be double flashing, someone would be walking around the halls, helping out. If management was out, the nurses wouldn't be sitting in the conference room not doing work, the nurses would be engaged and getting things done. So people would be helping you, people would be actually doing their job, people would be answering call lights if management wasn't guaranteed to be sitting in an office with their door closed." (RN)
- "Yeah! Not only can they help, but when they help, then the other staff are just a little more motivated to get up and help too." (RN)

Moral Distress

Another reason for missing nursing care identified by the interviewees was moral distress. The interviewees said that the stress of continually not being able to give the care they think they should accumulates and eventually leads to compassion fatigue or burnout. In those circumstances, they say they miss elements of nursing care.

- "I think sometimes you just don't take pride in your job anymore and there's a feeling of... I don't care. I'm going to get a paycheck whether or not I do my mouth care." (RN)
- "I don't know if this even counts or if this makes any sense... but I would say a reason care doesn't get done is because I've had, like where you're so overwhelmed where you literally just say 'F' it, I'm not going to do it, to be honest. Or literally like I put so much effort into this day, I'm so overwhelmed like literally, I'm not doing it. I'm going to choose not to do this. I don't know if that's evil." (RN)
- "I already feel like I've done so much today that I'm just, I just can't, like I have nothing else to give in this 12 hours. Because maybe I just spent two hours with an anxious family who's getting a first time chemo and is a new lymphoma, you know what I mean? And you're like, really, and this person didn't get up to the chair today? Like, that's like the least of my concerns. Or like, I just coded a patient." (RN)

In other cases, the nurses expressed a great amount of concern because the care that was ordered was not appropriate, in their opinion. For example, in the case that the patient will clearly not recover and the ordered care would have caused them further pain, a nurse may miss care.

> "I think when you feel like the only thing you're doing is torturing the patients by turning them or getting them up and out of bed. That patient I told you was on ECMO for about 290 days. We tried everything. We stood her on ECMO. We tried to get her to walk on ECMO. We literally were so invested in her, and her lungs were not, for a period of time they were recovering and then they didn't recover. The staff felt the patient was uncomfortable. You could see it, she mouthed words to us. And it was very hard for them when she wasn't doing well and you had to just push her. It was hard on everybody. So you get missed care because nurses are feeling an ethical dilemma about pushing." (Unit Supervisor)

Documentation Load

There were many comments that the burden of documenting was so heavy it sometimes interfered with giving care and lead to missed nursing care. They noted that the amount of documenting grows with time and the electronic health record (EHR) actually adds to the time required.

- "Some people say that they are nursing the computer and not the patient anymore. From my personal perspective, you have people that are proficient with technology and others that are not, and that does not reflect their nursing care. Some are just faster, better, or they are not. Regardless, documentation takes time, and it takes time away from the patient. And so, that leads 1) they either ignore the charting or 2) they ignore the patient." (RN)
- "It is a lot more involved to chart now. More time consuming. A lot more areas to login to, to chart with passwords, programs, etc." (RN)
- "Oh I miss things all the time. There are so many different pieces you chart on and you look at it and you think, 'Oh it's done,' but you may have missed something because there are so many different places. It is not all in front of you. So you think that you did it and later you go back and you are like, 'Oh, I never put that in there.'" (RN)

Large Number of Inexperienced Staff

One key reason for missed nursing care, according to the interviewees, was that new nurses are more likely to either forget or not know that care is needed. When any subset of the nursing staff has less experience, it increases the amount of missed nursing care on a unit. Being new to nursing was the most common reason given for lacking experience, but nurses who floated or were temporary on the unit were also described as being inexperienced.

- "I think the biggest issue for us a lot of times is just education and experience. The less experiential knowledge you have sometimes you don't foresee things happening. If you have seen it before, you can take the steps to do things appropriately. That's just part of learning for all nurses." (RN)

- "So if you have a lot of new grads, like a lot of medical–surgical units do because that is where nurses typically start, they literally don't have the skills to help each other out. They are just trying to get through their day. Just treading water." (RN)

- "If you do not have that rehab mind state, looking at the big picture of teaching, education, all of the things that are involved in the day-to-day care that you learn over time, things get missed. We lost a lot of our seniority and all those seasoned rehab nurses that know all of this. And now we are working with a lot of young, inexperienced nurses and they do not have that rehab concept under their belt yet and there is not as many senior people to ask or orient them. They are being oriented by people who are just one or two years out of orientation and aren't seasoned nurses. There is a lot that happens when you lose those vital pieces of care." (RN)

- "A lot of [nurses] are right out of college, the other day we had to bathe a person and the nurse didn't know how to bathe. She believed that it was the tech's job." (RN)

- "When you're a brand new nurse you're supposed to be focusing on your clinical skills, but because we are so short-staffed all the time your focus is split. Because you don't know what you don't know, and it is really difficult. That's why I'm really glad that I'm leaving in two months." (RN)

Complacency

Most nurses believe it is most important that they keep their mind on the task at hand when they are working. However, when a person does the same job all the time, they can become complacent. Complacency is a feeling of being satisfied with how things are and not caring to try to make them better. It is assumed that the work will always be done the same way and turn out with the same results, so there is no need to change or pay attention to new things. Although everyone does get complacent with things they have done over and over at some point, this way of thinking can become very detrimental, because if the nurse is not thinking about what they are doing, their behavior will not change to meet the needs of the current patient and situation.

Neuroscientists have traced our habit-making behaviors to a part of the brain called the basal ganglia, which also plays a key role in the development of emotions, memories, and pattern recognition. Decisions, meanwhile, are made in a different part of the brain called the prefrontal cortex. But as soon as a behavior becomes automatic, the decision-making part of the brain slows down. Charles Duhigg (2012) writes in his book, *The Power of Habit: Why We Do What We Do in Life and Business*, that the brain can almost completely shut down. He points out that this is a real advantage, because it means you have mental activity you can devote to something else. When you drive to work every day, you don't have to think. But if on one day you are going to the airport instead, you may find yourself at your work because you did not think. It happens to all of us. This is also why you can have a conversation while driving, watch television while eating, and observe a patient while talking to them. Duhigg points out that a person can do complex behaviors without being mentally aware of it at all because of the capacity of our basal ganglia to take a behavior and turn it into an automatic routine. Studies have shown that people will perform automated behaviors—like brushing teeth—the same way every single time, if they're in the same environment. But if they take a vacation, the behavior will probably change because the cues have changed. It's not just individual habits that become automated. Duhigg says there are studies that show organizational habits form among workers working for the same company.

An example is helping patients avoid falling by adopting such safety habits as moving their eyes before they move their hands, feet, body, or car; testing their footing or grip before they commit their weight to it; and looking at their "second foot" as they step over a cord or something on which they could trip (it is usually the second foot that is not being paid attention to that gets caught or hung up).

Complacency also causes problems with decision-making. One of these problems is with trusting something important—especially something that is critical from a quality or safety perspective—to your memory. This can be as simple as forgetting to change the IV tubing or to wash your hands. In some cases, the consequences are just wasted time or wasted money. At other times, the consequences can be deadly. In nursing, the latter is more likely to be the case than in many other work situations.

So when we say to ourselves, "I've got to remember this" or "I can't forget to do that," we need to realize that right now is your last best chance to do something to aid your memory (a note in line of vision, an alarm on the phone, etc.). But, once again, complacency can get in the way. Because we don't always forget or, worse, hardly ever forget, it's very easy for us to get complacent about doing something else to aid our memory, especially if whatever we need to do takes a bit of effort or seems silly (such as putting a Post-It note on the IV bag).

The check lists that have become standard practice in operating rooms are an example of creating an aid to memory. But they are not foolproof since complacency sets in and staff members check off the items without really ensuring that the task has been completed. This accounts for the fact that there are still major mistakes made in operating rooms (such as removing the wrong leg).

Complacency also causes problems with recognizing change. People can talk and drive at the same time but it can be a distraction. Sometimes it's not too distracting (not too dangerous) and sometimes the conversation can be very preoccupying (very dangerous). In situations like these, it's easy to become complacent and rationalize that it is not dangerous and the risk is low. It only becomes a problem if the conversation starts to get more involved. But this can be difficult to recognize because now the focus is on whatever it is that's preoccupying attention, not on driving. So even though most people know driving when preoccupied is dangerous, complacency can lead them to do things that may easily become very dangerous without always recognizing it.

Another fairly obvious problem complacency causes is overconfidence. Many safety devices, procedures, or protocols are redundant if nobody makes a mistake. We all know you don't need a life jacket unless you fall in the water so a good swimmer might be less inclined to wear a life jacket. Healthcare professionals also can become complacent about using checklists or following policies for example. An RN may not tell the other staff that she is leaving for lunch and when she will be back. Patients can get complacent about holding the handrail, even if they have fallen going down the stairs before.

Therefore, we need to teach patients, for example, more than just the critical error reduction techniques but also how to compensate for complacency leading to our minds not being on task. The same applies to nursing staff. We need to teach not just what needs to be done but also the impact of not keeping our mind on the work. A deep respect for complacency and what it can do to decision-making needs to be emphasized.

Summary

In this chapter, we reviewed the reasons for missing nursing care: lack of nursing staff resources; lack of material resources (including medications); communication and teamwork issues; interruptions, multitasking, and task switching; fatigue and physical exhaustion; cognitive biases; lack of patient and family engagement; lack of human resources; leadership issues; moral distress and compassion fatigue; documentation load; large proportion of new nurses; and complacency. Potential solutions will be covered in later chapters.

References

Alhola, P., & Polo-Kantola, P. (2007). Sleep deprivation: Impact on cognitive performance. *Neuropsychiatric Disease and Treatment, 3*(5): 553–567.

American Psychological Association. (2006). Multitasking: Switching costs. Retrieved from https://www.apa.org/research/action/multitask.aspx

Arnsten, A. F. (1998). The biology of being frazzled. *Science, 280*(5370), 1711–1712.

Asch, S. E. (1955). Opinions and social pressure. *Scientific American, 193*(5), 31–35.

Asch, S. E. (1956). Studies of independence and conformity. A minority of one again a unanimous majority. *Psychological Monographs, 70*(9), 1–70.

Ausserhofer, D., Zander, B., Busse, R., Schubert, M. S., De Geest, S., Rafferty, A. M., … Schwendimann, R. (2014). Prevalence, patterns and predictors of nursing care left undone in European hospitals: Results from the multicountry cross-sectional RN4CAST study. *BMJ Quality & Safety*, 23(2), 126–135.

Baron, J., & Ritov, I. (1994). Reference points and omission bias. *Organizational Behavior and Human Decision Processes, 59*(3), 475–498.

Biron, A. D., Lavoie-Tremblay, M., & Loiselle, C. G. (2009). Characteristics of work interruptions during medication administration. *Journal of Nursing Scholarship, 41*(4), 330–336.

Brixey, J. J., Tang, Z., Robinson, D. J., Johnson, C. W., Johnson, T. R., Turley, J. P., Patel, V. L., & Zhang, J. (2008). Interruptions in a level one trauma center: A case study. *International Journal of Medical Informatics, 77*(4), 235–241.

Caruso, C.C. (2006). Possible broad impacts of long work hours. *Industrial Health, 44*(4), 531–536.

Cohen, D. A., Wang, W., Wyatt, J. K., Kronauer, R. E., Derk-Jan, D., Czeisler, C. A., & Klerman, E. B. (2010). Uncovering residual effects of chronic sleep loss on human performance. *Science Translational Medicine, 2*(14)14ra3. doi:10.1126/scitranslmed.3000458

Coiera, E. W., Jayasuriya, R. A., Hardy, J., Bannan, A., & Thorpe, M. E. (2002). Communication loads on clinical staff in the emergency department. *The Medical Journal of Australia, 176*(9), 415–418.

Connolly, T., & Zeelenberg, M. (2002). Regret in decision making. *Current Directions in Psychological Science, 11*(6), 212–216.

Cowan, N. (2001). The magical number 4 in short-term memory: A reconsideration of mental storage capacity. *Behavioral and Brain Sciences, 24*(1), 87–185.

Dean, G. E., Scott, L. D., & Rogers, A. E. (2006). Infants at risk: When nurse fatigue jeopardizes quality care. *Advances in Neonatal Care, 6*(3), 120–126.

Dembe, A. E., Erickson, J. B., Delbos, R. G., & Banks, S. M. (2005). The impact of overtime and long work hours on occupational injuries and illnesses: New evidence from the United States. *Occupational and Environmental Medicine, 62*(9), 588–597.

Dismukes, K., Young, G., & Sumwalt, R. (1998). Cockpit interruptions and distractions: Effective management requires a careful balancing act. *Aviation Safety Reporting System Directline, 10*. Retrieved from http://asrs.arc.nasa.gov/docs/dl/DL10.pdf

Drake, D. A., Luna, M., Georges, J. M., & Steege, L. M. (2012). Hospital nurse force theory: A perspective of nurse fatigue and patient harm. *Advances in Nursing Science, 35*(4), 305–314. doi: 10.1097/ANS.0b013e318271d104

Duhigg, C. (2012). *The power of habit: Why we do what we do in life and business.* New York, NY: Random House.

Ebright, P. R., Patterson, E. S., Chalko, B. A., & Render, M. L. (2003). Understanding the complexity of registered nurses work in acute care settings. *Journal of Nursing Administration, 33*(12), 630–638.

Fincham, F. D., & Jaspers, J. M. (1980). Attribution of responsibility: From man the scientist to man as lawyer. *Advances in Experimental Social Psychology, 13*, 81–138. doi:10.1016/S0065-2601(08)60131-8

Fukuda, K., & Vogel, E. K. (2009, July). Human variation in overriding attentional capture. *The Journal of Neuroscience, 29*(27), 8726–8733.

Gigerenzer, G., & Gaissmaier, W. (2011). Heuristic decision making. *Annual Review of Psychology, 62*, 451–482.

Grundgeiger, T., & Sanderson, P. (2009). Interruptions in healthcare: Theoretical views. *International Journal of Medical Informatics, 78*(5), 293–307.

Grundgeiger, T., Sanderson, P., MacDougall, H. G., & Venkatesh, B. (2010). Interruption management in the intensive care unit: Predicting resumption times and assessing distributed support. *Journal of Experimental Psychology: Applied, 16*(4), 317–334.

Harrison, Y., & Horne, J. A. (2000). The impact of sleep deprivation on decision making: A review. *Journal of Experimental Psychology, 31*(11), 2501–2509.

Hyman, I. E., Boss, S. M., Wise, B. M., McKenzie, K. E., & Caggiano, J. M. (2009). Did you see the unicycling clown? Inattention blindness while walking and talking on a cell phone. *Applied Cognitive Psychology, 24*(5), 597–607.

Izawa, C., & Ohta, N. (Eds.). (2005). *Human learning and memory: Advances in theory and application: The 4th Tsukuba International Conference on Memory.* (pp. 155–175). Mahwah, NJ: Erlbaum.

Josephs, R. A., Larrick, R. P., Steele, C. M., & Nisbett, R. E. (1992). Protecting the self from the negative consequences of risky decisions. *Journal of Personality & Social Psychology. 62*(1), 26–37.

Kahneman, D. (2011). *Thinking fast and slow.* New York, NY: Farrar, Straus, and Giroux.

Kahneman, D., & Tversky, A. (1979). Prospect theory: An analysis of decision under risk. *Econometrica, 47*(2), 263–291.

Kahneman, D., & Tversky, A. (1982). The psychology of preferences. *Scientific American, 246*(1), 160–173.

Kalisch, B. J. (2006). Missed nursing care: A qualitative study. *Journal of Nursing Care Quality, 21*(4), 306–313.

Kalisch, B. J. (2009). Nurse and nurse assistant perceptions of missed nursing care: What does it tell us about teamwork? *Journal of Nursing Administration, 39*(11), 485–493.

Kalisch, B. J., & Aebersold, M. (2010). Interruptions and multitasking in nursing care. *The Joint Comission Journal on Quality and Patient Safety, 36*(3), 126–132.

Kalisch, B. J., Landstrom, G., & Williams, R. A. (2009). Missed nursing care: Errors of omission. *Nursing Outlook, 57*(1), 3–9.

Kalisch, B. J., Tschannen, D., Lee, H., & Friese, C. (2011). Hospital variation in missed nursing care. *American Journal of Medical Quality, 26*(4), 291–299.

Kalisch B. J., & Williams, R. A. (2009). Development and psychometric testing of a tool to measure missed nursing care (*MISSCARE Survey*). *The Journal of Nursing Administration, 39*(5), 211–219.

Killgore, W. D. (2010). Effects of sleep deprivation on cognition. *Progress in Brain Research, 185*, 105–129. doi: 10.1016/B978-0-444-53702-7.00007-5

Kosits, L. M., & Jones, K. (2011). Interruptions experienced by registered nurses working in the emergency department. *Journal of Emergency Nursing, 37*(1), 3–8.

Kowinsky, A. M., Shovel, J., McLaughlin, M., Vertacnik, L., Greenhouse, P. K., Martin, S. C., & Minnier, T. E. (2012). Separating predictable and unpredictable work to manage interruptions and promote safe and effective work flow. *Journal of Nursing Care Quality, 27*(2), 109–115.

Laxmisan, A., Hakimzada, F., Sayan, O. R., Green, R. A., Zhang, J., & Patel, V. L. (2007). The multitasking clinician: Decision-making and cognitive demand during and after team handoffs in emergency care. *International Journal of Medical Informatics, 76*(11–12), 801–811.

McElree, B. (2001). Working memory and focal attention. *Journal of Experimental Psychology: Learning, Memory, and Cognition, 27*(3), 817–835.

McGillis Hall, L., Pedersen, C., Hubley, P., Ptack, E., Hemingway, A., Watson, C., & Keatings, M. (2010). Interruptions and pediatric patient safety. *Journal of Pediatric Nursing, 25*(3), 167–175.

Miller, D. T., & Taylor, B. R. (1995). Counterfactual thought, regret, and superstition: How to avoid kicking yourself. In N. J. Roese and J. M. Olson (Eds.), *What might have been: The social psychology of counterfactual thinking* (pp. 305–331). Hillsdale, NJ, England: Lawrence Erlbaum Associates, Inc.

Muecke, S. (2005). Effects of rotating night shifts: Literature review. *Journal of Advanced Nursing, 50*(4), 433–439.

Nass, C. (2013). The myth of multitasking. NPR. Retrieved from http://www.npr.org/2013/05/10/182861382/the-myth-of-multitasking

Papastavrou, E., Andreou, P., Tsangari, H., Schubert, M., & De Geest, S. (2014). Rationing of nursing care within professional environmental constraints: A correlational study. *Clinical Nursing Research, 23*(3), 314–335.

Potter, P., Wolf, L., Boxerman, S., Grayson, D., Sledge, J., Dunagan, C., & Evanoff, B. (2005). Understanding the cognitive work of nursing in the acute care environment. *The Journal of Nursing Administration, 35*(7–8), 327–335.

Raafat, R. M., Chater, N., & Frith, C. (2009). Herding in humans. *Trends in Cognitive Sciences, 13*(10), 420–428.

Rajaratnam, S. M., Howard, M. E., & Grustein, R. R. (2013). Sleep loss and circadian disruption in shift work: Health burden and management. *Medical Journal of Australia, 199*(8), S11–S15.

Reason, J. T. (1990). *Human error.* New York, NY: Cambridge University Press.

Reb, J., & Connolly, T. (2009). Myopic regret avoidance: Feedback avoidance and learning in repeated decision making. *Organizational Behavior and Human Decision Processes, 109*(2), 182–189.

Ritov, I., & Baron, J. (1990). Reluctance to vaccinate: Omission bias and ambiguity. *Journal of Behavioral Decision Making, 3,* 263–277.

Rivera-Rodriguez, A. J., & Karsh, B. T. (2010). Interruptions and distractions in healthcare: Review and reappraisal. *Quality and Safety in Health Care, 19*(4), 304–312.

Rogers, A. E., Hwang, W. T., & Scott, L. D. (2004). The effects of work breaks on staff nurse performance journal of nursing administration. *The Journal of Nursing Administration, 34*(11), 512–519.

Rogers, A. E., Hwang, W. T., Scott, L. D., Aiken, L. H., & Dinges, D. F. (2004). The working hours of hospital staff nurses and patient safety. *Health Affairs, 23*(4), 202–212.

Rothschild, J. M., Keohane, C. A., Rogers, S., Gardner, R., Lipsitz, S. R., Salzberg, C. A., … Landrigan , C. P. (2009). Complications by attending physicians after nighttime procedures. *Journal of the American Medical Association, 302*(14),1565–1572.

Schubert, M., Clarke, S. P., Aiken, L. H., & De Geest, S. (2012). Associations between rationing of nursing care and inpatient mortality in Swiss hospitals. *International Journal for Quality in Health Care, 24*(3), 230–238.

Schumacher, E. H., Seymour, T. L., Glass, J. M., Fencsik, D. E., Lauber, E. J, Kieras, D. E., & Meyer, D. E. (2001). Virtually perfect time sharing in dual-task performance: Uncorking the central cognitive bottleneck. *Psychological Science, 12*(2), 101–108.

Scott, L. D., Arslanian-Engoren, C., & Engoren, M. C. (2014). Association of sleep and fatigue with decision regret among critical care nurses. *American Journal of Critical Care, 23*(1), 13–23. doi: 10.4037/ajcc2014191

Scott, L. D., Hofmeister, N., Rogness, N., & Rogers, A. E. (2010). An interventional approach for patient and nurse safety: A fatigue countermeasures feasibility study. *Nursing Research, 59*(4): 250–258. doi: 10.1097/NNR.0b013e3181de9116

Scott, L. D., Hwang, W. T., Rogers, A. E., Nysse, T., Dean, G. E., & Dinges, D. F. (2007). The relationship between nurse work schedules, sleep duration, and drowsy driving. *Sleep, 30*(12), 1801–1806.

Scott, L. D., Rogers, A. E., Hwang, W. T., & Zhang, Y. (2006). Effects of critical care nurses' work hours on vigilance and patients' safety. *American Journal of Critical Care, 15*(1), 30–37.

Shimanoff, S. B. (1984). Commonly named emotions in everyday conversations. *Perceptual and Motor Skills*, 58, 514. doi: 10.2466/pms.1984.58.2.514

Simmons, B., Lanuza, D., Fonteyn, M., Hicks, F., & Holm, K. (2003). Clinical reasoning in experienced nurses. *Western Journal of Nursing Research, 25*(6), 701–719.

Spranca, M., Minsk, E., & Baron, J. (1991). Omission and commission in judgment and choice. *Journal of Experimental Social Psychology, 27*, 76–105.

Stimpfel, A. W., Sloane, D. M., & Aiken, L. H. (2012). The longer the shifts for hospital nurses, the higher the levels of burnout and patient dissatisfaction. *Health Affairs, 31*(11), 2501–2509.

Trinkoff, A. M., Johantgen, M., Storr, C. L., Gurses, A. P., Liang, Y., & Han, K. (2011). Nurses' work schedule characteristics, nurse staffing, and patient mortality. *Nursing Research, 60*(1), 1–8.

Tucker, A. L., & Spear, S. J. (2006). Operational failures and interruptions in hospital nursing. *Health Services Research, 41*(3 Pt 1), 643–662.

Verhaeghen, P., & Basak, C. (2005). Ageing and switching of the focus of attention in working memory: Results from a modified N-Back task. *The Quarterly Journal of Experimental Psychology Section A: Human Experimental Psychology, 58*(1), 134–154.

Verhaeghen, P., & Hoyer, W. J. (2007). Aging, focus switching, and task switching in a continuous calculation task: Evidence toward a new working memory control process. *Aging, Neuropsychology and Cognition, 14*(1), 22–39.

Walter, S. R., Li, L., Dunsmuir, W. T., & Westbrook, J. I. (2014). Managing competing demands through task-switching and multi-tasking: A multi-setting observational study of 200 clinicians over 1000 hours. *BMJ Quality and Safety, 23*(3), 231–241.

Weigl, M., Muller, A., Vincent, C., Angerer, P., & Sevdalis, N. (2012). The association of workflow interruptions and hospital doctors' workload: A prospective observational study. *BMJ Quality and Safety, 21*(5), 399–407.

Westbrook, J. I., Coiera, E., Dunsmuir, W. T., Brown, B. M., Kelk, N., Paoloni, R., & Tran, C. (2010). The impact of interruptions on clinical task completion. *Quality and Safety in Healthcare, 19*(4), 284–289. doi:10.1136/qshc.2009.039255

Westbrook, J. I., Duffield, C., Li, L., & Creswick, N. J. (2011). How much time do nurses have for patients? A longitudinal study quantifying hospital nurses' patterns of task time distribution and interactions with health professionals. *BMC Health Services Research, 11*, 319.

Westbrook, J. I., Woods, A., Rob, M. I., Dunsmuir, W. T. M., & Day, R. O. (2010). Association of interruptions with an increased risk and severity of medication administration errors. *Archives of Internal Medicine, 170*(8), 683–690.

Woloshynowych, M., Davis, R., Brown, R., & Vincent, C. (2007). Communication patterns in a UK emergency department. *Annals of Emergency Medicine, 50*(4), 407–413.

Zeelenberg, M. (1999). Anticipated regret, expected feedback and behavioral decision making. *Journal of Behavioral Decision Making, 12*(2), 93–106.

4

Variations in Reports of Missed Nursing Care by Role

In this section, we discuss the differences we found in the reports of nurses versus nursing assistants and between nursing staff and nurse leaders.

Nurses versus Nursing Assistants

Nursing care in acute care hospital settings is organized into teams of nursing personnel that include RNs, LPNs, and NAs. Since these nursing staff members work side-by-side caring for patients, it seems logical that they would have similar reports on incomplete nursing care. The survey asked them to rate the entire unit, not just their own care.

Elements of Nursing Care

We compared RNs' and NAs' perceptions of elements of missed care and reasons for missing care, collecting the data from 11 hospitals (RNs, n = 3535; NAs, n = 1012) (see Table 4.1). The RNs in this study were primarily women (92%) between the ages of 26 and 44 (58.5%) and worked full time (82.3%). The average RN had greater than 5 years of experience (40%) and held a baccalaureate degree (57.2%). The NAs sampled were predominately women (84.2%), younger than 44 years (78.7%), working full time (76.1%), and with the highest education being a high school diploma (64%). Most NAs had between 6 months and less than 5 years of experience (74.9%).

Significant differences in demographic characteristics between RNs and NAs can be seen in Table 4.1; gender (more male NAs), age (NAs younger), shift (more NAs working evenings due to 12-hour shifts worked by RNs), experience (RNs have more), education (NAs grade school, RNs baccalaureate), and overtime (RNs have more). There were no significant differences in type of patient unit worked on or amount of absenteeism.

Although RNs and NAs should be working together as a team to care for patients, the general practice is that RNs are responsible for certain tasks and NAs for others; there are, however, some responsibilities that are shared. The overall findings of the study showed that RNs (mean, 1.58 [SD, 0.39]) reported more missed care than NAs (mean, 1.41 [SD, 0.42]) ($t = 12.57, p < .001$).

In order to understand these differences in ratings of missed nursing care between the two groups, the 24 elements of care in Part A of the *MISSCARE Survey* were categorized as RN, NA, and combined responsibilities. As can be seen in Table 4.2, RNs reported that elements of nursing care that were typically completed by the NA (e.g., bathing, vital signs, etc.) and those shared between RNs and NAs were missed more than the NAs felt they were, with the exception of bedside glucose monitoring. The perceptions of missed care were similar between RNs and NAs for only 3 of 24 elements of care (two RN-only responsibilities and one NA-only responsibility; i.e., PRN medication requests addressed within 15 minutes, focused reassessments according to the patient's condition, and bedside glucose monitoring). RNs reported significantly more missed care than NAs in all remaining elements of care: ambulation, mouth care, intravenous or central line care, documentation, patient bathing or skin care, toileting patients, feeding patient while food is warm, turning, assessing response to medications, providing emotional support, monitoring intake and output, providing wound care, performing vital signs, responses to call lights and monitors, hand washing, medication administration, patient assessment, patient teaching and discharge planning, and attending interdisciplinary conferences (all $p < 0.001$). On the other hand, NAs did not identify any areas where they believed more care was missed than RNs.

Table 4.1.   **Demographic characteristics of RNs (n = 3535) vs. NAs (n = 1012).**

		RNs n (%)	NAs n (%)	$\chi2$	p
Education	Grade school or less	33(.9)	650 (64)	2464.61	<.001
	Associate degree	1465 (41.8)	222 (21.9)		
	Bachelor's degree or higher	2005 (57.2)	143 (14.1)		
Gender	Male	217 (8)	155 (15.8)	57.51	<.001
	Female	3187 (92)	849 (84.2)		
Age	Under 25 years	386 (10.9)	284 (28)	189.76	<.001
	26 to 34 years	1136 (32.2)	300 (29.6)		
	35 to 44 years	930 (26.3)	214 (21.1)		
	Over 45 years	1079 (20.6)	216 (21.3)		
Full-time equivalency	Part time	625 (17.7)	243 (23.9)	19.67	<.001
	Full time	2904 (82.3)	773 (76.1)		
Shifts	Days	1723 (48.9)	512 (50.4)	82.56	<.001
	Evenings	230 (6.5)	150 (14.8)		
	Nights	1304 (37)	292 (28.8)		
	Rotating	269 (7.6)	61 (6.0)		
Working Experience	Up to 6 months	249 (7.1)	118 (11.7)	99.83	<.001
	6 months to 2 years	992 (28.3)	388 (38.4)		
	2 years to 5 years	865 (24.6)	250 (24.8)		
	5 years to 10 years	701 (20)	151 (15)		
	Greater than 10 years	703 (20)	103 (10.2)		
Overtime	None	964 (27.2)	417 (40.9)	70.05	<.001
	Yes	2574 (72.8)	602 (59.1)		
Absenteeism	None	1562 (44.1)	419 (41.1)	2.95	0.086
	Yes	1976 (55.9)	600 (58.9)		

The results of this study underscore previous findings that there are problems in the working relationships of RNs and NAs (Barter, McLaughlin, & Thomas, 1997; Chaboyer, McMurray, & Patterson, 1998; Chang, Lam, & Lam, 1998; Huber, Blegen, & McCloskey, 1994; Keeney, Hasson, McKenna, & Gillen, 2005; McKenna, Hasson, & Keeney, 2004). Mather and Bakas (2002) identified the lack of teamwork as a barrier to appropriate continence care for nursing home patients. This

TABLE 4.2. **Comparison of elements of missed nursing care identified by RNs vs. NAs (Mean ± SD).**

	RN (n = 3535)	NA (n = 1012)	t	p
Overall	1.58 ± .39	1.41 ± .42	12.57	<.001
Nursing care usually done by RN alone				
Attend interdisciplinary care rounds whenever held	2.12 ± .93	1.66 ± .82	13.30	<.001
Full documentation of all necessary data	1.75 ± .73	1.46 ± .66	11.61	<.001
Patient teaching about procedures, tests, and other diagnostic studies	1.75 ± .73	1.48 ± .68	9.54	<.001
Medications administered within 30 minutes before or after scheduled time	1.81 ± .75	1.56 ± .70	8.27	<.001
Assess effectiveness of medications	1.63 ± .67	1.41 ± .63	8.27	<.001
IV/central line site care and assessments according to hospital policy	1.44 ± .63	1.23 ± .52	9.43	<.001
PRN medication requests acted on within 5 minutes	1.50 ± .64	1.57 ± .73	−2.50	.012
Skin/wound care	1.38 ± .56	1.25 ± .54	6.21	<.001
Patient discharge planning and teaching	1.31 ± .58	1.22 ± .51	4.27	<.001
Focus on reassessments according to patient condition	1.31 ± .55	1.27 ± .55	1.64	.102
Patient assessments performed each shift	1.11 ± .39	1.20 ± .54	−4.45	<.001
Nursing care usually done by NA				
Ambulation three times per day or as ordered	2.16 ± .78	1.87 ± .80	10.15	<.001
Mouth care	1.96 ± .81	1.66 ± .79	10.17	<.001
Turning patient every 2 hours	1.80 ± .72	1.50 ± .67	11.82	<.001
Feeding patient when the food is still warm	1.81 ± .74	1.50 ± .69	11.15	<.001
Assist with toileting needs within 5 minutes of request	1.64 ± .68	1.38 ± .63	10.73	<.001
Monitoring intake/output	1.71 ± .79	1.46 ± .69	9.92	<.001
Patient bathing/skin care	1.58 ± .65	1.38 ± .64	8.33	<.001
Setting up meals for patients who feed themselves	1.49 ± .68	1.27 ± .59	9.63	<.001
Bedside glucose monitoring as ordered	1.17 ± .45	1.14 ± .51	1.78	.076
Nursing care done by both RN and NA				
Vital signs assessed as ordered	1.32 ± .56	1.23 ± .55	4.46	<.001
Emotional support to patient and/or family	1.58 ± .71	1.39 ± .66	7.92	<.001
Hand washing	1.35 ± .59	1.26 ± .61	4.43	<.001
Response to call light is initiated within 5 minutes	1.66 ± .72	1.54 ± .74	4.47	<.001

TABLE 4.3.   **Reasons for missed nursing care: RNs versus NAs (n=4557).**

	RNs (n = 3535)		NAs (n = 1012)			
	Mean	SD	Mean	SD	t	p
Staffing resources	3.07	0.63	2.91	0.71	6.84	0.001**
Inadequate number of staff	2.91	0.94	3.00	0.95	−2.76	0.006 **
Urgent patient situations	3.07	0.89	2.72	1.00	10.66	0.001**
Unexpected rise in patient volume and/or acuity on the unit	3.23	0.89	2.98	0.95	8.11	0.001**
Inadequate number of assistive and/or clerical personnel	3.08	0.90	3.04	0.96	1.17	0.039 *
Heavy admission and discharge activity	2.09	0.89	2.82	1.00	7.95	0.001**
Material resources	2.62	0.66	2.38	0.79	9.80	0.001 **
Medications were not available when needed.	3.06	0.82	2.55	0.97	15.10	0.001 **
Supplies/equipment not available when needed	2.51	0.82	2.35	0.91	5.09	0.001 **
Supplies/equipment not functioning properly when needed	2.29	0.83	2.27	0.94	0.63	0.530
Communication/ teamwork	2.28	0.56	2.26	0.65	0.87	0.385
Unbalanced patient assignments	2.74	0.88	2.67	1.00	2.17	0.034 *
Inadequate hand-off from previous shift or sending unit	2.33	0.75	2.33	0.89	−0.13	0.895
Other departments did not provide the care needed	2.27	0.78	2.22	0.88	1.63	0.101
Lack of back-up support from team members	2.22	0.87	2.39	1.00	−5.25	0.001**
Tension or communication breakdowns with ancillary/ support departments	2.17	0.81	2.19	0.93	−0.37	0.715
Tension or communication breakdowns within the nursing team	2.09	0.84	2.24	0.98	−4.77	0.001 **
Tension or communication breakdowns with the medical staff	2.26	0.83	2.18	0.93	2.53	0.011 **
Nursing assistant did not communicate that care was not done	2.49	0.90	2.15	0.90	10.33	0.001**
Caregiver off unit or unavailable	1.98	0.82	1.95	0.89	1.05	0.296

Note: ** , p < .01; *, p < .05

study also documented a perception that RNs do not listen to NAs or include them in the planning of care. In interviews with 13 RNs and 9 NAs in an acute care hospital, Potter and Grant (2004) identified a lack of trust and respect in the RN–NA relationships, validating findings by other investigators (Salmond, 1995; Spilsbury & Meyer, 2004).

In a qualitative study of the impact of RN–NA relationships on quality and safety, seven themes emerged (Kalisch, 2011):

1. Lack of role clarity (e.g., RNs feel that the NAs do not understand the requirements of their role; NAs don't see RNs as leaders of the team; NAs feel RNs don't assume accountability for all patient care no matter who provides it; etc.)

2. Lack of working together as a team (e.g., responsibilities divided into RN work and NA work; lack of backup; etc.)

3. Inability to deal with conflict (e.g., problems with confrontation and feedback, etc.)

4. RNs do not engage NAs in decision-making (e.g., NAs don't get reports from RNs; RNs don't listen to the NAs; RN's command is seen as disrespectful; etc.)

5. Deficient delegation (e.g., RN does not create buy-in for the NA; RNs do not retain accountability and follow through; unclear directions; etc.)

6. More than one boss (e.g., NA reports to two or more RNs, etc.)

7. "It's not my job syndrome" (e.g., it's aides work; it's RNs work)

With this type of working relationship, it is not uncommon for nursing care to be missed.

Reasons

When the reasons for missed care were compared between those reported by RNs and those reported by NAs, labor resources were identified as the greatest reason for missed care by both RNs and NAs, with material resources next and communication last (as can be noted in Table 4.2 and Figure 4.3). RNs (mean, 3.19 [SD, 0.57]) felt that labor resources were more of a cause for missing care than did NAs ($p < .01$). RNs identified an unexpected rise in patient volume, urgent patient situations, and a heavy volume of admissions and discharges more frequently than NAs ($p < .001$). RNs and NAs did not vary significantly on two reasons for missing care—level of staffing and the number of assistive personnel.

RNs attributed missed care to gaps in material resources more frequently than NAs ($p < 0.001$). While RNs perceived medications, supplies, and equipment availability as a more significant reason for missed care than NAs ($p < 0.05$), NAs and RNs agreed (no significant difference) on the equipment functioning properly. Although there were no significant differences between RNs and NAs on the overall communication and teamwork subscale as a reason for missed nursing care, several individual items were identified as problems by RNs more often than NAs: other departments did not provide the care needed; nursing assistant did not communicate that care was not done; and unbalanced patient assignments. NAs reported more problems with lack of back-up support from team members and tension or communication breakdowns within the nursing team than RNs (Table 4.3).

In order to understand more completely the differences in ratings by RNs and NAs, we conducted follow-up focus groups with the staff members who completed the survey (Kalisch, 2009). The following key findings from the quantitative study reported above were presented to the focus group participants:

- RNs reported significantly more missed care than did NAs.
- RNs felt that nursing care activities that were typically completed by the NA or shared with the NAs were missed more frequently than the NAs felt they were.
- Perceptions of missed care were similar between RNs and NAs for only 5 (of 24) elements of care, all of which were typically RN responsibilities.
- NAs did not identify any areas where they believed more care was missed than did RNs.
- RNs rated labor resources as more of a cause for missing care than did NAs.
- RNs identified an unexpected rise in patient volume, urgent patient situations, and heavy admissions and discharges more frequently than did NAs.
- RNs attributed missed care to gaps in material resources more frequently than NAs.
- RNs rated "nursing assistant did not communicate that care was not done" significantly more often than did the NAs.
- NAs cited communication breakdowns within the nursing team as more of a reason for missed care than did the RNs.

Focus group members were asked to provide their explanations and insights about these study findings. A free flow of ideas was encouraged and issues that emerged were examined fully. The following reasons emerged from the RN focus groups:

- Not enough staff (in regard to both RNs and NAs, but especially the number of NAs).

- NAs do not know or have the knowledge base so they do not value the importance of certain care.

- NAs sometime refuse to do what the RNs ask them to do.

- NAs are not always motivated to do a good job and will sometimes simply skip care.

- There is little to no communication between staff members before or during the shift.

- RNs feel they are too busy to follow up to see if the care is actually completed.

- RNs feel that NAs' work should be done without their involvement, and if they engage in it, they will not be able to get their own work done.

- NAs do not give a complete report to the RN ("We have tried everything, even check lists, but they still don't give us a complete report").

The themes that emerged from the NA focus group participants were the following:

- They do the care, but the RN does not believe them.

- They do not always have the time to do everything for the patient.

- The RNs do not listen to them and do not respect them ("I will tell them a patient has a reddened area or the patient is in pain, and they do nothing").

- The RNs call them to do the "simplest thing, like getting a patient water" instead of doing it themselves, thus taking valuable time they could spend completing other care.

- The NAs receive late patient reports or none at all (since they do not attend report).

- Little to no contact occurs between the RNs and NAs during the shift.

- Little to no communication between the RN and NA as to what aspects of care have been completed and what care is left that needs to be done.

Nursing Staff versus Nurse Leaders

In another study, we compared nursing staff and nursing leaders (i.e., managers, clinical nurse specialists, advanced practice nurses; Kalisch & Lee, 2012). A comparison of sample characteristics of the two groups revealed that, as expected, nursing staff were less educated, less experienced, younger, and less likely to work full time than were nursing leaders. The gender of nursing staff were similar to nursing leaders, largely female.

The mean missed nursing care score for nursing staff was 1.55 (SD, 0.41) compared with 1.62 (SD, 0.34) for nursing leaders (midway between rarely missed [1] and occasionally missed [2]). As noted in Table 4.4 and Figure 4.1, nursing staff reported lower overall missed nursing care than did nursing leaders, but it was only marginally significant ($t = -1.80$, $p = .074$). Nursing staff responded that labor resources ($t = -5.72$, $p = .000$) and material resources ($t = 2.13$, $p = .036$) were

TABLE 4.4.   **Overall missed nursing care and reasons for missed nursing care: Differences between staff and leaders (n = 4519).**

Variable	Staff (Mean ± SD)	Leader (Mean ± SD)	t	p
Overall missed nursing care	1.55 ± .41	1.62 ± .34	−1.80	.074
Communication	2.29 ± .58	2.20 ± .51	1.68	.097
Labor resources	3.04 ± .65	2.67 ± .69	5.72	.000
Material resources	2.57 ± .70	2.44 ± .60	2.13	.036

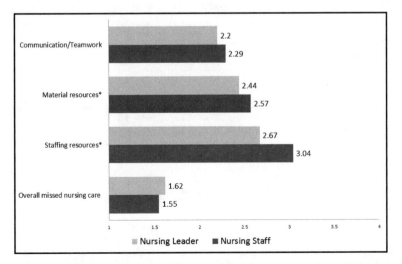

FIGURE 4.1.   **Overall missed nursing care and reasons for missed nursing care: Differences between staff and leaders (n = 4519).**
Note: *$p < .05$

more prevalent as reasons for missed nursing care than did nursing leaders. Communication issues as a cause of missed nursing care were not significantly different between nursing staff and leaders.

Although nursing staff reported lower scores (less missed nursing care) on all but two elements of nursing care (glucose monitoring and attending interdisciplinary rounds). Of the specific elements of missed nursing care, only 6 of 24 elements of nursing care were identified by nursing staff to be missed significantly less than reported by nurse leaders (Table 4.5, Figures 4.2 and 4.3). These six elements were full documentation, patient teaching, emotional support, hand washing, patient discharge planning, and medication effectiveness assessment. Nursing staff reported marginally less missed care on glucose monitoring, PRN (as needed) medications administration, and skin and

TABLE 4.5. Elements of missed nursing care: Nurse leaders vs. nursing staff (n = 4519).

Variable	Missed Care?	Staff (n = 4415) n (%)	Leader (n = 104) n (%)	χ2	p
Ambulation	No	978(24.0)	19 (19.2)	1.22	.270
	Yes	3102 (76.0)	80 (80.8)		
Turning	No	1812 (41.4)	37 (36.3)	1.08	.300
	Yes	2566 (58.6)	65 (63.7)		
Feeding	No	1705 (42.6)	35 (35.0)	2.34	.127
	Yes	2293 (57.4)	65 (65.0)		
Meal set up	No	2610 (65.2)	60 (60.0)	1.17	.280
	Yes	1392 (34.8)	40 (40.0)		
Timely medication administration	No	1634 (40.4)	36 (36.0)	.79	.375
	Yes	2410 (59.6)	64 (64.0)		
Vital signs	No	3278 (75.4)	75 (74.3)	.07	.797
	Yes	1071 (24.6)	36 (25.7)		
Monitoring I/O	No	2248 (51.3)	44 (43.1)	2.69	.101
	Yes	2130 (48.7)	58 (56.9)		
Full documentation	No	1972 (45.7)	21 (20.6)	25.30	.000
	Yes	2347 (54.3)	81 (79.4)		
Patient teaching	No	1843 (44.7)	32 (31.4)	7.16	.007
	Yes	2280 (55.3)	70 (68.6)		
Emotional support	No	2511 (57.7)	45 (44.1)	7.56	.006
	Yes	1838 (42.3)	57 (55.9)		
Bathing	No	2382 (55.0)	52 (51.0)	.65	.419
	Yes	1948 (45.0)	50 (49.0)		

Variable	Missed Care?	Staff (n = 4415) n (%)	Leader (n = 104) n (%)	$\chi2$	p
Mouth care	No	1587 (36.5)	35 (34.3)	.20	.656
	Yes	2766 (63.5)	67 (65.7)		
Hand washing	No	3184(72.7)	55 (54.5)	16.32	.000
	Yes	1198 (27.3)	46 (45.5)		
Patient discharge planning	No	2992 (75.6)	64 (62.7)	8.76	.003
	Yes	968 (24.4)	38 (37.3)		
Glucose monitoring	No	3721 (86.6)	95 (93.1)	3.75	.053
	Yes	578 (13.4)	7 (6.9)		
Assessment each shift	No	3776 (90.6)	91 (89.2)	.22	.638
	Yes	392 (9.4)	11 (10.8)		
Focused reassessments	No	3034 (74.0)	68 (67.3)	2.25	.134
	Yes	1068 (26.0)	33 (32.7)		
IV/Central line site care	No	2668 (65.7)	62 (61.4)	.82	.366
	Yes	1392 (34.3)	39 (38.6)		
Call-light response	No	2186 (50.1)	50 (49.5)	.02	.900
	Yes	2174 (49.9)	26 (50.5)		
PRN meds administration	No	2345 (57.5)	49 (48.5)	3.24	.072
	Yes	1734 (42.5)	52 (51.5)		
Meds effectiveness assessment	No	2050 (50.7)	40 (39.6)	4.83	.028
	Yes	1996 (49.3)	61 (60.4)		
Attend interdisciplinary care conferences	No	1303 (34.5)	41 (41.0)	1.85	1.74
	Yes	2479 (65.5)	59 (59.0)		
Assist with toileting	No	2230 (51.2)	48 (48.0)	.40	.529
	Yes	2127 (48.8)	52 (52.0)		
Skin/Wound care	No	2855 (67.5)	59 (58.4)	2.24	.134
	Yes	1373 (32.5)	42 (41.6)		

Note: No = rarely missed; Yes = occasionally, frequently, or always missed

wound care than did nurse leaders (p = .053, p = .072, and p = .054, respectively). The remaining 15 elements of nursing care, which were not rated significantly different between nursing staff and leaders, included ambulation, turning, feeding, meal setup, timely medication administration, vital signs, monitoring intake and output, bathing, mouth care, patient assessment, focused reassessment, intravenous and central line site care, call-light response, interdisciplinary care, rounds attendance, and toileting assistance.

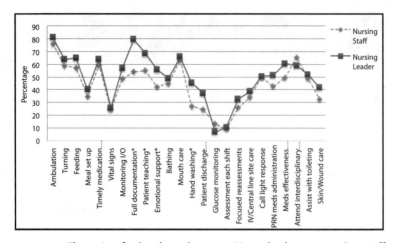

FIGURE 4.2. **Elements of missed nursing care: Nurse leaders vs. nursing staff (n = 4519).**

Note: *$p < .05$

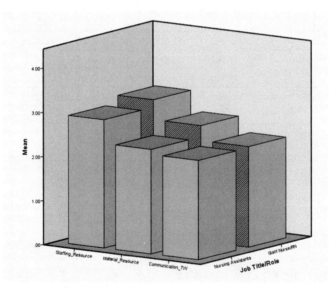

FIGURE 4.3. **Comparison with reasons for missed nursing care between RNs and NAs (n = 4547).**

The findings of this study show a lack of congruence between nurse leaders and nursing staff members. Nurses report fewer instances of missed care than leaders, and nursing staff list more problems with access to adequate material and labor resources than leaders.

Among leadership theories, the leader–member exchange (LMX) framework has been gaining momentum in recent years (Brown & Trevino, 2009). LMX focuses on the relationship between follower and leader. High-quality exchanges are characterized by trust, respect, mutual obligation, and reciprocal influence between leader and follower. In contrast, other leadership theories focus on the leader (e.g., traits, behavioral approaches, etc.) or the follower (e.g., empowerment approaches; Graen & Uhl-Bien, 1995).

Gerstner and Day (1997) reviewed 164 LMX studies from 1974 to 1996 in order to examine leader–member agreement and the correlation between these studies. The authors reported that LMX was significantly related to job performance, satisfaction with supervision, overall satisfaction, commitment, role clarity, member competence, and turnover intentions (Gerstner & Day, 1997). According to LMX theory and from the vantage point of the nurses, leaders are overestimators of the amount of missed nursing care and underestimators of the availability of staffing and material resources (including medications) that lead to missed nursing care.

The impact of the lack of congruence between the nurse leaders and staff members has serious consequences for these individuals and the organization. Research has consistently demonstrated that a low level of congruence between leaders and followers results in negative outcomes, including lower job satisfaction (Cogliser, Schriesheim, Scandura, & Gardner, 2009; Fix & Sias, 2006), lack of role clarity (Gerstner & Day, 1997), low levels of trust (Scandura & Pellegrini 2008), higher turnover (Gerstner & Day, 1997), lower job performance (Cogliser et al., 2009; Gerstner & Day, 1997; Vidyarthi, Liden, Anand, Erdogan, & Ghosh, 2010), diminished organizational commitment (Abu Bakar, Dilbeck, & McCroskey, 2010; Gerstner & Day, 1997), increased resistance to change (Furst & Cable, 2008), and less citizen behavior (discretionary behaviors which contribute to organizational effectiveness, which are not part of the job description, and are performed by the employee as a result of personal choice; Ilies, Nahrgang, & Morgeson, 2007; Vidyarthi et al., 2010). This lack of congruence between nursing staff members and their leaders often leads to distrust and disrespect between them. Because trust and respect have been identified as essential elements of performance, contentment with supervision, and overall satisfaction, a lack of these components in the workplace may result in nursing staff and leaders not working effectively together as a team (Kalisch & Begeny, 2005; Salas, Sims, & Burke, 2005). Instead, an adversarial relationship may develop.

Using perceptions of staffing adequacy as an example, if leaders feel—based on their experience with staff members—that no matter how many personnel are provided, it will not be considered sufficient by the nurses, then they stop listening to these complaints and dismiss them as illegitimate. The nursing staff, on the other hand, may believe that leaders are holding back from providing needed staff because they are trying to save money or appeal to those above them. Nurses may then feel that they are not listened to or that their opinions are unimportant. This can be aggravated by the nursing staff members focusing on those shifts that are short-staffed and not on those that are well-staffed. A similar process can occur related to other issues. For example, if leaders fail to recognize the lack of adequate supplies, equipment, and medications, they may not recognize the need to develop interventions to address these issues.

Summary

In this chapter, the reports of missed nursing care by RNs were compared to those reports by NAs. The perceptions of missed care were similar between RNs and NAs for only 3 of 24 elements of care (two RN-only responsibilities and one NA-only responsibility; i.e., PRN medication requests addressed within 15 minutes, focused reassessments according to patient condition, and bedside glucose monitoring). RNs reported significantly more missed care than NAs in all remaining elements of care. On the other hand, NAs did not identify any areas where they believed more care was missed than RNs. Also, nursing staff were contrasted with nurse leaders as to their reports of missed nursing care. Although nursing staff reported lower scores (less missed care) on all but two (i.e., glucose monitoring and attending interdisciplinary care rounds) of the specific elements of missed nursing care, only 6 of 24 elements of missed nursing care were identified by nursing staff to be missed significantly less than reported by nurse leaders. The findings of this study show a lack of congruence between nurse leaders and nursing staff members. Nurses report less missed care than do leaders, and nursing staff list more problems with having adequate material and labor resources than do leaders.

References

Abu Bakar, H., Dilbeck, K., & McCroskey, J. (2010). Mediating role of supervisory communication practices on relations between leader–member exchange and perceived employee commitment to workgroup. *Communication Monographs, 77*(4), 637–656.

Barter, M., McLaughlin, F., & Thomas, S. (1997). Registered nurse role changes and satisfaction with unlicensed assistive personnel. *The Journal of Nursing Administration, 27*(1), 29–38.

Brown, M. E., & Trevino, L. K. (2009). Leader–follower values congruence: Are socialized charismatic leaders better able to achieve it? *The Journal of Applied Psychology, 94*(2), 478–490.

Chaboyer, W., McMurray, A., & Patterson, E. (1998). Unlicensed assistive personnel in the critical care unit: What is their role? *International Journal of Nursing Practice, 4*(4), 240–246.

Chang, A. M., Lam, L., & Lam, L. W. (1998). Nursing activities following the introduction of health care assistants. *Journal of Nursing Management, 6*(3), 155–163.

Cogliser, C. C., Schriesheim, C. A., Scandura, T. A., & Gardner, W. L. (2009). Balance in leader and follower perceptions of leader–member exchange: Relationships with performance and work attitudes. *The Leadership Quarterly, 20*(3), 452–465.

Fix, B., & Sias, P. M. (2006). Person-centered communication, leader–member exchange, and job satisfaction. *Communication Research Reports, 23*(1), 35–44.

Furst, S. A., & Cable, D. M. (2008). Employee resistance to organizational change: Managerial influence tactics and leader–member exchange. *Journal of Applied Psychology, 93*(2), 453–462.

Gerstner, C. R., & Day, D. V. (1997). Meta-analytic review of leader–member exchange theory: Correlates and construct issues. *Journal of Applied Psychology, 82*(6), 827–844.

Graen, G. B., & Uhl-Bien, M. (1995). Relationship-based approach to leadership: Development of leader–member exchange (LMX) theory of leadership over 25 years: Applying a multi-level multi-domain perspective. *The Leadership Quarterly, 6*(2), 219–247.

Huber, D. G., Blegen, M. A., & McCloskey, J. C. (1994). Use of nursing assistants: Staff nurse opinions. *Nursing Management, 25*(5), 64–68.

Ilies, R., Nahrgang, J. D., & Morgeson, F. P. (2007). Leader–member exchange and citizenship behaviors: A meta-analysis. *Journal of Applied Psychology, 92*(1), 269–277.

Kalisch, B. (2009). Nurse and nurse assistant perceptions of missed nursing care: What does it tell us about teamwork? *Journal of Nursing Administration, 39*(11), 485–493.

Kalisch, B. (2011). The impact of RN–UAP relationships on quality and safety. *Nursing Management, 42*(9), 16–22.

Kalisch, B., & Begeny, S. M. (2005). Improving nursing unit teamwork. *The Journal of Nursing Administration, 35*(12), 550–556.

Kalisch, B., & Lee, K. (2012). Congruence of perceptions among nursing leaders and staff regarding missed nursing care and teamwork. *Journal of Nursing Administration, 42*(10), 473–477.

Keeney, S., Hasson, F., McKenna, H., & Gillen, P. (2005). Nurses', midwives' and patients' perceptions of trained health care assistants. *Journal of Advanced Nursing, 50*(4), 345–355.

Mather, K. F., & Bakas, T. (2002). Nursing assistants' perceptions of their ability to provide continence care. *Geriatric Nursing, 23*(2), 76–81.

McKenna, H. P., Hasson, F., & Keeney, S. (2004). Patient safety and quality of care: The role of the health care assistant. *Journal of Nursing Management, 12*(6), 452–459.

Potter, P., & Grant, E. (2004). Understanding RN and unlicensed assistive personnel working relationships in designing care delivery strategies. *The Journal of Nursing Administration, 34*(1), 19–25.

Salas, E., Sims, D. E., & Burke, C. S. (2005). Is there a "big five" in teamwork? *Small Group Research, 36*(5), 555–599.

Salmond, S. (1995). Models of care using unlicensed assistive personnel. Part I: Job scope, preparation and utilization patterns. *Orthopaedic Nursing, 14*(5), 20–30.

Scandura, T. A., & Pellegrini, E. K. (2008). Trust and leader–member exchange: A closer look at relational vulnerability. *Journal of Leadership and Organizational Studies, 15*(2), 101–110.

Spilsbury, K., & Meyer, J. (2004). Use, misuse and non-use of health care assistants: Understanding the work of health care assistants in a hospital setting. *Journal of Nursing Management, 12*(6), 411–418.

Vidyarthi, P. R., Liden, R. C., Anand, S., Erdogan, B., & Ghosh, S. (2010). Where do I stand? Examining the effects of leader–member exchange social comparison on employee work behaviors. *Journal of Applied Psychology, 95*(5), 849–861.

5

Missed Nursing Care in Magnet Hospitals

by
Beatrice Kalisch, PhD, RN, FAAN
and Kyung Hee Lee, PhD, RN

The American Nurses Credentialing Center (ANCC) serves in the role of evaluating nursing organizations for the quality of nursing care as well as the nature of the work environment for nursing staff. Those that meet the criteria are designated Magnet hospitals. As such, these hospitals, in addition to providing desirable working environments for nurses, are believed to offer a higher quality of nursing care. The aim of this chapter is to report how Magnet versus non-Magnet hospitals are comparable in regards to the amount, type, and reasons for missed nursing care.

Background
In the mid-1980s, members of the American Academy of Nursing conducted a study where they identified hospitals that were considered a have a good environment for the practice of nursing (Aiken, 1981; Aiken, Havens, & Sloane, 2000). The emphasis was on the organization's ability to recruit and retain nurses. After several steps where hospitals were nominated and examined as to their work environments, they identified 41 hospitals, which became the first Magnet hospitals.

Previous Studies

Most of the studies of Magnet facilities have focused on and quality of the work environment for nursing staff. Researchers have found that Magnet hospital nurses are more satisfied (Brady-Schwartz, 2005; Laschinger, Heather, Almost, & Tuer-Hodes, 2003; Schmalenberg & Kramer, 2008; Ulrich, Buerhaus, Donelan, Norman, & Dittus, 2007; Upenieks, 2002), have less emotional exhaustion (Aiken et al., 2000; Aiken & Sloane, 1997; Friese, 2005), more collegial physician–nurse relationships (Laschinger et al., 2003), better teamwork among the nursing staff (Ulrich et al., 2007), enhanced work environments (Friese, 2005), more opportunity to influence decisions and empowerment (Laschinger et al., 2003; Ulrich et al., 2007), more acceptable workloads (Lacey et al., 2007), and a higher level of staffing (Friese 2005; Lake, Shang, Klaus, & Dunton, 2010). Magnet hospital nursing staff also report more intent to stay in their position (Lacey et al., 2007), more facilitative managers (Friese, 2005), and healthier work environments (Kramer & Schalenberg, 2004). For example, in 2000, 13 of the original Magnet hospitals were compared with 7 hospitals who had received Magnet recognition more recently. The results of this study showed that nurses in the more recently designated Magnet hospitals had even lower burnout rates and higher levels of job satisfaction than the original Magnet hospital comparison group (Aiken et al., 2000).

Fewer studies have examined the difference in quality of nursing care and patient outcomes between Magnet hospitals and non-Magnet organizations. The initial studies of quality and outcomes were conducted by Aiken and colleagues. In 1994, this research team compared the original Magnet hospitals with 195 control hospitals selected from all non-Magnet hospitals to determine if the quality of care was still higher in Magnet organizations. After adjusting for differences in predicted mortality, the Magnet hospitals were found to have a 4.6% lower mortality rate (Aiken, Smith, & Lake, 1994). Later, in 1999, Aiken, Sloane, Lake, Sochalski, and Weber compiled another study comparing the 30-day mortality rate and satisfaction with care in 40 dedicated AIDS units, some of which were in hospitals with Magnet status. They found that dedicated units and Magnet hospitals combined resulted in lower mortality odds within 30 days of admission and higher patient satisfaction. On nursing units where practice environments were positive, patients were more than twice as likely to be highly satisfied with their nursing care than were patients in units with a less desirable work setting (Aiken et al., 1999). More recently, Lake and colleagues compared fall rates in Magnet versus non-Magnet hospitals using the National Database of Nursing Quality Indicators data from 5,388 facilities and found that the fall rate was 5% lower in Magnet hospitals (Lake et al., 2010).

Other studies have relied on perceptions of nursing staff to assess the quality of care (Aiken et al., 2000; Friese, 2005; Laschinger, Shamian, & Thomson, 2001). These studies have shown that nurses in Magnet facilities perceive that the care is of a higher quality than nursing care in non-Magnet hospitals. Ulrich and colleagues asked nursing staff to evaluate the extent to which their organization emphasizes quality of care and found that Magnet hospitals and those working toward the designation reported higher scores on this question (Ulrich et al., 2007).

In addition to these studies, which have directly tested the relationship between quality variables and Magnet status, many studies have linked the work environment variables found in a greater degree in Magnet facilities with better patient outcomes. The variables include staffing levels, where lower patient mortality, fewer adverse events, and reduced lengths of stay are associated with a higher level of nurse staffing (Aiken, Clarke, Sloane, Sochalski, & Silber, 2002; Cho, Ketefian, Barkauskas, & Smith, 2003; Kovner, Jones, Zhan, Gergen, & Basu, 2002; Needleman, Buerhaus, Mattke, Stewart, & Zelevinsky, 2002).

We did not find studies which have examined the differences in the process of nursing care between these two types of institutions (Magnet vs. non-Magnet). In fact, as noted in previous chapters, little research has investigated the process of nursing care that would explain the relationship between structure variables (e.g., staffing levels, Magnet status, hospital size, teaching intensity, nurse characteristics, etc.) and patient outcomes (e.g., mortality, falls, pressure ulcers, readmissions, infection rates, etc.) that have been uncovered in numerous research studies.

In this chapter, we report on the relationship between the structure variable of Magnet on missed nursing care and reasons for missing that care. We also examine the relationships between unit characteristics (i.e., type of unit and Case Mix Index [CMI]), staffing variables (Hours per Patient Day [HPPD], nursing education, and experience), and missed nursing care.

Study Methods
Research Questions
The research questions for this study were as follows:

1. Does the amount and type of missed nursing care differ between patient care units within designated Magnet versus non-Magnet hospitals?
2. How do reasons identified by nursing staff for missing nursing care vary in Magnet versus non-Magnet hospitals?
3. Does the level of staffing differ between patient care units within designated Magnet versus non-Magnet hospitals?
4. Does Magnet status predict missed nursing care controlling for staffing levels (i.e., HPPD, nursing education, and experience), and unit characteristics (CMI and type of unit)?

Sample and Setting
This study utilized a cross-sectional, descriptive design. It was conducted in 124 medical–surgical, intermediate, intensive care, and rehabilitation units in 11 hospitals located in the Midwest and Western regions of the United States. Unit inclusion criteria were: (1) an average patient length of stay greater than 2 days and (2) a patient population greater than 18 years of age. All patient care units in the eleven study hospitals that met the inclusion criteria participated in the study. Four of the eleven study hospitals were designated Magnet and the other seven were non-Magnet. Among the 124 units, 62 units (50%) were in Magnet hospitals. A total of 4,412 nursing staff (i.e., Registered Nurses [RN], Licensed Practical Nurses [LPN], and nursing assistants [NA]) completed the *MISSCARE Survey*. The overall response rate was 57.3%, with a range of 34.4% to 99.6% by patient care unit.

Study Variables
The dependent variable of this study was Magnet status; independent variables were missed nursing care, reasons for missed nursing care, nurse staffing (i.e., HPPD, RN HPPD, and skill mix), and unit characteristics. These variables are defined below.

> **Magnet status.** Magnet status is an award given by the ANCC, an affiliate of the American Nurses Association, which recognizes excellence for hospital organizations that foster not only a positive work environment for nurses but also a higher level nursing care and patient outcomes.
>
> **Missed nursing care and reasons of missed nursing care.** The *MISSCARE Survey* was utilized to measure nursing staff

perceptions of both missed care (Part A) and the reasons for missed care (Part B). In Part A, RNs, LPNs, and NAs were asked to identify how frequently nursing care elements are missed on their unit. Respondents were instructed to check the best response: always missed, frequently missed, occasionally missed, or rarely missed. In Part B (reasons for missed care), nursing staff members were asked to indicate the reasons nursing care is missed. Respondents were asked to grade the relative importance for each reason: significant reason, moderate reason, minor reason, or not a reason for missed care. Exploratory and confirmatory factor analysis yielded three factors: labor resources, material resources, and communication. Validity and reliability of the *MISSCARE Survey* has been published elsewhere (Kalisch & Williams, 2009).

Nursing staffing measures. Nursing staffing indicators included HPPD, RN HPPD, skill mix, nursing education, and experience.

HPPD and RN HPPD. HPPD refers to the overall time expended by the RNs, LPNs, and NAs working on the unit per patient day. HPPD was calculated as the sum of total nursing hours worked by nursing staff (RN, LPN, and NA) divided by the number of patient days. RN HPPD is the time spent by the RNs alone per patient day. RN HPPD was calculated as total RN hours per day divided by patient days.

Skill mix. Skill mix is defined as the proportion of RNs working on the unit. The skill mix value was calculated as the number of productive hours worked by the RNs divided by the total number of productive hours worked by nursing staff (RN, LPN, and NA).

Nursing education. Nurses were asked to identify their highest degree earned in their profession or occupation. This variable was dichotomized as 1) associate degree or lower and 2) baccalaureate degree or higher.

Experience. Experience levels referred to the number of years the respondent had been working in the profession or occupation (i.e., RN, LPN, and NA).

Unit characteristics. Unit characteristics included patient acuity (CMI) and type of unit.

Case Mix Index (CMI). CMI is the average diagnosis-related group (DRG) weight for all Medicare patients on a given patient care unit. CMI, although it does not measure patient acuity directly, serves as a proxy for acuity by accounting for the relative differences in resources expended for patient care.

Type of Unit. Type of unit was categorized as follows: (1) intensive care unit (ICU), and (2) non-ICU unit, which included intermediate units, medical–surgical units, and rehabilitation units.

Data Analysis

Data were coded, entered into the Statistical Package for the Social Sciences (SPSS) 17.0, and verified. For the first three research questions, the missed nursing care mean score on the individual level, which was collected via the *MISSCARE Survey*, was aggregated to the missed nursing care mean score on a unit level. The three reasons for missed nursing care mean scores were calculated in a similar fashion as the missed nursing care variable. Independent *t*-tests were completed to establish significant differences between Magnet and non-Magnet hospital units on missed nursing care, reasons for missed nursing care, and staffing levels.

The fourth research question was addressed by hierarchical linear modeling (HLM). Because of the data structure, in which individuals (Level-1 data) were nested within patient units (Level-2 data), a multilevel regression model was applied using the HLM software package (Scientific Software International, Inc.). Nesting within hospitals was not accounted for in this analysis because the sample size was small (n = 11) and trends in frequency of missed care were similar across these hospitals (Kalisch, Landstrom, & Williams, 2009; Kalisch, Tschannen, Lee, & Friese, 2011). The dependent variable was the missed nursing care mean score; independent variables were experience (years of experience), education (0 = associated degree or lower, 1 = BSN or higher), Magnet (0 = non-Magnet, 1 = Magnet), type of unit (0 = non-ICU, 1 = ICU), HPPD, and CMI. Model specifications of the 2-level HLM regression are as follows:

Level-1:
Missed nursing care $= \beta_{0j} + \beta_{1j} (\text{Experience})_{ij} + \beta_{2j} (\text{Education})_{ij} + \gamma_{ij}$

Level-2:
$\beta_{0j} = \gamma_{00} + \gamma_{01} (\text{Magnet})_j + \gamma_{02} (\text{Type of unit})_j + \gamma_{03} (\text{HPPD})_j + \gamma_{04} (\text{CMI})_j + \mu_{0j}$

$\beta_{1j} = \gamma_{10}$

$\beta_{2j} = \gamma_{20}$

In these models, missed nursing care was modeled as a function of the years of experience and the level of education at Level-1 (individual) and the unit characteristics (Magnet, type of unit, HPPD, and CMI) at Level-2 (unit). Continuous variables (i.e., experience, HPPD, and CMI) were grand-mean centered because grand-mean centering could reduce multicollinearity between levels (Cronbach, 1987).

Study Findings

There were 124 units in the study, of which 54.8% were medical–surgical units, 25.8% intensive care units, 13.7% intermediate units, and 5.6% rehabilitation units. Among 124 units, 62 were Magnet hospital units (50%) and the rest were non-Magnet hospital units.

Missed nursing care differences. As can be seen in Table 5.1, Magnet unit staff reported significantly less overall missed nursing care than staff on patient care units in non-Magnet hospitals ($t = 2.20$, $p = 0.03$). Ten of the twenty-four specific elements of nursing care were missed significantly more often in non-Magnet hospitals than in Magnet designated facilities, namely: turning, feeding, meal set up, full documentation, patient teaching, mouth care, IV and central line site care, call-light and monitor response, medication effectiveness assessment, and skin and wound care. Hand washing and PRN medication administration showed marginally significant differences by Magnet status ($p = .06$ and $p = .08$, respectively). The remaining 12 elements of nursing care, which were not significantly different by Magnet status, included: ambulation, timely medication, vital signs, monitoring intake and output, emotional support, bathing, patient discharge planning, glucose monitoring, assessment each shift, focused reassessments, interdisciplinary rounds attendance, and toileting assistance. There were no elements of nursing care which were missed more in Magnet than non-Magnet hospitals.

Reasons for missed nursing care. As noted in Table 5.1, Magnet unit staff reported that lack of communication ($t = 2.49$, $p = .014$) and labor resources ($t = 3.31$, $p = 0.01$) were significantly less prevalent in Magnet hospitals versus non-Magnet facilities. There were no differences relative to material resources between the two categories of hospitals.

Staffing differences. No staffing differences were found between Magnet hospitals and non-Magnet hospitals (Table 5.2). Specifically, HPPD, RN HPPD, and skill mix were not different by Magnet status ($t = 0.44$, $p = .66$; $t = 0.19$, $p = .85$; $t = -0.04$, $p = .97$, respectively).

Predictors of missed nursing care. The result of HLM regression is presented in Table 5.3. R^2 indicates that level-2 variables (i.e., Magnet, type of unit, HPPD, and CMI) account for 15% of the variance of missed nursing care, and level-1 variables (i.e., experience and education) account for only 4.6%. Magnet status was negatively associated with the missed nursing care mean score. Specifically, Magnet units had a lower missed nursing care score than non-Magnet units after adjusting for other variables ($\gamma_{01} = -0.074$, $p = .015$). In addition,

TABLE 5.1. **Amount and reasons for missed nursing care differences by Magnet status.**

| Variable | Magnet status | | t | p |
	Yes (Mean ± SD)	No (Mean ± SD)		
Overall missed nursing care	1.50 ± .21	1.57 ± .15	2.20	.03
Ambulation	2.03 ± .36	2.13 ± .28	1.57	.12
Attend interdisciplinary care conferences	1.99 ± .28	2.05 ± .50	.83	.41
Mouth care	1.81 ± .32	1.93 ± .31	2.02	.05
Timely medication administration	1.76 ± .33	1.79 ± .24	.55	.58
Turning	1.65 ± .31	1.77 ± .23	2.34	.02
Feeding	1.65 ± .26	1.82 ± .30	3.34	.00
Patient teaching	1.62 ± .25	1.72 ± .22	2.24	.03
Full documentation	1.60 ± .29	1.73 ± .24	2.72	.01
Monitoring I/O	1.59 ± .40	1.65 ± .38	.78	.44
Call-light response	1.54 ± .31	1.67 ± .29	2.38	.02
Assist with toileting	1.54 ± .24	1.60 ± .23	1.40	.17
Meds effectiveness assessment	1.52 ± .25	1.63 ± .20	2.65	.01
Bathing	1.50 ± .27	1.56 ± .22	1.22	.22
Emotional support	1.47 ± .25	1.53 ± .22	1.53	.13
PRN meds administration	1.45 ± .25	1.52 ± .21	1.75	.08
Meal set up	1.35 ± .27	1.47 ± .22	2.65	.01
IV/Central line site care	1.32 ± .26	1.47 ± .18	3.79	.00
Skin/Wound care	1.32 ± .26	1.39 ± .15	1.99	.05
Patient discharge planning	1.29 ± .28	1.31 ± .14	.47	.64
Focused reassessments	1.28 ± .27	1.29 ± .15	.18	.86
Vital signs	1.27 ± .29	1.29 ± .17	.54	.59
Hand washing	1.27 ± .27	1.35 ± .19	1.88	.06
Glucose monitoring	1.14 ± .32	1.17 ± .13	.90	.37
Assessment each shift	1.11 ± .29	1.12 ± .10	.28	.78
Reasons for missed nursing care				
Communication	2.23 ± .18	2.32 ± .20	2.49	.014
Labor resource	3.00 ± .29	3.12 ± .18	3.31	.001
Material resource	2.56 ± .22	2.61 ± .23	1.37	.174

TABLE 5.2   **Staffing differences by Magnet status.**

Variable	Magnet status		t	p
	Yes (Mean ± SD)	No (Mean ± SD)		
HPPD	10.94 ± .18	11.30 ± 4.98	0.44	.662
RN HPPD	8.71 ± 4.17	8.86 ± 4.58	0.19	.847
Skill mix	0.781 ± .14	0.780 ± .18	−0.04	.969

TABLE 5.3.   **Hierarchical regression result summary.**

Variable	Coefficient	Robust S.E.	t ratio
Intercept	1.530**	0.040	37.775
Individual-level predictors			
Experience	0.044**	0.005	8.961
Education (BS or higher)	0.088**	0.014	6.374
Unit-level predictors			
Magnet (Magnet)	−0.074*	0.030	−2.471
Type of unit (ICU)	0.077	0.159	0.484
HPPD	−0.022	0.012	−1.827
CMI	−0.002	0.021	−0.104
Level-1 R^2	4.6%		
Level-2 R^2	15.0%		

Note: S.E. standard error; *$p < 0.05$. **$p < 0.01$

experience was positively associated with missed nursing care; staff that held BSN degree or higher reported more missed nursing care than staff that held associate degrees or less.

The results of this study offer evidence that Magnet hospitals provide a higher level of nursing care; they also help explain the findings of studies that have shown a significant relationship between Magnet status and patient outcomes (i.e., falls, staff perceptions of quality). There was less missed nursing care in Magnet facilities.

In an examination of the specific elements of nursing care missed or not missed in the two categories of nursing organizations, we found that turning, feeding, meal set up, full documentation, patient teaching, mouth care, IV and central line site care, call-light and monitor response, medication effectiveness assessment, and skin and wound care were completed more often in the Magnet hospitals than others.

On the other hand, there were no differences between the two types of organizations in the extents to which the following elements of care were missed: ambulation, timely medication, vital signs, monitoring intake and output, emotional support, bathing, hand washing, patient discharge planning, glucose monitoring, assessment at the beginning of each shift, focused reassessments, PRN medication administration, interdisciplinary conference attendance, and toileting assistance. It is interesting that several of these nursing actions are among the most missed elements of care (i.e., ambulation and interdisciplinary round attendance) or the least missed aspects of care (i.e., vital signs, glucose monitoring, assessment at the beginning of each shift, and patient discharge planning). While this finding suggests that there are certain nursing actions that are completed in every hospital regardless of the quality of nursing care, there are also other nursing interventions, such as ambulation, timely medications, and hand washing, that are also universally missed across hospital types.

Looking specifically at the lack of patient ambulation, which we have found to be the most prevalent element of missed care across facilities, suggests that there is something inherent in all settings or all nurses that interferes with this nursing action. This could be accounted for by the length of time it typically takes to ambulate patients, the need to rely on colleagues to assist them, or the belief that it is not important. In regard to timely medications, this finding may be related to the fact that there were no significant differences between Magnet and non-Magnet hospitals; both were able to access material supplies, while medication was identified as the most problematic to attain. Emotional support is reported to be missed equally between Magnet and non-Magnet hospitals, which may suggest that there is not time, or the perception that there is not time, to provide this care, even in well-staffed and managed nursing organizations.

The findings that show less education and more experience are associated with fewer instances of identified missed care suggest that, perhaps, baccalaureate-prepared nurses have a higher standard of care. The fact that those nursing staff members with more experience often do not recognize missed care could be due to an acceptance of norms of care that have been in place for some time.

The differences in the reasons for missing nursing care show that Magnet hospitals are considered by nursing staff to have better communication and teamwork. Additionally, there is the belief that staffing is more adequate in Magnet hospitals. However, a comparison of actual HPPD uncovered no significant differences in staffing levels between Magnet and non-Magnet organizations, even though the staff perceived the former to be better. This suggests that it is not staffing levels alone which account for the differences in positive patient and staff outcomes, but rather the hospital and patient unit culture (e.g., safety, quality, physician and nurse relationships, teamwork among nursing staff members, management, participation in decision-making, etc.) that makes the difference.

Summary

The findings of this study highlight the value of hospital nursing organizations working toward and achieving Magnet status. It appears that the level of staffing in a hospital is an important but not sufficient element in achieving excellence in nursing care. It is critical that nursing organizations work toward the creation and maintenance of the type of culture promoted by the Magnet program, which includes strong leadership, empowerment of the staff, respect, integrity, collaboration, recognition, and recruitment of the highest quality nursing staff. Also evaluated by the Magnet program is the presence of exemplary professional practice and the continuous application of new knowledge.

References

Aiken, L. H. (1981). Nursing priorities for the 1980s: Hospitals and nursing homes. *The American Journal of Nursing, 81*(2), 324–330.

Aiken, L. H., Clarke, S. P., Sloane, D. M., Sochalski, J., & Silber, J. H. (2002). Hospital nurse staffing and patient mortality, nurse burnout, and job dissatisfaction. *Journal of the American Medical Association, 288*(16), 1987–1993.

Aiken, L. H., Havens, D. S., & Sloane, D. M. (2000). The Magnet nursing services recognition program: A comparison of two groups of Magnet hospitals. *The American Journal of Nursing, 100*(3), 26–36.

Aiken, L. H., & Sloane, D. M. (1997). Effects of organizational innovations in AIDS care on burnout among urban hospital nurses. *Work and Occupations, 24*(4), 453–477.

Aiken, L. H., Sloane, D. M., Lake, E. T., Sochalski, J., & Weber, A. L. (1999). Organization and outcomes of inpatient AIDS care. *Medical Care, 37*(8), 760–772.

Aiken, L. H., Smith, H. L., & Lake, E. T. (1994). Lower Medicare mortality among a set of hospitals known for good nursing care. *Medical Care, 32*(8), 771–787.

Brady-Schwartz, D. C. (2005). Further evidence on the Magnet recognition program: Implications for nursing leaders. *Journal of Nursing Administration, 35*(9), 397–403.

Cho, S. H., Ketefian, S., Barkauskas, V. H., & Smith, D. G. (2003). The effects of nurse staffing on adverse events, morbidity, mortality, and medical costs. *Nursing Research, 52*(2), 71–79.

Cronbach, L. J. (1987). Statistical tests for moderator variables: Flaws in analyses recently proposed. *Psychological Bulletin, 102*(3), 414–417.

Friese, C. R. (2005). Nurse practice environments and outcomes: Implications for oncology nursing. *Oncology Nursing Forum, 32*(4), 765–772.

Kalisch, B. J., Landstrom, G., & Williams, R. A. (2009). Missed nursing care: Errors of omission. *Nursing Outlook, 57*(1), 3–9.

Kalisch, B., Tschannen, D., Lee, H., & Friese, C. (2011). Hospital variation in missed nursing care. *American Journal of Medical Quality, 26*(4), 291–299.

Kalisch, B. J., & Williams, R. A. (2009). Development and psychometric testing of a tool to measure missed nursing care. *Journal of Nursing Admimistration, 39*(5), 211–219.

Kovner, C., Jones, C., Zhan, C., Gergen, P. J., & Basu, J. (2002). Nurse staffing and postsurgical adverse events: An analysis of administrative data from a sample of U.S. hospitals, 1990–1996. *Health Services Research, 37*(3), 611–629.

Kramer, M., & Schalenberg, C. (2004). Essentials of a magnetic work environment, part 1. *Nursing, 34*(6), 50–54.

Lacey, S. R., Cox, K. S., Lorfing, K. C., Teasley, S. L., Carroll, C. A., & Sexton, K. (2007). Nursing support, workload, and intent to stay in Magnet, Magnet-aspiring, and non-Magnet hospitals. *Journal of Nursing Administration, 37*(4), 199–205.

Lake, E. T., Shang, J., Klaus, S., & Dunton, N. E. (2010). Patient falls: Association with hospital Magnet status and nursing unit staffing. *Research in Nursing & Health, 33*(5), 413–425.

Laschinger, S., Heather, K., Almost, J., & Tuer-Hodes, D. (2003). Workplace empowerment and Magnet hospital characteristics: Making the link. *Journal of Nursing Administration 33*(7/8), 410–422.

Laschinger, S. H., Shamian, K., J., & Thomson, D. (2001). Impact of Magnet hospital characteristics on nurses' perceptions of trust, burnout, quality of care, and work satisfaction. *Nursing Economics, 19*(5), 209–219.

Needleman, J., Buerhaus, P., Mattke, S., Stewart, M., & Zelevinsky, K. (2002). Nurse-staffing levels and the quality of care in hospitals. *New England Journal of Medicine, 346*(22), 1715–1722.

Schmalenberg, C., & Kramer, M. (2008). Essentials of a productive nurse work environment. *Nursing Research, 57*(1), 2–13.

Ulrich, B. T., Buerhaus, P. I., Donelan, K., Norman, L., & Dittus, R. (2007). Magnet status and registered nurse views of the work environment and nursing as a career. *Journal of Nursing Administration, 37*(5), 212–220.

Upenieks, V. V. (2002). Assessing differences in job satisfaction of nurses in Magnet and nonmagnet hospitals. *Journal of Nursing Administration, 32*(11), 564–76.

Endnote

This manuscript was published previously and is reprinted here with permission of Nursing Outlook. Kalisch, B., & Lee, K. (2012). Missed nursing care: Magnet versus non-Magnet Hospitals. *Nursing Outlook, 60*(5), 32–39.

— 6 —

International Missed Nursing Care

by
Beatrice Kalisch, Boqin Xie,[1] Helga Bragadóttir,[2] Myrna Dounit,[3] Kerri Holzhauser and Liz Burmeister,[4] Eunjoo Lee,[5] Fusun Terzioglu,[6] and Annamaria Ferraresi[7]

Previous Studies

There have been several studies comparing the quality of nursing care across countries. Aiken and colleagues (2001) studied nursing in Canada, England, Scotland, Germany, and the United States. They surveyed 43,000 nurses in over 700 hospitals from 1998 to 1999. The nurse survey included questions on a variety of issues related to the nurses' perceptions of their working environments, the quality of nursing care being delivered in their hospitals, care left undone, job satisfaction, career plans, and job burnout. Care left undone was measured in three of the five countries. The findings showed that German nurses reported less missed oral care (10%) than the United States and Canada (about 20%). The United States and Canada reported more missed skin care (30% to 34%) than in Germany (13%). Teaching patients was missed similarly across all three countries (26% to 29%). Comforting and talking with patients was missed the least in the United States (40%), more in Canada (44%), and the most in Germany (54%). Care planning was reported to be missed from 34% in Germany to 47% in Canada. Discharge preparation was very similar across the three countries (13% to 14%).

In another study comparing the United States, England, Scotland, and Canada, 10,319 nurses working on medical and surgical units in 303 hospitals completed a survey which dealt with job satisfaction, burnout, and quality of care (Aiken, Clarke, Sloane, Sochalski, & Silber, 2002). The higher the number of patients assigned to nurses, the higher the risk-adjusted 30-day mortality, failure to rescue rates, and burnout.

Nurse work environments in the United States, China, South Korea, Thailand, Japan, New Zealand, United Kingdom, Canada, and Germany (98,116 nurses in 1,406 hospitals) were surveyed with the Nursing Work Index Practice Environment Scale (PES of the NWI) and four outcome variables were reported by nurses. Of the four outcomes, two were related to nurse outcomes—job dissatisfaction and Maslach Burnout Inventory—and two involved nurses' assessments of quality of care in their hospitals—readiness of patients for discharge and overall quality (Aiken et al., 2011). In most of the countries studied, a third or more of hospital nurses were dissatisfied with their jobs. Nurse burnout was high in almost all countries with over a third or more of bedside care nurses scoring in the high burnout range. In all countries, more than 1 in 10 nurses reported that care was either fair or poor, and in 3 of 4 Asian countries studied, nurses' ratings of fair or poor care were much more frequent. Almost half or more than half of nurses in all countries (except Germany) reported concern about their patients' ability to care for themselves following discharge from the hospital.

Aiken and colleagues (2012) conducted another study surveying 33,659 nurses and 11,318 patients in Europe along with 27,509 nurses and more than 120,000 patients in the United States. Participating nurses were from 488 hospitals in Europe and 617 in the United States, and the patient subjects were from 210 European and 430 U.S. hospitals. Outcomes of nursing that were studied include: hospital staffing, work environment burnout, dissatisfaction, intention to leave their job in the next year, patient safety, and quality of care. Patient outcomes that were measured include: satisfaction, nursing care overall, and willingness to recommend their hospitals. The percentage of nurses reporting poor or fair quality patient care varied substantially by country, from 11% in Ireland to 47% in Greece, as did percentages of nurses who gave their hospital a poor or failing safety rating (4% in Switzerland to 18% in Poland). Results uncovered varying rates of nurse burnout (from 10% in the Netherlands to 78% in Greece), job dissatisfaction (11% in the Netherlands to 56% in Greece), and intention to leave (14% in the United States to 49% in Finland and Greece).

Patients' high satisfaction ratings of their hospitals also varied considerably (35% in Spain to 61% in Finland and Ireland), as did the rates of patients willing to recommend their hospital (53% in Greece to 78% in Switzerland). Improved work environment and reduced ratios of patients to nurses were associated with increased quality of care and patient satisfaction. In European hospitals, after adjusting for hospital and nurse characteristics, nurses with better work environments were half as likely to report poor or fair quality of care (adjusted odds ratio 0.56, 95% confidence interval 0.51 to 0.61) and give their hospitals poor or failing grades on patient safety (0.50, 0.44 to 0.56). Each additional patient per nurse increased the odds of nurses reporting poor or fair quality of care (1.11, 1.07 to 1.15) and poor or failing safety grades (1.10, 1.05 to 1.16). Patients in hospitals with better work environments were more likely to rate their hospital highly (1.16, 1.03 to 1.32) and recommend their hospitals (1.20, 1.05 to 1.37), whereas those with higher ratios of patients to nurses were less likely to rate them highly (0.94, 0.91 to 0.97) or recommend them (0.95, 0.91 to 0.98). Results were similar in the United States. Nurses and patients agreed on which hospitals provided good care and could be recommended.

Ausserhofer and colleagues (2014) investigated the extent and type of nursing care left undone across 12 European countries (Belgium, England, Finland, Germany, Greece, Ireland, The Netherlands, Norway, Poland, Spain, Sweden, and Switzerland). The sample was 33,659 nurses in 488 hospitals. The data for the study was obtained from the RN4CAST nurse questionnaire (Ball, Pike, Griffiths, Rafferty, & Murrells, 2012). The following issues were investigated: nursing care left undone, the quality of the nurse work environment, nurse staffing levels, the amount of non-nursing duties, and nurse and hospital characteristics. The survey was translated into the languages of the countries involved in the study. In addition, the PES of the NWI was administered to study work environment variables. The most frequent nursing care activities left undone included: comfort or talk with patients (53%), developing or updating nursing care plans and care pathways (42%), and educating patients and families (41%). In hospitals with more favorable work environments ($\beta = -2.19$; $p < 0.0001$), lower patient to nurse ratios ($\beta = 0.09$; $p < 0.0001$), and lower proportions of nurses frequently carrying out non-nursing tasks ($\beta = 2.18$; $p < 0.0001$), fewer nurses reported missed nursing care. Nursing care left undone was prevalent across all European countries and was associated with nurse-related organizational factors. Similar patterns of missed nursing care were evident across the study hospitals.

Current Study

The study reported in this chapter is a comparison of missed nursing care in seven countries, namely: Australia, Iceland, Italy, South Korea, Lebanon, Turkey, and the United States. This study adds to our understanding of variations in the delivery of nursing care internationally, specifically, what care is provided and what is not, as well as the quality of care. The United States and South Korea have been studied in the work of Aiken and colleagues (2011), but we were unable to find studies which compared the extent of missed nursing care in the other countries.

Research Questions

The purpose of this study was to compare the amounts of missed nursing care and the reasons for missed care across seven countries. The specific research questions were:

1. Do the amounts of missed nursing care differ across these countries?
2. What are the specific elements of nursing care that are missed the most and the least across these countries?
3. How do the reasons for missed nursing care differ across these countries?

Methods

Design, samples, and settings

A cross-sectional design was used for this study. The sample was comprised of 6,212 RNs who provided direct patient care in the seven study countries. The nurses who completed the survey in all of the countries were drawn from medical–surgical, rehabilitative, intermediate, and intensive care patient units in acute care hospitals. The Australian sample was made up of RNs (n = 364) working on 5 units in 1 hospital (830 beds). The return rate was 31%. In Iceland, the RN subjects (n = 344) worked on 27 units in 8 hospitals (ranging in size from 8 to 670 beds). These hospitals comprised all hospitals in the country. The return rate was 69.3%. For Italy, the study sample was comprised of RNs (n = 887) working on 67 units in 5 hospitals (ranging in size from 450 to 1,407 beds) with a return rate of 81.3%. In South Korea, RNs (n = 555) working on 73 units in 2 academic medical centers and 1 teaching hospital made up the sample, with a return rate of 87%. For Lebanon, RNs (n = 118) working on 18 units in 1 large teaching hospital (250 beds) with a return rate of 44.4% made up the sample. RNs (n = 406) working in 2 university hospitals (913 and 1,053 beds) on 82 patient care units made up the sample in Turkey. The return rate was 80%. The U.S. sample (n = 3538) came from 11 hospitals (ranging in size from 60 to 913 beds) and 126 patient care units. The return rate was 59%.

Measures

The *MISSCARE Survey—English* was used to measure nursing staff perceptions of the amount of missed care (Part A) and the reasons for missed care (Part B). As presented in Chapter 2, the *MISSCARE Survey* is a five-point Likert-type scale with 23 items in Part A and 17 items in Part B. In Part A, RNs were asked to identify how frequently elements of nursing care were missed on their unit (e.g., ambulation three times a day, on-time medication administrations, repositioning and turning, patient assessment, IV site care, patient education, etc.; Kalisch & Williams, 2009). Nursing staff were asked to check the most accurate response: never or rarely missed, occasionally missed, frequently missed, or always missed. In Part B, nursing staff identified the reasons why nursing care was missed ranging from not a reason to a significant reason.

The English version of the *MISSCARE Survey* was used in the United States, Australia, and Lebanon. For the other countries—Iceland, Italy, South Korea, and Turkey—the survey was translated from English into Icelandic, Italian, Korean, and Turkish using a step-by-step translation process including preparation, translation, back translation, adjudication, pretest, revision, and test–retest. The process utilized was designed to ensure the meaning was not lost or changed during the translation. The preparation step gave an overview of the methods, background of the study, definition of key terms, and a general paraphrase summary of each question. The translation was done by three bilingual translators in each country and the back translation was completed by one bilingual translator. The adjudication process involved an expert team of three individuals that reviewed both the English, Icelandic, Italian, Korean, and Turkish surveys and revised in accordance to the original meaning of each item. The resulting *MISSCARE Survey—Icelandic, MISSCARE Survey—Italian, MISSCARE Survey—Korean,* and *MISSCARE Survey—Turkish* utilized the same basic structure of the *MISSCARE Survey—English.*

The reliability and validity of the English version of the *MISSCARE Survey* has been reported previously (Kalisch & Williams, 2009), as has the Icelandic version (Bragadóttir, Kalisch, Smáradóttir, & Jónsdóttir, 2014) and the Turkish version (Kalisch, Terzioglu, & Duygulu, 2012). For the United States, the content validity index was 0.89 and test–retest reliability for Part A was 0.88 ($p < .001$). Exploratory and confirmatory factor analyses on Part B revealed a three-factor solution: staffing resources, material resources, and communication/teamwork with a range of factor loadings from 0.35 to 0.85 and a range of Cronbach α coefficients from 0.71 to 0.86.

Cronbach's α coefficients for the *MISSCARE Survey* Part A in the countries of Australia, Iceland, Italy, Lebanon, Turkey, South Korea, and the United States were 0.91, 0.89, 0.94, 0.91, 0.91, 0.93, and 0.92 respectively. The internal consistency reliability of the *MISSCARE Survey*—Part A was acceptable across all countries. The subscales in Part B—staffing resources, material resources and communication/teamwork—ranged from 0.50 to 0.93.

Procedures

After acquiring the approval of institutional review boards at the participating hospitals in each country, survey packets that contained a letter explaining the study and ensuring confidentiality, the *MISSCARE Survey,* and a return envelope were placed in each nursing staff member's mail box. Nurses were asked to place completed surveys in locked boxes located on their respective units or put the envelope in the mail.

Data Analysis

After data cleaning, frequencies were calculated to explore the distribution of missed care and reasons for missed care. The overall missed care score was the average amount of missed care identified for each of the elements of nursing care for each participant. Higher scores indicated more missed nursing care. To examine the percentage of missed care for each specific element of care (e.g., turning, mouth care, medications on time, etc.), the items were categorized as dichotomous variables. As described in the previous chapter, elements of care were considered missed if frequently missed or always missed was reported. One-way analysis of variance (ANOVA) was calculated to examine the differences in the amounts of missed care and reasons for missed care across countries. Bonferroni correction was used for multiple comparisons. Each outcome variable (the amount of missed care and reasons for missed care) constituted a family of the post-hoc comparison. The family-wise error rate after the Bonferroni correction was 0.05.

Study Findings

The sample was comprised of 6,212 RNs in seven countries. The participants were largely female (90.7%), aged 26 to 44 years (62.7%), and worked 30 hours or more (85%) per week. The nurses holding a baccalaureate or higher degree were 52.2% and the other 41.4% held an associate degree or its equivalent. The day shift was the most frequently reported working shift (36.9%), followed by rotating shifts (33.9%), nights (24.2%), and evenings (5%). The percentage of nurses with work experience greater than 10 years was 36.2%, followed by 5 to 10 years (20.8%), 2 to 5 years (20.7%), 6 months to 2 years (17.7%), and less than 6 months (4.5%). The details are displayed in Table 6.1. Table 6.2 contains the mean number of patients cared for during the last shift, admissions, and discharges. A comparison across countries indicated a significant difference in mean patient load.

The amount of missed nursing care by country

There were significant differences in the total amount of missed nursing care among the seven countries (F = 28.91, p < .001) with Italy reporting the most missed care (1.59 ± .59), and the United States next (Figure 6.1). RNs in Lebanon reported the least amount of missed nursing care (1.28 ± .33). The amounts of missed care reported by RNs in the other countries are contained in Tables 6.3, 6.4, and Figure 6.1. This is confusing, given the fact that the United States has much richer staffing than Italy for example (Table 6.3). Even though we found that the better the staffing levels, the less the missed care in a study conducted in the United States (Kalisch, Tschannen, & Lee, 2011; Chapter 11), these results did not hold up in this international study. There are a number of possible explanations but this requires further study.

The elements of missed nursing care by country

Table 6.4 displays the percentages of each element of nursing care that were reported missed across the study countries. Ambulation is missed a great deal in every country, ranging from 19% in Iceland to 53% in Italy. It was either the most or the second most missed element of nursing care in all of the countries studied. Another prevalent element of missed nursing care was oral care, which ranged from 10% missed in Iceland and Turkey to 28% in Italy. Turning patients also had a high level of missed care in most of the countries except for Iceland, which was 6.3%. Italy, on the other hand, reported missing turning 44% of the time and South Korea followed behind at 33%. Hand washing was

TABLE 6.1. Demographic characteristics of study participants by country (n = 6212).

	Australia %	Iceland %	Italy %	Korea %	Lebanon %	Turkey %	United States %
Under 35 years of age	50.3	34.6	30.7	91.4	91.5	—*	43.1
Education (university graduate)	91.9	87.4	40.3	7.8	95.8	2.1	57.2
5–9 years of experience in nursing	20.1	20.5	22.7	21.8	32.2	30.5	18.7
10 or more years of experience in nursing	43.7	48.7	49.7	9.4	9.6	30.5	36.6
Full time	85.4	74.3	94	100+	100+	92.9	82.3
Female	87.8	98.8	78.1	98	63.6	95.8	92.5

Note: *Data were not collected in this country. +All of nurses in Korea and Lebanon worked full time

TABLE 6.2. Mean number of patients cared for, admissions, and discharges during last shift: A comparison across countries (Mean ± SD) (n = 6212).

	United States	Iceland	Australia	Lebanon	Korea	Italy	F	p
Patients cared for	4.10 ± 1.74a	5.81 ± 3.01b	5.31 ± 3.01b	4.12 ± 2.60a	9.87 ± 7.30c	13.25 ± 4.07d	1190.5	<.001
Admissions	1.09 ± 1.13a	1 ± 1.86a	2.03 ± 2.71bc	1.57 ± 2.28ab	2.38 ± 3.39c	3.49 ± 2.84d	202.2	<.001
Discharges	0.83 ± 1.16a	0.95 ± 1.89a	1.67 ± 2.48b	1.34 ± 2.12ab	2.10 ± 3.34c	3.03 ± 2.48d	185.3	<.001

Note: SD, standard deviation. Means that do not share subscripts differ at $p < .05$ using the Bonferroni correction

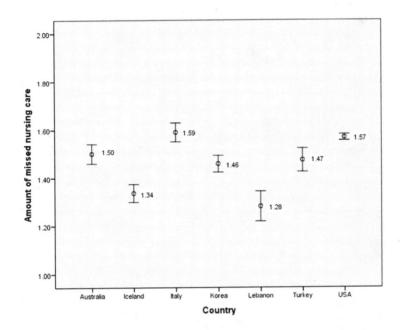

FIGURE 6.1. **The amount of overall missed nursing care (n = 6212).**
Note: Each bar line indicates 95% confidence interval

TABLE 6.3. **A comparison of missed nursing care and reasons for missed nursing care across countries (n = 6212).**

		Reasons for missed care		
	Missed Care M (SD)	Staffing Resources M (SD)	Material Resources M (SD)	Communication/ Teamwork M (SD)
Australia (n = 364)	1.50 ± .40	2.77 ± .66	2.46 ± .66	2.11 ± .56
Iceland (n = 344)	1.34 ± .35	3.18 ± .94	2.44 ± 1.32	2.18 ± 1.14
Italy (n = 887)	1.59 ± .59	3.42 ± .58	2.55 ± .84	2.55 ± .75
S. Korea (n = 555)	1.46 ± .42	3.33 ± .53	2.61 ± .67	2.39 ± .59
Lebanon (n = 118)	1.28 ± .33	3.17 ± .61	2.91 ± .74	2.59 ± .71
Turkey (n = 406)	1.47 ± .51	3.64 ± .38	3.48 ± .70	2.97 ± .72
USA (n = 3538)	1.57 ± .39	3.07 ± .63	2.62 ± .66	2.28 ± .56
F	28.91	105.73	98.93	96.59
p	<.001	<.001	<.001	<.001

TABLE 6.4.   The percentage of elements of nursing care reported "frequently" or "always" missed by country (n = 6212).

	Australia %	Iceland %	Italy %	S. Korea %	Lebanon %	Turkey %	United States %
Ambulation	37.3	18.5	52.8	29.4	23	23	35.1
Turning patient	18.3	6.3	44.0	33.3	15	18	16.3
Feeding	11.1	7.6	17.9	17.7	9.3	24.7	18.4
Setting up meal	7.8	5.2	27.9	25.8	4.6	13.5	9.0
Medications administered	9.3	7.6	14.6	5.0	1.8	13.1	18.5
Vital signs	2.8	2.9	7.5	2.5	0	7.3	4.1
Intake/Output	25.6	5.8	9.4	2.3	7.1	7.6	18.8
Documentation	22.3	11.7	16.1	4.0	8.0	6.8	15.3
Patient teaching	19.2	16.1	16.4	6.5	15.9	13.1	16
Emotional support	12.4	10.5	17.6	12.3	16.7	22.2	12.4
Bathing	3.9	2.1	10.8	28.2	0	14.6	8.1
Mouth care	27.8	10.0	28.1	27.1	12.5	10.4	27
Hand washing	5.8	4.7	12.7	4.5	9.2	5.3	5.4
Discharge planning	10.2	13.5	22.7	4.7	4.5	16.1	5.1
Bedside glucose	1.6	1.2	8.0	2.9	0.9	10.2	2.0
Patient assessment	6.0	4.4	12.2	2.5	2.6	6.2	1.8
Reassessment	5.8	3.0	12.9	2.9	1.8	—*	3.9
IV care	8.0	8.2	11.5	2.2	1.8	5.4	6.6
Call light answered	11.6	2.1	9.1	5.6	2.7	12.0	13.7
PRN medication	3.0	1.8	8.6	3.4	3.6	10.3	7.2
Assess effectiveness of medication	10.3	9.0	9.7	4.3	7.1	10.6	10.3
Toileting	8.5	2.1	12.8	10.6	6.3	13.1	10.7
Skin/Wound care	4.7	1.2	8.8	9.2	2.7	7.2	3.4

Note: *Data was not collected in this country

reported to be missed about 5% of the time, except for Italy (13%) and Lebanon (9.2%). Bedside glucose monitoring was missed from 0.9% in Lebanon to 10.2% in Turkey. Vital signs missed ranged from 0% in Lebanon to 7.3% in Turkey and 7.5% in Italy. Skin and wound care was also one of the least missed aspects of nursing care across all seven countries (1.2% in Iceland to 9.2% in South Korea).

Documentation was reported to be missed very little in South Korea (4%), while Australia reported 22.3% missed. Discharge planning was missed around 5% in Lebanon, the United States, and Korea, but 23% in Italy and 16% in Turkey. In the United States, patient assessment at the beginning of each shift was missed very little (1.8%), but Italian nurses reported missing it 12.2% of the time, and Turkey and Australia, 6%. Bathing showed a wide range of being missed from none in Lebanon and 2% in Iceland to 28% in Korea and 15% in Turkey. Emotional support was missed most in Italy and Turkey (18% and 22%). Monitoring intake and output ranged from a low of 5.3% in South Korea to 26% in Australia. Medications were reported to not be given or given late from 2% in Lebanon to 19% in the United States and 15% in Italy.

The reasons for missed nursing care by country
Although the reasons for missed nursing care differed, inadequate staffing was the top reason for missed care reported by RNs across the seven countries. Inadequate communication/teamwork scored the lowest (yet still was substantial) of the three reported reasons (Table 6.2 and Figure 6.2). Inadequate staffing levels were identified the most in Turkey and Italy and the least in Australia. RNs working in Turkey, Lebanon, South Korea, and Italy cited communication/teamwork as more of a problem than the other countries. In terms of the shortage of material resources, Turkey and Lebanon had the highest percentages.

Discussion
The results of this study lend evidence to the belief that there is a problem with missed nursing care internationally. Nurses in all countries reported missing standard, required nursing care. Even though there were certain elements of nursing care that were missed more often, such as ambulation, turning, and mouth care, and others that tended not to be missed, such as patient assessment, vital signs, and bedside glucose testing, there are differences between countries as to which elements of nursing care are being missed.

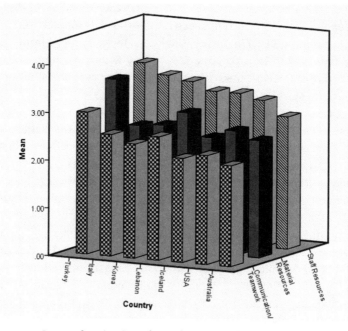

FIGURE 6.2. **Reasons for missed care (means) by countries (n = 6212).**

While the summary scores provide an overall view of missed nursing care in a given country, it does not tell the whole story. The nurses in a country may miss less care in one area and more in another, which averages the score out. Therefore, it is necessary to review the individual elements of care to get a better idea of differences across countries. As far as the individual elements of nursing care are concerned, Italy missed the most ambulation, turning, setting up meals, hand washing, discharge planning, patient assessments, reassessments, and IV care. Turkey missed feeding, emotional support, bathing, bedside glucose monitoring, and PRN medications the most. Australia and the United States had similar scores on ambulation, turning, intake and output monitoring, documentation, patient teaching, mouth care, hand washing, answering call lights, and toileting. Except for patient teaching (missed 16.1%), Iceland had the least of amount of missed care in all categories.

In general, these findings are similar to those uncovered by other researchers who have conducted international comparisons. Since the elements of nursing care that were measured have differed from study to study, it is not possible at this point to make a direct comparison of specific findings.

There are a number of limitations of this study. Sampling was completed on a convenience basis. Therefore, making generalizations of the findings to the country level cannot be done. The study does not account for differences in practice customs or patient acuity in the seven countries. For example, in Turkey and Lebanon, patient families are in the hospital with the patient and complete part of the nursing care that is the sole responsibility of the nursing staff in other countries. The level of documentation required in the countries may vary considerably, and thus may influence the answers to this question and the time available to provide aspects of nursing care. Another limitation is the sampling of only one hospital in Lebanon (which has a reputation for being one of the highest quality organizations in that country) and one in Australia.

However, the focus of the questions on specific nursing actions mitigates these problems somewhat. In other words, in all likelihood, such common nursing actions (e.g., vital signs, bathing, etc.) are universally understood by nurses. The achievement of good test–retest reliability is also a positive indication of the clarity of the survey items. Each country had expert panels who reviewed the instrument (before and after translation) to ensure that it represented nursing practice in their country as well.

Summary

In this chapter, the results of an international study of missed nursing care in seven countries are reported. There were significant differences in the total amount of missed nursing care among the countries with Italy reporting the most missed care. Inadequate staffing resources was the top reason for missed care reported by RNs across the countries. Inadequate communication/teamwork scored the lowest, yet was still identified as a substantial reason for missed nursing care in each of the seven countries.

References

Aiken, L. H., Clarke, S. P., Sloane, D. M., Sochalski, J. A., Busse, R., Clarke, H., ... Shamian, J. (2001). Nurses' reports on hospital care in five countries. *Health Affairs, 20*(3), 43–53.

Aiken, L. H., Clarke, S. P., Sloane, D. M., Sochalski, J. A., & Silber, J. H. (2002). Hospital nurse staffing and patient mortality, nurse burnout, and job dissatisfaction. *Journal of the American Medical Association, 288*(16), 1987–1993.

Aiken, L. H., Sermeus, W., Van den Heede, K., Sloane, D. M., Busse, R., McKee, M., ... Kutney-Lee, A. (2012). Patient safety, satisfaction, and quality of hospital care: Cross sectional surveys of nurses and patients in 12 countries in Europe and the United States. *BMJ, 344*, e1717. doi: 10.1136/bmj.e1717

Aiken, L. H., Sloane, D. M., Clarke, S., Poghosyan, L., Cho, E., You, L., ... Aungsuroch, Y. (2011). Importance of work environments on hospital outcomes in nine countries. *International Journal for Quality in Health Care, 23*(4), 357–364.

Ausserhofer, D., Zander, B., Busse, R., Schubert, M., De Geest, S., Rafferty, A. M., ... Schwendimann, R. (2014). Prevalence, patterns and predictors of nursing care left undone in European hospitals: Results from the multicountry cross-sectional RN4CAST study. *BMJ Quality & Safety, 23*(2), 126–135.

Ball, J., Pike, G., Griffiths, P., Rafferty, A., & Murrellls, T. (2012). RN4CAST nurse survey in England. *International Journal of Nursing Studies, 50*(2), 264–273.

Bragadóttir, H., Kalisch, B. J., Smáradóttir, S. B., & Jónsdóttir, H. H. (2014). Translation and psychometric testing of the Icelandic version of the MISSCARE Survey. *Scandinavian Journal of Caring Sciences*. Advance online publication. doi: 10.1111/scs.12150

Kalisch, B. J., Doumit, M., Lee, K.H., & Zei, J. E. (2013). Missed nursing care, level of staffing, and job satisfaction: Lebanon versus the United States. *Journal of Nursing Adminstration, 43*(5), 274–279.

Kalisch, B. J., Terzioglu, F., & Duygulu, S. (2012). The MISSCARE Survey-Turkish: Psychometric properties and findings. *Nursing Economics, 30*(1), 29–37.

Kalisch, B. J., Tschannen, D., & Lee, K. (2011). Do staffing levels predict missed nursing care? *International Journal for Quality in Health Care, 23*(3), 1–7.

Kalisch, B. J., & Williams, R. A. (2009). Development and psychometric testing of a tool to measure missed nursing care. *Journal of Nursing Administration, 39*(5), 211–219.

Siqueira, L. D., Caliri, M. H., Kalisch, B., & Dantas, R. A. (2013). Cultural adaptation and internal consistency analysis of the *MISSCARE Survey* for use in Brazil. *Revista Latino-Americana de Enfermagem, 21*(2), 610–617.

Endnotes

1   University of Michigan School of Nursing, Ann Arbor, Michigan, U.S.

2   University of Iceland Faculty of Nursing & Landspitali University Hospital, Reykjavik, Iceland

3   American University of Lebanon, Beirut, Lebanon

4   Princess Alexandra Hospital, Brisbane, Australia

5   Kyngpook National University, Daegu, South Korea

6   Hacettepe Universtiy, Ankara, Turkey

7   On behalf of the Italian Missed Care Study Group: Annamaria Ferraresi, Luisa Sist, Anna Bandini, Stefania Bandini, Carla Cortini, Massa Licia Massa, and Roberta Zanin. Research program, Regione Emilia-Romagna Università, Italy

— 7 —

Missed Nursing Care in the Operating Room

by
AkkeNeel Talsma, PhD, RN, FAAN and
Margaret McLaughlin, PhD, MPH, RN

More than any other area in a hospital, the operating room (OR) is a convergence of resources uniting people, equipment, and time. The perioperative environment is also important for quality improvement initiatives, as errors with grave consequences are apt to occur in the OR (Institute of Medicine, 2000).

The persistent global nursing shortage causes some unease about the availability of skilled, experienced OR nursing staff who have experience with the complexities of procedures, collaboration, preparation, and task management inherent in surgical processes (Gillespie, Wallis, & Chaboyer, 2008; Mitchell et al., 2011). An estimated 30.2 million surgical procedures and 21.2 million nonsurgical procedures occurred in short-stay hospitals in the United States in 2010 (Centers for Disease Control and Prevention, 2012). In an 85-year lifetime, an average American might expect to have nearly six surgical procedures in an OR (Lee & Gawande, 2008). A population that is living longer and an upsurge in patients insured through the Patient Protection and Affordable Care Act (PPACA) are expected to increase the demand for surgical services in the United States (Etzioni, Liu, Maggard, & Ko, 2003; Sheldon, 2010; Jim, Owens, Sanchez, & Rubin, 2012; Munnich &

Parente, 2014). Growth in surgical volume brings additional patient care handoffs, increased surgical team workload, and higher expectations to master complex surgical processes, all of which raise the risk of missed nursing care resulting in adverse events and suboptimal patient outcomes.

Patient Safety in the Operating Room

The Joint Commission (TJC) tracks wrong site, wrong procedure, and wrong person surgeries as unexpected occurrences that may involve death or serious physical or psychological injury (The Joint Commission, 2001) (Table 7.1). Root cause analysis of 126 reported cases of wrong-site, wrong-person, or wrong-procedure surgery identified risks for adverse surgical events, including emergency cases, unusual physical patient characteristics, extreme time pressures, equipment and set up, and multiple surgeons or procedures in a case. Many factors contributed to the occurrence of sentinel events (i.e., an unexpected occurrence involving death or serious physical or psychological injury, or the risk thereof). In surgery, the most common were communication breakdowns, lack of policy about preoperative patient preparation, and incomplete preoperative patient assessment (TJC, 2001). In its review of sentinel events occurring in 2013, TJC identified human factors, communication, and leadership as the most frequent root causes (TJC, 2014b).

Other studies have linked communication failures to avoidable perioperative mishaps. An analysis of 60 surgical cases that had communication breakdowns leading to patient harm indicated that most breakdowns (64%) involved verbal communications between two people (Greenberg et al., 2007). The authors noted that common factors contributing to communication breakdowns included status asymmetry concerning unequal rank or authority among surgical team members, ambiguity about responsibilities, roles, and leadership, and handoffs between providers (Greenberg et al., 2007). The study recommended structured handoff processes and reading back transmitted information as solutions to prevent communication breakdowns (Greenberg et al., 2007). Lingard and colleagues (2004) tallied communication failures within about 30% of relevant exchanges between surgical team members. Many of those breakdowns included content that was not timely, accurate, and inclusive (Lingard et al., 2004). More than one third of those miscommunications led to disruptions within the surgical team and to increased tension and cognitive load (Lingard et al., 2004). Human factor issues,

TABLE 7.1. Overview of Preoperative Safety Bundle and Specified Associated Guidelines.

Preoperative Safety Bundle Items	Patient Identification	Site Marking	Allergy Verification	Operative Consent Confirmation	History and Physical Confirmation	Time-out or Pre-procedure Briefing Completed
The Joint Commission's Universal Protocol	NPSG.01.01.01: "Use at least two patient identifiers when providing care, treatment, and services."	UP.01.02.01 "Mark the procedure site."		UP.01.01.01 "Conduct a pre-procedure verification process." Element of Performance 2. "Relevant documentation (for example,...signed procedure consent form)."	UP.01.01.01 "Conduct a pre-procedure verification process." Element of Performance 2. "Relevant documentation (for example, history and physical...)."	UP.01.03.01 "A time-out is performed before the procedure."
World Health Organization's Surgical Safety Checklist	X	X	X	X		X
AORN's Comprehensive Surgical Checklist	X	X	X	X	X	X
Potential Reasons for Missed Care	Absence of at least two identifiers; patient not involved in identification; name alerts not recognized.	Site mismarked; patient not involved in site marking process; site not marked by operating surgeon or approved designee.	Cross-allergies not noted; allergies not noted on history and physical; family history of allergies not noted.	Consent incomplete (e.g., not signed, not dated); preoperative change in intended procedure; emergency and unavailability of patient designee.	Physical exam incomplete; H and P overlooked on patient chart; document not updated and completed within time frame indicated by policy.	Checklist fatigue; lack of commitment to structured, collective briefings; surgical team attitudes, knowledge deficit as regards correct implementation.

displayed in disruptive behavior such as yelling or calling names, are prominent in the operating room and negatively affect communication and teamwork. A total of 4,530 nurses, physicians, and administrators responded to a survey to assess the significance and impact of disruptive behaviors. More than two-thirds of respondents connected disruptive behaviors to adverse events and medical errors (Rosenstein & O'Daniel, 2008). In this study, operating rooms were among the clinical settings most likely to exhibit disruptive behaviors, and 80% of respondents agreed that disruptive behaviors impaired information transfer (Rosenstein & O'Daniel, 2008).

In addition to communication breakdowns, factors contributing to missed nursing care in the OR include the lack of policies and procedures (Talsma, McLaughlin, Bathish, Sirichorachai, & Kuttner, 2014), specifically staff noncompliance with existing policies and procedures (Michaels et al., 2007), work culture related to hierarchy that prevents staff from speaking up in case of an error (Sexton, Thomas, & Helmreich, 2000; TJC, 2013a; Weissman et al., 2007), and inexperience (Gawande, Zinner, Studdert, & Brennan, 2003). Work pressures arising from time constraints and unfamiliarity with the surgical procedure may also contribute to missed nursing care in the OR (TJC, 2001; Kalisch, 2006).

Omissions of perioperative care also persist (Kalisch, Landstrom, & Williams, 2009). Wrong-patient, wrong-site, wrong-procedure errors and unintended retention of a foreign body were among the sentinel events most often reviewed by TJC in 2013 (TJC, 2014a). Such surgical never-events (events that should never occur) are a costly burden to the American economy, amounting to some $1.3 billion in malpractice payments between 1990 and 2010 (Mehtsun, Ibrahim, Diener-West, Pronovost, & Makary, 2013). Increased care coordination and adherence to protocols have been two of the adjustments made to improve patient safety (Auerbach, Staiger, Muench, & Buerhaus, 2013).

Nursing Care in the Operating Room

Even before a patient's arrival into the surgical suite, multiple care providers have prepared by coordinating the efforts of nursing, surgeons, and anesthesia professionals. A surgical team typically involves at least one surgeon, one anesthetist or anesthesiologist, and nursing staff including a circulating registered nurse (the RN circulator), and a scrub person. It is the position of the Association of periOperative Registered Nurses (AORN) that the circulator in every operative or invasive procedure be a perioperative RN (Association of periOperative Registered Nurses, 2014a). The scrub person may be an RN, a surgical technologist, or a Licensed Practical Nurse (LPN) (AORN, 2014b). The RN circulator works outside the sterile field, whereas the scrub person dons sterile attire, yet both advocate for the anesthetized patient. Working in tandem, the RN circulator and the scrub person prepare solutions and supplies for the surgical procedure, safeguard the sterile field, manage specimens, prevent retained surgical items (RSIs), anticipate surgical team needs, and complete other indispensable perioperative activities. Although each provider's role is distinct, the OR's team-focused environment shapes the extent and quality of care that is provided—or left undone—at each step of a surgical procedure.

A pair or group of at least one circulator and one scrub person remains in the surgical suite for the entirety of most procedures. From case to case, or even within one case, the circulator and the scrub person may be relieved temporarily for breaks or for the remainder of the shift and will hand over patient responsibility to their replacement. Throughout a patient's OR experience, the RN circulator perceives and implements measures supporting patient preparedness for procedures using sound clinical judgment and knowledge about anatomy, physiology, and pharmacology to champion the surgical patient's well-being (AORN, 2014a). Nurses regulate their practice in this specialized perioperative environment by paying particular heed to time and techniques, such as setting up instrumentation for a surgical case, meeting patient needs through advocacy, and applying knowledge of surgical processes (Riley & Manias, 2002). A scrub person is expected to have expertise managing the sterile field throughout the surgical procedure, applying knowledge of human anatomy, surgical processes, and technologies to ensure a safe OR environment while facilitating successful performance of invasive and diagnostic procedures (AORN, 2011b; Association of Surgical Technologists, 2014). The scrub person is responsible for setting up the sterile field with selected instruments and supplies, and preparing instruments, sutures, dressings, and other items in a timely fashion (Goodman & Spry, 2014, p. 8).

Missed nursing care in the OR may be viewed in terms of failure to perform required standard nursing care as defined by the Perioperative Nursing Data Set (PNDS), which contains a listing of perioperative nursing actions aimed to protect patients and support quality outcomes (AORN, 2011a; Petersen, 2011; Kalisch et al., 2009). Potential missed nursing care activities in the perioperative setting are derived from select activities outlined in the PNDS. Examples of essential activities that exemplify missed OR nursing care are shown in Table 7.2.

TABLE 7.2.   **Examples of perioperative nursing care subject to being missed.**

Perioperative Nursing Care Subject to Being Missed
Patient not identified correctly
Patient consent form absent or incomplete
Patient's allergies not checked
Preoperative verification process not followed per organizational guidelines
Perioperative teaching not completed
Equipment, instrumentation, and supplies improperly set up and monitored
Inadequate patient positioning supports provided
Surgical item count not performed
Sterile field not monitored to maintain sterility
Surgical specimens mishandled
Unpreparedness to treat cardiac, respiratory, and other crises
Team roles and scope of practice not understood
Perioperative events not documented

Note: Adapted from the *Perioperative Nursing Data Set*, 3rd Edition, 2011

Preoperative Patient Safety Bundle Items

The Preoperative Safety Bundle, developed by the Perioperative Outcomes Initiative (POI, see www.poi-cqi.org) in consultation with OR nurses, consists of safety checks that are included within TJC's Universal Protocol for Preventing Wrong Site, Wrong Procedure, and Wrong Person Surgery™ (TJC, 2015), the World Health Organization's (WHO) Surgical Safety Checklist©, and the AORN Comprehensive Surgical Checklist©. The Preoperative Safety Bundle© was developed by the POI staff (Talsma, McLaughlin, Bathish, Sirichorachai, & Kuttner, 2014) and derived from the literature, recommended practices and regulations, and careful review of available data from POI. The circulating RN, the scrub person, the anesthetist or anesthesiologist, and the surgeon to be involved in each procedure are accountable for verifying the completion of each item of the Safety Bundle, which includes: (1) allergies checked; (2) patient identified; (3) site marked; (4) surgical consent completed; (5) history and physical available and checked; and (6) time-out completed. These items will be described in more detail below.

Organizations Standards

The preoperative safety bundle is built on various organization recommendations for preventing surgical adverse events.

The Association of periOperative Registered Nurses

The AORN Comprehensive Surgical Checklist©, a resource included in AORN's Correct Site Surgery Tool Kit, is a one-page document that incorporates safety checks required by WHO and TJC (AORN, 2012a). The AORN Comprehensive Surgical Checklist©, designed for use in inpatient and outpatient ORs and physician offices, reinforces surgical team communication and preparedness throughout the perioperative process (AORN, 2012a).

The Joint Commission

TJC approved the Universal Protocol for Preventing Wrong Site, Wrong Procedure, and Wrong Person Surgery™ in July 2003, to address these issues occurring on a regular basis in TJC-accredited hospitals, ambulatory care, and office-based surgery facilities. The Universal Protocol is based on broad consensus about feasible measures that healthcare facilities may take to prevent surgery involving the wrong patient, procedure, and site, by addressing discrepancies and missing information before the start of a surgical procedure. There are three distinct steps—pre-procedure verification, surgical site marking, and a time-out (or pause) directly before making the incision—that are included in the Universal Protocol (TJC, 2015).

The World Health Organization

WHO developed its Surgical Safety Checklist© as a focused, actionable, verbal, and unified strategy for preventing adverse surgical events (WHO, 2009). The Checklist covers 19 items in three stages of the surgical procedure: before anesthesia induction, before surgical incision, and before the patient leaves the OR (WHO, 2009). Many protocols to improve surgical outcomes target events occurring before a patient is brought into the surgical suite and prior to the surgical incision. Policies in the OR aim to counteract missed care have been established, yet the persistence of adverse events in perioperative care indicates the need to further develop practice guidelines. Perioperative nurses are responsible for counting surgical items, positioning the patient with appropriate positioning supports, educating the patient, applying surgical skin antisepsis, making a thorough preoperative patient assessment, and communicating with the patient and family.

A review of the literature confirms these recommended practices should take place prior to the initiation of the procedures and confirms the importance of communication as a validated safety measure to help prevent the occurrence of an adverse event. In addition, the literature also indicates that missed OR care items concur with human factors analyses and safety science concepts of conducting specific steps and building hard stops into a high-risk process to ascertain all items have been completed in a satisfactory fashion. Although not all items are fully supported by science, the endorsements and recommended practices from accreditation and professional organizations have led to the consensus that they should be implemented for all surgical procedures to assure patient safety and optimal outcomes.

Elements of the Preoperative Safety Bundle

As indicated above, the preoperative safety bundle is made up of six actions. Each of these will be further explained below.

Allergy verification

Anaphylactic reactions to agents used in the perioperative period can be lethal. The threat of serious anaphylactic reactions to latex in gloves and various devices used during surgical procedures signals the need for healthcare professionals to question patients about rubber allergies (Tomazic, Withrow, Fisher, & Dillard, 1992). Concordance among healthcare providers about patient allergy information is an important feature of preoperative safety measures (Burda, Hobson, & Pronovost, 2005). Surgical team members have tools available to identify patients at risk for anaphylaxis due to allergies such as latex during surgery (Laxenaire, Mertes, & Groupe d'Etudes des Réactions Anaphylactoïdes, 2001). As Espin, Lingard, Baker, and Regehr reported, those on surgical teams agree that subjecting an allergic patient to an allergy-triggering medication represents a breach of professional practice standards (Espin et al., 2006). A descriptive study of the near-miss experiences of perioperative nurses indicated that inconsistent information about patient allergies was a frequent problem in the OR setting, and that lapses in communication about cross-allergic reactions to latex contributed to near-misses (Cohoon, 2011).

Patient identification

In surgical and invasive procedures, wrong-patient operations persist despite the institution of preoperative verification protocols (Clarke, Johnston, & Finley, 2007). A multidisciplinary and concurrent approach to confirming the patient's identity is required, involving several forms of pre-incision verification. Wherever possible, the patient identification process should actively involve patients and use at least two patient identifiers such as birth date and name (WHO,

2007). The RN circulator has multiple opportunities to prevent the surgical team from operating on the wrong patient. As a member of the patient's surgical team, the RN circulator supports multidisciplinary engagement in implementing collaborative risk reduction strategies to prevent wrong-patient events (AORN, 2011b). Serving as a patient advocate in the preoperative holding area, the surgical suite, and the OR, the RN circulator confirms the patient's identity to ensure that the surgical procedure proceeds with the correct patient on the operating table (Clarke et al., 2007).

Operative consent confirmation

Before a surgical or other invasive procedure, a surgeon is legally and ethically bound to discuss with the patient the risks of the intended procedure and alternative treatment options (American College of Surgeons, 2008). The informed consent discussion "must be presented fairly, clearly, accurately, and compassionately" (ACS, 2008). Education in the form of informed consent allows patients and surgeons to engage in a dialogue that fosters knowledgeable and voluntary decisions about treatment (Brenner, Brenner, & Horowitz, 2009). Nurses, too, have an ethical duty relative to informed consent and patient rights to make autonomous decisions about care (American Nurses Association, 2001). In verifying the correctness and completeness of surgical informed consent, the RN circulator secures a critical link between patient rights and patient safety (Cook, 2014). It is often the perioperative nurse who is the last care provider to check the signed operative consent for completeness and correctness, and to verify that the patient has been duly informed about the surgical procedure (Brazell, 1997).

History and physical confirmation

Perioperative nurses coordinate the surgical team to complete the pre-procedure verification process, which includes confirming the presence and accuracy of the history and physical available in the medical record (AORN, 2012a). A critical component of each patient's perioperative evaluation, the history and physical provide information about preexisting conditions, past surgical history, and physical status that may indicate perioperative risks to which the surgical team should be alerted (Tinkham, 2012). Verifying a patient's history and physical status are critical components of preoperative risk assessment (Smetana, 1999).

Site marking

Alarming rates of wrong-site surgery have prompted professional organizations to initiate protocols for indicating the correct surgical site, level, and side. Inconsistent compliance with site marking protocols contributes to adverse surgical events that occur before incision (TJC Center for Transforming Healthcare, 2013). Surgical site marking should take place for procedures where there is ambiguity about the intended site. Surgical site marking must be completed in procedures including but not limited to those involving laterality (left or right side), multiple body parts (e.g., fingers and toes), or a specified level (e.g., spine surgery). TJC recommends that, when possible, the patient be involved in the process of identifying and marking the surgical site (2013b). Also, the patient should agree on the surgical site before receiving narcotics, sedation, or anesthesia (ACS, 2002).

Time-out or pre-procedure briefing completed

TJC has established guidelines to help accredited hospitals improve communication before surgical procedures in the form of a time-out. During the time-out, information about the patient and procedure is confirmed by the members of the patient's operating team who will be actively participating in the procedure. The time-out occurs before the incision or initiation of the procedure. One surgical team member is designated to lead the time-out, and all other activities will cease throughout duration of the time-out. At the time of this collective briefing, each team member is expected to actively participate and verbally recognize any discrepancies that arise as the items included in the time-out list are reviewed. Among the items reviewed are patient name and identity, procedure name, side, site, allergies, and anticipated equipment and supplies required during the case. When possible, the patient or patient representative is asked to verify his or her name, the intended procedure, and the surgical site (TJC, 2013b). Checklists and briefings designed to enhance surgical safety have demonstrated lower death and complication rates (Lee, 2010; Haynes et al., 2009), improved attitudes about safety (Haynes et al., 2011), and decreased unplanned hospital readmissions (Lepänluoma, Takala, Kotkansalo, Rahi, & Ikonen, 2014).

Case Studies of Missed OR Nursing Care

There are numerous opportunities to miss nursing care prior to the surgical incision. The concept of missed OR nursing care must take into account that every surgical procedure occurs through the coordinated efforts of a surgical team whose membership may change. Therefore, several caregivers may be involved in episodes—such as communication failures or noncompliance with protocols—that lead to missed nursing care in the OR. In this section, we include case studies that exemplify each of the six components of the Preoperative Safety Bundle and attributes of missed nursing care that may occur when these actions are not completed.

Allergies Not Verified

A five-year-old with a latex allergy is scheduled for strabismus surgery. The child's father does not mention the latex allergy during the preoperative assessment because "none of the nurses asked [him] about this." In the OR, the nursing staff are setting up for the case and they put latex items on the sterile field, thereby creating a risk to the patient of intraoperative anaphylaxis caused by latex. Just as the scrub person and RN circulator finish the baseline surgical item count, the anesthesia resident enters the room and announces that she is ready to bring the patient in and that the patient has a latex allergy. The circulator and scrub person scramble to disassemble the sterile field and remove all of the surgical items that have been set out, gather fresh instruments and supplies, and once again prepare the OR, this time with latex-free items. The circulator informs the preoperative holding area and the surgeon that the case will be delayed for about 25 minutes while the room is being set up (Kalisch, McLaughlin, & Dabney, 2012).

Operative Consent Not Confirmed

While verifying preoperative paperwork, the RN circulator overlooks the surgical consent form, not noticing that it is missing from the patient's chart. The circulator informs the anesthesiologist that the patient is ready; the patient is brought into the OR and anesthesia induction commences. When the resident arrives, he mentions that he had the consent form in his pocket, having forgotten to put it on the patient's chart. The circulator notices that the consent form has not been signed. She is aware that the patient may not have received proper informed consent information about the operation, but by this time the patient is anesthetized.

History and Physical Not Confirmed

During the preoperative patient interview, the RN circulator notices that there is no history and physical documentation for the patient. The patient has a family history of adverse anesthetic reactions and is susceptible to malignant hyperthermia, a life-threatening disorder. However, this family history is not acknowledged during the preoperative assessment. Therefore, the potential for malignant hyperthermia is not brought forward within the surgical team, nor do the circulator and anesthesiologist communicate about the provision of non-triggering anesthetics. During anesthesia induction, the patient experiences tachypnea and muscle rigidity, initial signs of malignant hyperthermia crisis, and the surgical procedure has to be canceled (Kalisch, Xie, & Dabney, 2013).

Patient Misidentified

An RN circulator is giving report to the relief nurse during change of shift. The patient for the upcoming procedure, a laparoscopic hysterectomy, has a name similar to that of another patient scheduled for surgery that day. The incoming circulator, unfamiliar with the procedure, has many questions about the equipment to be used during the case. In the midst of relating how to prepare supplies preferred by the surgeon, the outgoing circulator forgets to signal the patient's name alert. The relief circulator goes to the preoperative holding area, reads a patient's name band as "Marguerite Obrian," as opposed to "Margaret O'Brian," and takes the wrong patient into the OR. Only after Ms. Obrian is brought to the recovery room after undergoing the laparoscopic hysterectomy does the surgeon learn that she has operated on the wrong patient.

Wrong Site Marked

A patient is scheduled for anterior cruciate ligament (ACL) reconstruction on the right side. The surgeon puts an "X" on the left knee to indicate that surgery should *not* be done on the left side. When the patient is brought into the OR suite, the scrub nurse says to the patient, "We're going to be working on your left knee, right?" The patient is nervous and responds, "Yes." During the time-out, the scrub nurse announces that the surgical site is the left knee. The circulator does not read the consent, which specifies a right-sided ACL repair. The left leg is prepped and draped prior to the surgery. When the surgeon arrives, she does not notice that it is the patient's left leg that has been draped nor that the chart indicates a right-knee procedure, so surgery proceeds on the wrong leg.

Time-out Completed Incorrectly

A surgical team including an RN circulator, a scrub nurse, an anesthesiologist, and an attending surgeon are assembled in the OR. Before skin incision, the RN circulator is leading the time-out when a surgical resident comes into the OR. The resident begins talking to the attending surgeon, who is scrubbed and gowned. Not wanting to interrupt the attending surgeon, the circulator proceeds with the time-out. The attending surgeon, deep in conversation with the surgical resident, does not speak up when the nursing staff and anesthesiologist verbally confirm that the intended procedure is a thoracotomy and complete the time-out. When the attending surgeon is finished with his conversation, he removes his gown, announcing that he has to check on another patient. He instructs the surgical resident to scrub in, telling him to go ahead and make the skin incision. As he takes the scalpel, the surgical resident asks about the procedure, and the anesthesiologist responds, "This is a thoracotomy." Later, while the surgical resident is putting the dressing on the thoracotomy site, the attending surgeon returns to the OR, asking how the laparotomy went. The resident responds that this patient had a thoracotomy, not a laparotomy. Upon hearing that the patient had a thoracotomy, the attending surgeon tells the surgical team that this patient was scheduled to have a laparotomy and wonders aloud why nobody on the surgical team caught this before the wrong procedure was performed.

In summary, the content described thus far has shown the patient implications of missed OR care and identified a number of common practices that are subject to being missed or skipped when preparing for a procedure. The case studies highlight the miscommunication, misinterpretation, time constraints, and work pressure that may influence surgical staff to miss a critical item. Common practices and protocols from accreditation and professional organizations support the utilization of the Preoperative Safety Bundle items as part of the missed OR nursing care discussion.

Study of Missed OR Care

The next section of this chapter presents a study that highlights the occurrence of the missed OR nursing items described earlier in this chapter. The research question explored the prevalence of missing components of the preoperative safety bundle.

Study Design and Sample

A cross-sectional cohort study was developed to evaluate the adherence to the Preoperative Safety Bundle. The study was conducted using the data available from the POI, a BlueCross BlueShield of Michigan (BCBSM)/BlueCare Network (BCN) funded collaborative quality initiative (CQI) (www.valuepartnerships.com). POI aims to improve the quality of care in the perioperative area for best patient outcomes. A total of 17 Michigan acute care hospitals were included in this initial baseline study. The hospitals have participated in the POI CQI program since 2011. Inclusion criteria require that the hospital has implemented a mature electronic health records (EHR) system and has a data warehouse available that captures perioperative data, staffing information, charges, and other pertinent administrative data. The participating hospitals submit perioperative data to a secure server and data are subsequently prepared for analyses.

Methods and Procedures

The study relies on clinical data pertaining to general surgical cases. The case (patient) level and outcomes data are obtained from the Michigan Surgical Quality Collaborative (MSQC) network, which uses the National Surgical Quality Improvement Program (NSQIP) data collection approach. The MSQC data are collected at the hospital site by a nurse with special training and are entered into a database for analyses. The POI data pertaining to general surgical cases have been merged with MSQC case level data for the purposes of the study.

The POI Data Dictionary©, derived from the AORN Perioperative Standards and Recommended Practices (AORN, 2012b), defines the data elements used for the Preoperative Safety Bundle. It captures key perioperative nursing practices. When initially establishing the database, specifications were communicated with each participating hospital IT staff. For the purpose of this study, a number of patient populations were examined. Performance on the Preoperative Safety Bundle is presented for the following patient populations: (1) all cases included, (2) breast cancer, (3) colon, (4) gallbladder, (5) abdominal hysterectomy, and (6) hip prosthesis surgery.

The requested data for this study were uploaded using a secure file transfer protocol (FTP) for all participating hospitals. An SQL™ server database captured all data elements and the following data validation protocols were used for reporting purposes. The site coordinator at each of the POI hospitals received training as to the identification and selection of the specific data elements, and submitted data were reviewed for completeness, odd values, and other irregularities by the project staff. Hospitals resubmitted their data if there was a problem with completeness and coding issues that hampered the interpretation of performance reports. The specific variables evaluated for this study are those in the Preoperative Safety Bundle described above.

Results
Descriptive analyses were conducted to compare cases in which *yes the safety step was taken* and was selected compared with those cases in which there was a *missing data* element or *no* was chosen. The *no* and *missing data* were combined in the *no* category. Figures 7.1 through 7.6 represent the Preoperative Safety Bundle for six patient groups: all surgical cases, breast procedures, colon surgery, gallbladder, abdominal hysterectomy, and hip prosthesis. The procedures represent varying specialties, laterality, and complexity. For all procedures, except for hip prosthesis (77%), the time-out element of nursing care was completed most often: 83% for gallbladder and 88% for colon and abdominal hysterectomy. The item most often missed was site marking, with the completion percentage ranging from 29% (abdominal hysterectomy) to 73% (breast surgery and hip prosthesis). The procedures that did not involve bilaterality were less likely to be completed; however, the rate for breast cancer and hip prosthesis was not documented for all cases.

Average Preoperative Safety Bundle scores were calculated (not weighted) and provided a range between 64.3% to 73.8% completion, and conversely, a Missed OR Care score of 35.7% to 26.2% missed. Gallbladder procedures showed the greatest number of missing OR care items, especially site marking, which is not specifically recommended in the literature. Breast cancer procedures showed the fewest missed OR care items. For the procedures that did not have a bilateral component, completion of the time-out was least often missed (15.2%) and health and physical completion was missed most often (41.2%).

Although national guidelines recommend that all sites be marked, hospitals may have different policies and accountability practices. For instance, procedures that do not involve bilaterality, such as colon surgery, do not require site marking before the procedure, a common practice across U.S. hospitals. These hospital policies and local practices are reflected in the rates for site marked. The rates reported here reflect both the completion of this Preoperative Safety Bundle item and the documentation that this item was completed. Although the actual completion of these items by clinicians may be higher, failure

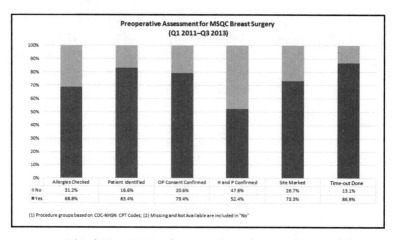

FIGURE 7.1.   **Missed OR care rate of Preoperative Safety Bundle items (All Cases, n = 25482).**

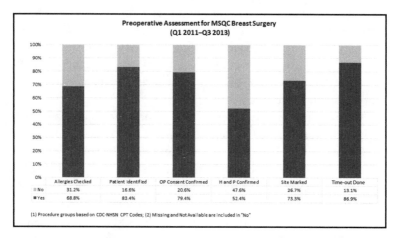

FIGURE 7.2.   **Missed OR care rate of Preoperative Safety Bundle items (Breast Surgery, n = 2510).**

to document the completion of a Bundle item will be interpreted as a missed item.

This study of the extent to which required elements of care are missed in the OR shows that there is considerable variation between the diverse procedures and that there is substantive room for improvement. Results from this study demonstrate that substantive improvements of all items are necessary to ascertain that a patient does not experience the consequences of missed OR care, such as anaphylactic

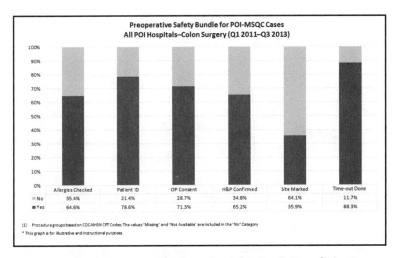

FIGURE 7.3. **Missed OR care rate of Preoperative Safety Bundle items (Colon Surgery, n = 3554).**

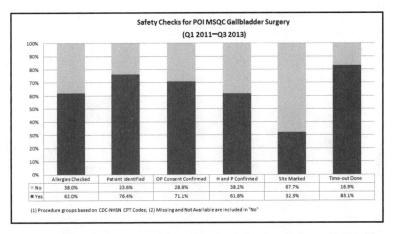

FIGURE 7.4. **Missed OR care rate of Preoperative Safety Bundle items (Gallbladder Surgery, n = 7101).**

shock if allergy information is missed, or the risk of a wrong-site surgery if the site is not clearly marked. Though these measures are not reported on a national basis, it is concerning that, on average, 31% of them were missed in this study despite the inclusion of these items in The Joint Commission's Universal Protocol (TJC, 2005) as required actions (Figures 7.1–7.6).

The item most likely to be missed was site marking, with distinct differences for procedures with bilateral possibilities, such as hernia

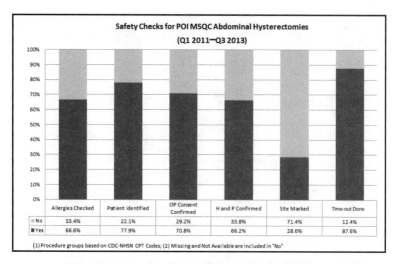

FIGURE 7.5. **Missed OR care rate of Preoperative Safety Bundle items (Abdominal Hysterectomy Surgery, n = 2836).**

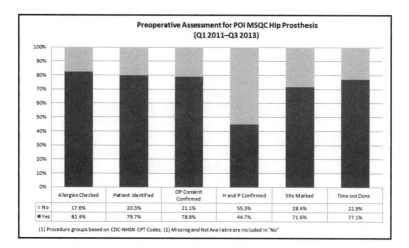

FIGURE 7.6. **Missed OR care rate of Preoperative Safety Bundle items (Hip Prosthesis Surgery, n = 380).**

and breast surgery. Site marking was determined to occur the least for abdominal hysterectomy procedures (28%) and hernias (50%). The highest rate of site marking was found for breast surgeries, where 73% of all cases had proper site marking documented. The average rate of site marking for the total study population was 53%, reflecting a substantial population of cases where the procedure cannot be bilateral (e.g., gallbladder removal) and does not require site marking per current guidelines. The average rate of all six Preoperative Safety Bundle items combined is 69.5%, confirming the prevalence of missed OR care. There is an urgent need to communicate current performance and improve adherence to guidelines to guarantee safe patient care.

Implications
This study provides valuable insights into the actual missed OR elements of care. The results suggest that problem areas targeted by TJC and other organizations have certainly begun to be remedied in the OR. However, it shows that OR performance has room for improvement. As the items included in the Preoperative Safety Bundle are not mandatorily reported, staff members are unaware of performance that is lacking and items that are missed for a surgical patient, which hampers awareness of the urgency to address the missed care items.

The variation in missed items between reported procedures is noted, especially for the site marking items, which can have either a lateral or a bilateral component. However, even with procedures that have a bilateral component (e.g., breast surgery), a gap in the performance of site marking has been shown, leading to the necessity of targeted efforts for sustained improvement. The association between missed OR nursing care and patient outcomes needs to be studied. It is important to determine whether missing elements of nursing care contribute to delays in the OR or to unsafe care circumstances.

Another implication of this study is that the data can provide managers and staff with an understanding of their safety practices. In order to improve performance, the current status needs to be better understood. The presentation of the data empowered the OR directors to speak to staff members about the issue, using the results as a tool to communicate opportunities for improvement.

Future efforts should include the development of a Preoperative Safety Bundle Score that summarizes all required items. A Preoperative Safety Bundle Score would present a concise measure of the status of missed OR care as well as the status of safe patient care delivery. Any safety events that do occur can be evaluated in light of adherence to the Preoperative Safety Bundle. Additional attention should be focused on variation among hospitals, systems, and staffing arrangements to understand the role of local cultures, consistency in staffing, patient characteristics, etc., as these issues may contribute to the presence or absence of OR elements of care. For example, studies have shown that noncompliance with implementing structured pre-procedure briefings is related to surgical team culture and attitudes about implementing checklists (Saturno, Soria-Aledo, Gama, Lorca-Parra, & Grau-Polan, 2014), which leads to lapses in covering all checklist items (Ockerman & Pritchett, 2000), checklist fatigue, and ultimately, the need for behavioral change on the part of many individuals within a group (Vijayasekar & Steele, 2009).

The results from this preliminary study suggest that despite the implementation of the safety measures as part of the Universal Protocol, many items are missed and require substantial improvement-related activities. The widespread adoption of the EHR and accompanying data warehouses will provide OR leadership and staff with transparency about the actual implementation and documentation of commonly accepted safety practices. Information about actual adherence to the Preoperative Safety Bundle provides a powerful message for OR directors in their efforts to provide a safe patient care environment. The missed OR care concept provides a valuable perspective in the continuing effort to maintain a safe OR and ascertain adherence to widely adopted preoperative safety practices.

Summary

In this chapter, we described the care that OR nurses provide to patients and the safety implications of not completing that care. Using the Preoperative Safety Bundle made up of six required actions (allergies checked, patient identified, operative consent, health and physical completed, site marked, and time-out performed), we studied a number of surgical patient populations and found a considerable amount of missed care. Case studies were presented to illustrate the problems that can occur when these actions are not completed. Our goal is to further develop and evaluate the utility of the Preoperative Safety Bundle to reduce the amount of missed OR nursing care.

References

American College of Surgeons. (2002). [ST-41] Statement on ensuring correct patient, correct site and correct procedure surgery. Retrieved from http://www.facs.org/fellows_info/statements/st-41.html

American College of Surgeons. (2008). *Statements on principles.* Retrieved from http://www.facs.org/fellows_info/statements/stonprin.html#anchor171960

American Nurses Association. (2001). *Code of ethics for nurses with interpretive statements.* Retrieved from http://www.nursingworld.org/MainMenuCategories/EthicsStandards/CodeofEthicsforNurses/Code-of-Ethics-For-Nurses.html

Association of periOperative Registered Nurses. (2010). *Comprehensive surgical checklist.* Retrieved from http://www.aorn.org/Clinical_Practice/ToolKits/Correct_Site_Surgery_Tool_Kit/Comprehensive_checklist.aspx

Association of periOperative Registered Nurses. (2011a). *Perioperative nursing data set—The perioperative nursing vocabulary* (3rd ed.). Denver, CO: AORN.

Association of periOperative Registered Nurses. (2011b). *AORN position statement on allied health care providers and support personnel in the perioperative practice setting.* Retrieved from http://www.aorn.org/Clinical_Practice/Position_Statements/Position_Statements.aspx

Association of periOperative Registered Nurses. (2012a). Correct site surgery tool kit—comprehensive surgical checklist. Retrieved from https://www.aorn.org/Secondary.aspx?id=21152&LangType=1033

Association of periOperative Registered Nurses. (2012b). *Perioperative standards and recommended practices.* Denver, CO: AORN.

Association of periOperative Registered Nurses. (2014a). *AORN position statement on one perioperative registered nurse circulator dedicated to every patient undergoing an operative or other invasive procedure.* Retrieved from http://www.aorn.org/Clinical_Practice/Position_Statements/Position_Statements.aspx

Association of periOperative Registered Nurses. (2014b). *AORN position statement on perioperative safe staffing and on-call practices.* Retrieved from http://www.aorn.org/Clinical_Practice/Position_Statements/Position_Statements.aspx

Association of Surgical Technologists. (2014). Standards of practice. Job description: Surgical technologist. Retrieved from http://www.ast.org/uploadedFiles/Main_Site/Content/About_Us/Job%20Descriptions.pdf/

Auerbach, D. I., Staiger, D. O., Muench, U., & Buerhaus, P. I. (2013). The nursing workforce in an era of health care reform. *New England Journal of Medicine, 368*(16), 1470–1472.

Brazell, N. E. (1997). The significance and application of informed consent. *AORN Journal, 65*(2), 377–386.

Brenner, L. H., Brenner, A. T., & Horowitz, D. (2009). Beyond informed consent. Educating the patient. *Clinical Orthopaedics and Related Research, 467,* 348–351.

Burda, S. A., Hobson, D., & Pronovost, P. J. (2005). What is the patient really taking? Discrepancies between surgery and anesthesiology preoperative medication histories. *Quality and Safety in Health Care, 14*(6), 414–416.

Centers for Disease Control and Prevention. (2012). *National hospital discharge survey. Number, rate, and standard error of all-listed surgical and nonsurgical procedures for discharges from short-stay hospitals, by selected procedure categories: United States, 2010.* Retrieved from http://www.cdc.gov/nchs/data/nhds/4procedures/2010pro4_numberrate.pdf

Clarke, J. R., Johnston, J., & Finley, E. D. (2007). Getting surgery right. *Annals of Surgery, 246*(3), 395.

Cohoon, B. (2011). Causes of near misses: Perceptions of perioperative nurses. *AORN Journal, 93*(5), 551–565.

Cook, W. E. (2014). "Sign here": Nursing value and the process of informed consent. *Plastic Surgical Nursing, 34*(1), 29–33.

Espin, S., Lingard, L., Baker, G. R., & Regehr, G. (2006). Persistence of unsafe practice in everyday work: An exploration of organizational and psychological factors constraining safety in the operating room. *Quality and Safety in Health Care, 15*(3), 165–170.

Etzioni, D. A., Liu, J. H., Maggard, M. A., & Ko, C. Y. (2003). The aging population and its impact on the surgery workforce. *Annals of Surgery, 238*(2), 170–177.

Gawande, A. A., Zinner, M. J., Studdert, D. M., & Brennan, T. A. (2003). Analysis of errors reported by surgeons at three teaching hospitals. *Surgery, 133*(6), 614–621.

Gillespie, B. M., Wallis, M., & Chaboyer, W. (2008). Operating theater culture implications for nurse retention. *Western Journal of Nursing Research, 30*(2), 259–277.

Goodman, T., & Spry, C. (2014). *Essentials of perioperative nursing* (5th ed.). Burlington, MA: Jones & Bartlett Learning.

Greenberg, C. C., Regenbogen, S. E., Studdert, D. M., Lipsitz, S. R., Rogers, S. O., Zinner, M. J., & Gawande, A. A. (2007). Patterns of communication breakdowns resulting in injury to surgical patients. *Journal of the American College of Surgeons, 204*(4), 533–540.

Haynes, A. B., Weiser, T. G., Berry, W. R., Lipsitz, S. R., Breizat, A. H., Dellinger, E. P., ... Gawande, A. A. (2009). A surgical safety checklist to reduce morbidity and mortality in a global population. *New England Journal of Medicine, 360*(5), 491–499.

Haynes, A. B., Weiser, T. G., Berry, W. R., Lipsitz, S. R., Breizat, A. H., Dellinger, E. P., ... Gawande, A. A. (2011). Changes in safety attitude and relationship to decreased postoperative morbidity and mortality following implementation of a checklist-based surgical safety intervention. *BMJ Quality & Safety, 20*(1), 102–107.

Institute of Medicine. (2000). *To err is human: Building a safer health system.* Washington, DC: The National Academies Press.

Jim, J., Owens, P. L., Sanchez, L. A., & Rubin, B. G. (2012). Population-based analysis of inpatient vascular procedures and predicting future workload and implications for training. *Journal of Vascular Surgery, 55*(5), 1394–1400.

The Joint Commission. (2001). Sentinel event alert—A follow-up review of wrong site surgery. Retrieved from http://www.jointcommission.org/sentinel_event_alert_issue_24_a_follow-up_review_of_wrong_site_surgery/

The Joint Commission. (2013a). Sentinel event alert: Preventing unintended retained foreign objects. Retrieved from http://www.jointcommission.org/assets/1/6/SEA_51_URFOs_10_17_13_FINAL.pdf

The Joint Commission. (2013b). National patient safety goals effective January 1, 2014: Hospital accreditation program. *Joint Commission Perspectives, 33*(7). Retrieved from http://www.jointcommission.org/assets/1/18/jcp0713_announce_new_nspg.pdf

The Joint Commission. (2014a). *Sentinel event data: General information (1995–2013).* Retrieved from http://www.jointcommission.org/assets/1/18/General_Information_1995-2Q2013.pdf

The Joint Commission. (2014b). *Sentinel event data: Root causes by event type (2004-2014)*. Retrieved from http://www.jointcommission.org/Sentinel_Event_Statistics/

The Joint Commission. (2015). The universal protocol for preventing wrong site, wrong procedure, and wrong person surgery. Retrieved from http://www.jointcommission.org/assets/1/18/UP_Poster1.PDF

The Joint Commission Center for Transforming Healthcare. (2013). Facts about the wrong site surgery project [Fact sheet]. Retrieved from http://www.centerfortransforminghealthcare.org/news/press/wss.aspx

Kalisch, B. J. (2006). Missed nursing care: A qualitative study. *Journal of Nursing Care Quality, 21*(4), 306-313.

Kalisch, B. J., Landstrom, G., & Williams, R. A. (2009). Missed nursing care: Errors of omission. *Nursing Outlook, 57*(1), 3-9.

Kalisch, B. J., McLaughlin, M., & Dabney, B. W. (2012). Patient perceptions of missed nursing care. *The Joint Commission Journal on Quality & Patient Safety, 38*(4), 161-167.

Kalisch, B. J., Xie, B., & Dabney, B. W. (2013). Patient-reported missed nursing care correlated with adverse events. *American Journal of Medical Quality*. Advance online publication. doi:10.1177/1062860613501715

Laxenaire, M. C., Mertes, P. M., & Groupe d'Etudes des Réactions Anaphylactoïdes (GDE) (2001). Anaphylaxis during anaesthesia. Results of a two-year survey in France. *British Journal of Anaesthesia, 87*(4), 549-558.

Lee, P. H., & Gawande, A. A. (2008). The number of surgical procedures in an American lifetime in 3 states. *Journal of the American College of Surgeons, 207*(3), S75.

Lee, S. L. (2010). The extended surgical time-out: Does it improve quality and prevent wrong-site surgery? *The Permanente Journal, 14*(1), 19-23.

Lepänluoma, M., Takala, R., Kotkansalo, A., Rahi, M., & Ikonen, T. S. (2014). Surgical safety checklist is associated with improved operating room safety culture, reduced wound complications and unplanned readmissions in a pilot study in neurosurgery. *Scandinavian Journal of Surgery, 103*(1), 66-72.

Lingard, L., Espin, S., Whyte, S., Regehr, G., Baker, G. R., Reznick, R., ... Grober, E. (2004). Communication failures in the operating room: An observational classification of recurrent types and effects. *Quality and Safety in Health Care, 13*(5), 330-334.

Mehtsun, W. T., Ibrahim, A. M., Diener-West, M., Pronovost, P. J., & Makary, M. A. (2013). Surgical never events in the United States. *Surgery, 153*(4), 465-472.

Michaels, R. K., Makary, M. A., Dahab, Y., Frassica, F. J., Heitmiller, E., Rowen, L. C., ... Pronovost, P. J. (2007). Achieving the National Quality Forum's "never events": Prevention of wrong site, wrong procedure, and wrong patient operations. *Annals of Surgery, 245*(4), 526.

Mitchell, L., Flin, R., Yule, S., Mitchell, J., Coutts, K., & Youngson, G. (2011). Thinking ahead of the surgeon. An interview study to identify scrub nurses' non-technical skills. *International Journal of Nursing Studies, 48*(7), 818-828.

Munnich, E. L., & Parente, S. T. (2014). Procedures take less time at ambulatory surgery centers, keeping costs down and ability to meet demand up. *Health Affairs, 33*(5), 764–769.

Ockerman, J., & Pritchett, A. (2000). A review and reappraisal of task guidance: Aiding workers in procedure following. *International Journal of Cognitive Ergonomics, 4*(3), 191–212.

Petersen, C. (Ed.). (2011). *Perioperative nursing data set: The perioperative nursing vocabulary.* (3rd ed.). Denver, CO: AORN.

Riley, R., & Manias, E. (2002). Foucault could have been an operating room nurse. *Journal of Advanced Nursing, 39*(4), 316–324.

Rosenstein, A. H., & O'Daniel, M. (2008). A survey of the impact of disruptive behaviors and communication defects on patient safety. *The Joint Commission Journal on Quality and Patient Safety, 34*(8), 464–471.

Saturno, P. J., Soria-Aledo, V., Gama, Z. A. D. S., Lorca-Parra, F., & Grau-Polan, M. (2014). Understanding WHO surgical checklist implementation: Tricks and pitfalls. An observational study. *World Journal of Surgery, 38*(2), 287–295.

Sexton, J. B., Thomas, E. J., & Helmreich, R. L. (2000). Error, stress, and teamwork in medicine and aviation: Cross sectional surveys. *BMJ, 320*(7237), 745–749.

Sheldon, G. F. (2010). Access to care and the surgeon shortage: American Surgical Association forum. *Annals of Surgery, 252*(4), 582–590.

Smetana, G. W. (1999). Preoperative pulmonary evaluation. *New England Journal of Medicine, 340*(12), 937–944.

Talsma, A. N., McLaughlin, M., Bathish, M., Sirichorachai, R., & Kuttner, R. (2014). The quality, implementation, and evaluation model: A clinical practice model for sustainable interventions. *Western Journal of Nursing Research, 36*(7), 929–946.

Tinkham, M. R. (2012). The importance of the preoperative history and physical. *OR Nurse, 6*(3), 40–46.

Tomazic, V. J., Withrow, T. J., Fisher, B. R., & Dillard, S. F. (1992). Latex-associated allergies and anaphylactic reactions. *Clinical Immunology and Immunopathology, 64*(2), 89–97.

Vijayasekar, C., & Steele, R. J. C. (2009). The World Health Organization's surgical safety checklist. *The Surgeon, 7*(5), 260–262.

Weissman, J. S., Rothschild, J. M., Bendavid, E., Sprivulis, P., Cook, E. F., Evans, R. S., & Bates, D. W. (2007). Hospital workload and adverse events. *Medical Care, 45*(5), 448–455.

World Health Organization. (2007). Patient identification. *Patient Safety Solutions, 1*, solution 2. Retrieved from http://www.who.int/patientsafety/solutions/patientsafety/PS-Solution2.pdf?ua=1

World Health Organization. (2009). Surgical safety checklist. Retrieved from http://whqlibdoc.who.int/publications/2009/9789241598590_eng_Checklist.pdf?ua=1

Patient Reports of Missed Nursing Care

While the previous chapters contain reports of missed nursing care from nursing staff, this chapter focuses on missed nursing care as described by patients and families. Patients and their families have a unique perspective about their care; this information is needed by nursing staff and others to improve care for patients. As stated earlier, missed nursing care is a different concept than patient satisfaction. Patient satisfaction survey tools focus on how happy or satisfied the patients and families were with their hospital experience. The goal of measuring patients' reports of missed nursing care is to create a measure of actual nursing care provided (or not).

Qualitative Study: What Can Patients Report?

Since it was not clear what patients could report on with accuracy, we conducted a qualitative study to find out (Kalisch, McLaughlin, & Dabney, 2012). On the one hand, we concluded that there are certain aspects of nursing care that patients and families would have difficulty reporting on. For example, when a nurse enters the room and talks with the patient, he or she may not be aware of the evaluation (surveillance) the nurse is engaged in. On the other hand, patients (and/or family members who spend time with the patient during hospitalization) are readily able to report on aspects of missed nursing care such as bathing and feeding.

This qualitative study involved in-depth, semi-structured face-to-face interviews with 38 patients on medical–surgical inpatient units, older than 18 years of age, hospitalized for at least three days, English-speaking, and capable of engaging in an interview. Interviewees (patients) ranged in age from 29 to 89 years of age. Trained nurse interviewers completed the interviews in pairs, one conducting the interviews and the other recording the responses. The interview questions were open-ended and interactive.

Interviews were conducted until saturation was reached. Saturation ensures that enough data has been collected to sufficiently develop themes (Heidegger, 1962). This method involves theoretical sampling, a process whereby once themes become clear, subsequent areas are explored in additional interviews until no new information is forthcoming (Corbin & Strauss, 2008).

Once completed, the interview data were categorized into key themes. The research team members analyzed the data independently and then compared their results. When discrepancies were identified in the interpretation of the data, analyzers engaged in discussion until they could all support the categories and themes emerging from the data.

Three categories of missed nursing care were identified: (1) fully reportable or areas of nursing care that patients and families are able to report on; (2) partially reportable or elements of nursing care that patients are partly able to report on (e.g., they can state that they received medications but not always if they were the correct medications or at the appropriate time); and (3) not reportable, which refers to areas of nursing care that patients were unable to report on. In addition, a secondary objective of the study was to determine what particular aspects of nursing care the patients had experienced. These results are reported below with the quantitative data.

Fully Reportable

Every patient interviewed in the study was able to describe whether he or she received mouth care (or assistance with oral hygiene) and if they had the materials they needed to do it themselves. They were also able to convey whether the nursing staff checked to see if they were completing their own mouth care, if able. Patients could report on whether they were bathed or bathed themselves. Another element of nursing care that patients were able to report on was whether they received adequate and timely pain medication, with reassessment to determine if pain was relieved. Patients were readily able to report whether their call lights and beeping monitors were answered and the length of time it took to do so. They were able to state if they received their meals and whether they received the necessary assistance they needed. Patients could report if nursing staff listened to their concerns and questions, and whether or not they were focusing solely on tasks or on their individual needs. Patients were able to articulate whether the nursing staff kept them informed about their daily routine and goals for the day or shift, and what to expect during their hospital stay.

Partially Reportable
Hand washing was identifiable by patients if there was a sink or a sanitizer dispenser visible in the room (or if they asked the provider). If they could not see a sink or dispenser, they could not determine whether hand washing had taken place. However, a few patients said they assumed the nursing staff had washed their hands if they were rubbing them together when they approached them. Patients were able to report whether their vital signs were taken. Although some patients were also able to identify the timing of the vital signs, the majority of the patients were not able to assess whether the vital signs were completed according to an appropriate prescribed time frame. Repositioning was another task that patients could partially report on. Patients knew when they had been repositioned, but they were not able to accurately report if they were repositioned as often as ordered or per nursing standards.

Ambulation was also found to be partially identifiable by patients. They had no difficulty stating whether nursing staff ensured they got out of bed and walked or sat in a chair. Again, unless they were specifically informed as to how many times a day they were to be ambulated, they were not able to evaluate whether the standard care was provided. Patients who were able to ambulate on their own were also able to report on whether the staff checked to be sure they had done so—but were not generally aware that they needed to get out of bed at least three times a day or as ordered. Education was another area that patients were able to partially evaluate. Since they were often unaware of the needed depth and appropriateness required, they could not fully report on this nursing intervention.

Discharge planning is difficult for patients to identify because they do not always know what is meant by the term and/or its varying definitions. Most of the patients in this study voiced the opinion that discharge planning is a responsibility, not of nurses, but rather of other members of the healthcare team, such as physical therapists, occupational therapists, or hospital discharge planners. Patients viewed the nurse's role as confined to a review of the discharge summary and paperwork with them at discharge. Patients were also confused between discharge planning and patient education.

Although a few patients expressed some knowledge of intravenous (IV) care, those interviewed stated they were unable to determine if the correct solution and flow rate were in place and if the IV tubing had been changed at appropriate times. They said they were able to report on how often a nurse monitored the IV site area (unless they were sleeping) and if there was redness, swelling, pain, or elevated skin temperature. They understood what infiltration meant in lay terms. They were not aware that extravasation could be a serious complication. A few of the interviewees were able to determine when the nurse flushed (cleared) the line. They seemed more aware of the lack of attention to the IV when it was not in use.

The final element of nursing care that patients could partially provide information was medication administration. With the exception of pain medications, it was difficult for patients to evaluate accurately whether they received their medications at the appropriate times. Patients could give details as to whether they received medications in general but could not always evaluate if the timing and the particular medications were correct. On the other hand, they were very aware of medications that they administered to themselves at home and compared what was given to them in the hospital with their personal experience at home. Sometimes a generic medication was used, for example, which changed the appearance of the drug, and they reported asking the nurses about this discrepancy.

Not Reportable
Patients were unable to determine if they were adequately assessed and monitored by nursing staff or whether the staff had developed a plan of care. Patients did not have the clinical knowledge to know what is involved in a complete nursing assessment nor did they possess the skill to know how much surveillance is needed for their condition. They could report if a daily goal was listed on their white board but if there was no goal(s), they were not able to state that it was missing (because they did not know it was supposed to be there). In terms of skin assessment, patients could not verify, except in a few cases, whether or not the nursing staff were checking for skin reddening or

breakdown. Patients and families were able to evaluate nursing staff surveillance by reporting on how often nursing staff were in their room and what they did while there. However, with so many different providers and others coming and going, they voiced concern that they were not always sure who were their assigned nursing staff. Therefore, they were unable to comment as to how often the nurses came into their room or how often they should have come in their room. In hospitals with a standard of practice of hourly rounds, the patients would perhaps be better able to give an account of the times nursing staff were in their room.

MISSCARE Survey—Patient

The qualitative study gave us an idea about what nursing care was missed with a small group of patients but a survey tool was needed to measure it widely. Thus we developed a survey tool entitled *MISSCARE Survey—Patient*. Patients were asked to identify whether or not nursing care was provided during their current hospitalization. The *MISSCARE Survey—Patient* contains three sections: (1) demographic character-istics and health status (including patient age, sex, race, education, marital status, hospitalized days, health status, diagnosis, and disease history), (2) elements of nursing care, and (3) adverse events. The section of elements of nursing care contains 13 items and uses 5-point Likert-type scales for measurement of communication and basic care (1 = never, 2 = rarely, 3 = sometimes, 4 = usually, and 5 = always) and for measurement of timeliness (1 = <5 minutes, 2 = 5–10 minutes, 3 = 11–20 minutes, 4 = 21–30 minutes, and 5 = >30 minutes). The mean of all 13 items was used as a total score for the scale, and the potential range of scores was 1 to 5.

All the items were reverse coded so that higher scores indicated more missed nursing care. In the adverse events section, participants were asked the question "Did you experience any of the following problems during this hospitalization?" Problems included falls, skin breakdown/pressure ulcers, medication errors, infections, and intra-venous running dry or leaking into the skin of the patient. A general category called "other problems" was included, in which patients could write in additional items.

Reliability and validity studies of *MISSCARE Survey—Patient* were conducted. Nurses who worked on medical–surgical units (n = 23) and patients (n = 47) hospitalized on these types of units participated as members of expert panels to identify the survey questions as well as evaluate each question for clarity and relevance. As indicated above, a qualitative study of patients' ability to report on items of nursing care that were completed or not was conducted and the results of that study informed the selection of items for the survey. Once a draft was completed, the expert panels reviewed the *MISSCARE Survey— Patient* for clarity and relevance. The content validity index (CVI) for nursing staff was .89, and the CVI for patients was .88. These scores indicate a high level of clarity and relevance.

Convergent validity was examined by comparing the results of the *MISSCARE Survey—Patient* to a question regarding satisfaction with nursing care that was imbedded in the survey. It was found that higher ratings of global satisfaction with nursing care correlated with fewer instances of missed nursing care ($r = .25$, $p < .001$). Exploratory factor analysis was performed to evaluate construct validity. A three-factor solution emerged: (1) communication (five items), (2) time to respond (four items), and (3) basic care (four items). The factor loadings ranged from .605 to .869. These three factors explained 59.2% of the variance in patient perceptions of missed nursing care. The confirmatory factor analysis resulted in a good model fit (comparative fit index = .969 and root mean square error of approximation = .058).

Test–retest reliability was examined by administering the *MISSCARE Survey—Pateint* to a randomly selected group of 30 patients who had completed the survey while hospitalized and then again two weeks after discharge. The intra-rater test–retest reliability for the *MISSCARE Survey—Patient* coefficient was .818. Internal consistency measured by Cronbach α coefficient was .838, and the subscale alphas ranged from .708 to .834. In this study, the Cronbach α was .86, and *alpha* for communication, time to response, and basic care was .784, .803, and .771, respectively.

Qualitative Study: What Care is Missed?

After acquiring Institutional Review Board approval at the study institutions, the survey was completed by patients who met the inclusion criteria of being (1) hospitalized for at least three days, (2) on medical–surgical units in acute care hospitals, (3) 18 years or older, and (4) proficient in the English language. A family member who had spent at least 5 hours a day with the patient in the hospital could assist or complete the survey if the patient was unable to do so.

On any given shift, research assistants (RAs) went to the patient units and asked the charge nurse to assist them in determining which patients met the eligibility criteria. The RAs then approached eligible patients (and/or family members), asking them if they would be willing to participate in the study. If they were, they obtained written consent and then administered the survey.

Study Design and Sample

In this cross-sectional descriptive study, a total of 729 patients in two hospitals (estimated 900 beds and 1,000 beds) participated in the survey. Most (90%) patients had been hospitalized before. The average length of stay for the current hospitalization was 7.86 ± 8.83 days. The average patient age was 60 years. The majority of patients completed the survey by themselves (n = 639, 88.9%), while 11.1% of patients had a family member help them. The gender was almost equally distributed between males (51%) and females (49%), 80% were white, 14% were African American, and the remaining 6% were Hispanic or Asian. Over 60% had some amount of college education, and 50% were married. They were asked to describe their general health and the majority chose good (32%) or fair (33%) while 14% chose very good and 3% selected excellent. The remaining 18% said their health was poor. Previous illnesses were reported as follows: 58% hypertension, 34% heart disease, 33% cancer, 30% diabetes, 20% lung disease, 16% psychiatric problems, 13% rheumatoid arthritis, 9% stroke, and 4% substance abuse. According to the Centers for Disease Control and Prevention, these are among the most frequently found chronic diseases of residents living within the study region (Centers for Disease Control and Prevention, 2013). The study sample demonstrated characteristics typical of the populations generally served by the participating hospitals in terms of age, gender, and race.

Extent and Type of Missed Nursing Care

The patient reports of missed nursing care overall was 1.82 ± 0.62 (on a five-point scale) (Figure 8.1). Patients reported more missed nursing care in the subscale of basic care (2.29 ± 1.06), followed by communication (1.69 ± 0.71) and time to respond (1.52 ± 0.64). Figure 8.2 contains the percentages of the specific elements of nursing care that were missed. The five most frequently reported specific elements of missed care were:

1. Mouth care (50.3%)
2. Ambulation (41.3%)
3. Getting out of bed into a chair (38.8%)
4. Providing information about tests/procedures (27%)
5. Bathing (26.4%)

Basic care

These results show us that what we defined as basic care is being omitted the most often (Figure 8.1). In this study, this includes: (1) mouth care (50.3%); (2) ambulation (41.3%); (3) getting out of bed into a chair (38.8%); and (4) bathing (27%). We realize this is not a universal definition but the study data clustered these nursing actions together and we named the subscale "basic care." Pipe and colleagues (2012, p. 225) write that "As the work of nursing becomes increasingly more complex and significantly more technical in nature, nurses are beginning to find that the basic nursing interventions that were once the hallmark of good nursing care are being left behind." Other nurses and nurse leaders have also highlighted this as a problem and have noted that research in this area needs to be placed higher on the agenda (Adamsen & Tewes, 2000; Englebright, Aldrich, & Taylor, 2014; Williams, 1998).

Mouth care

In regards to mouth care, patients in the qualitative study described above uniformly reported not receiving adequate assistance. Most patients stated that nursing staff did provide the materials (toothbrush,

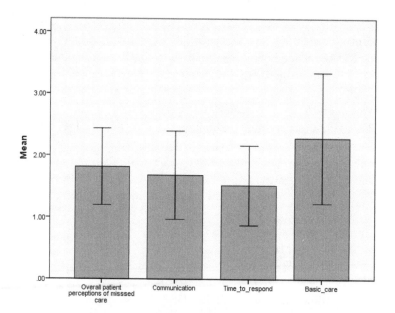

FIGURE 8.1. **Mean scores: Patient reports of missed nursing care (n = 729).**
Note: The solid bars represent the means of patient reports of missed care and the range lines represent the standard deviations.

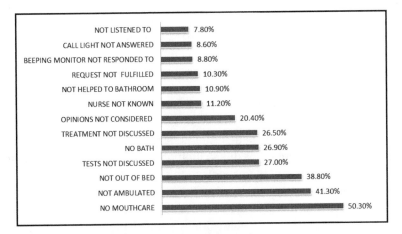

FIGURE 8.2. **Missed elements of nursing care (n = 729).**

toothpaste) for mouth care on admission to the unit. However, for most patients, that was the end of the nursing staff involvement with their mouth care. For a few patients, there was not even an offer of supplies. One patient reported that although she received the materials needed to brush her teeth, she did not receive assistance into the bathroom so that she could use them. Patients stated that the nurse would assist them if they asked but that nursing staff was not proactive about it. The interviewees indicated that mouth care was very important to them (more than we anticipated). In studies of nursing staff, they indicate that they feel they do not need to monitor mouth care since they are adults and should know to brush their teeth. The patients indicated that they value mouth care and viewed this as "missed care" when they did not receive it. Reports of more assistance with mouth care were found in the ICU. Rehabilitation patients indicated that occupational therapy assisted them with mouth care.

Ambulation and getting out of bed

The second highest element of missed nursing care was ambulation, followed closely by receiving assistance to get out of bed and into a chair. When patients stated that they walked on their own, they were asked if the nursing staff made sure they ambulated, and the answer was uniformly "no." Patients who did need help responded that they were not ambulated three times a day. Common themes were that patients were simply not asked or helped to ambulate and that the patients perceived that the nurses did not have enough time to help them ambulate. In other studies, nurses report patient resistance or refusal to get out of bed and walk. The nursing staff notes that it takes two or more staff members to assist most patients in this activity, which is often difficult to arrange.

Bathing

It is interesting that not taking a bath or being bathed came out as the sixth highest element of missed nursing care for patients. In the qualitative study of 38 patients, bathing was reported to be omitted in two patients, but it was due to their physical condition that did not permit it. The rest of the patients in this qualitative study stated that the nursing staff and their aides did ask each day if they needed to be bathed. However, confusion about the definition of bathing was uncovered in these interviews. Many patients did not consider that they had a bath if they did not have a shower or tub bath. The bath in a bag, or bathing kit, did not qualify as a real bath in the minds of many of the interviewees.

Communication

The second most frequently missed area of nursing care was the subscale of communication (after basic care) (Figure 8.1). Providing information to patients about tests and other procedures was missed 27% of the time, followed by discussing the treatment plan with patients (26.5% missed), considering the opinions of patients (20.4% missed), the patient knowing who their assigned nurse was (11.2% missed), and listening to the patient (7.8% missed). This is particularly troublesome in light of a recent editorial in *Health and Hospital Networks* that pointed out that patients are looking for human connection during their time of crisis. This serves to highlight studies that found that patients often depend more on healthcare providers for emotional support than their families (Bush, 2012).

Receiving information and discussing the treatment plan

The next most frequent element of missed nursing care was keeping patients informed about their care. Patients felt they were not kept informed about their care or treatment and that the nursing staff often failed to alleviate their concerns about events that occurred while they were in the hospital. For example, one very bothersome issue was the failure to check back with patients to update them on the expected time of tests or discharge. In some instances, patients were left to wait for hours with no update from the nursing staff about how much longer they could expect to wait. Nurses explained this phenomenon, pointing out that they were not kept updated by the other departments as to when the test or procedures would take place.

In some instances, patients wanted to learn more about their care but found that their requests were not recognized. Several patients felt that orientation to the unit and to the hospital environment was scant. In a new setting such as a hospital room, they report the need to receive more information about daily activities and the way things work on the unit. In those instances, patients noted that nurses did not communicate effectively with them about what to expect in the hospital.

Opinions not considered

Of all the patients included in this study, 20% did not feel that their opinions were considered. To a lesser extent but still impacting 8% of the study sample was the belief that they were not being listened to. Patients noted that the nurses often did not have sufficient time to make an emotional connection with them. Patients commented that the nursing staff seemed to be focused more on completing tasks related to their physical illness than on seeing them as individuals with emotional and social needs, as well.

Not knowing their nurse

One in five patients reported not knowing who their specific nursing staff members were. They noted that many different people came in and out of their room and they were all dressed similarly. They reported having difficulty reading the name tags that might tell them who was a nurse, nursing assistant, physician, housekeeper, etc. A number of the patients said that when the names were written on the white board, they could keep track of their caregivers, but that it was often not kept up to date.

Timely response

The third subscale of missed nursing care was timeliness in response (Figure 8.1). Well-timed help to the bathroom was missed 10.9% of the time, followed by fulfilling call-light requests (10.3% missed), and answering beeping monitors (8.8% missed) and call lights (8.6% missed). The importance of timely response for the avoidance of patient harm is readily apparent.

**Demographic Characteristics, Health Status,
and Hospital Differences**

A series of bivariate regression analyses were completed to find significant variations in overall patient reports of missed nursing care by using patient demographic characteristics and health status. Three variables were found to be significantly associated with missed nursing care: education, general health status, and history of a psychiatric diagnosis. Compared with patients whose education was high school or less, patients with some amount of college or earned degrees reported more missed care ($\beta = 0.10$, $p = 0.032$). Patients who had a poorer health status reported more missed care ($\beta = -0.08$, $p < 0.0001$). Patients who had ever been diagnosed or treated for a psychiatric problem also reported more missed care ($\beta = -0.19$, $p = 0.002$). Other demographic characteristics and health status variables were not significantly associated with patient reports of missed nursing care (e.g., race, marital status, gender, etc.).

There were no significant differences in overall missed care as perceived by patients, as well as missed communication between the two study hospitals. However, there was a significant difference in perceived response time between Hospital 1 and Hospital 2. Patients in Hospital 2 identified more delays in response time than patients in Hospital 1 ($p = 0.0006$) (Table 8.3). Patients in Hospital 2 reported significantly more missed timely assistance to the bathroom ($\chi^2 = 5.93$, $p = 0.015$). In addition, Hospital 1 reported more instances of missed basic care, which approached but did not quite reach significance ($p = 0.054$). Significant differences were found between Hospital 1 and Hospital 2 in reports of missed ambulation, getting patients out of bed and into a chair, and bathing. Patients in Hospital 2 reported more missed bathing ($\chi^2 = 7.09$, $p = 0.008$), and patients in Hospital 1 reported more missed mobilization, such as getting out of bed ($\chi^2 = 41.88$, $p < .0001$) and walking ($\chi^2 = 26.62$, $p < 0.0001$).

Adverse Events and Missed Nursing Care

The most frequently reported adverse event occurrences were IV running dry (12%) and infiltrating (15%). Hospital 1 had more IV-related problems than Hospital 2 ($p < .001$). Other reported adverse events were skin breakdown (6.3%), new infection, (6.1%), falls (2.3%), and medication errors (2.2%). Table 8.1 contains information regarding the occurrence of adverse events identified by patient reports of missed nursing care and the correlation with missed nursing care as reported by patients. The results indicate that patients who experienced skin

TABLE 8.1. Relationship between patient-reported adverse events and patient reports of missed nursing care (n = 729).

	Fall		Skin breakdown/ pressure ulcer		Medication administration error		New infection		IV running dry		IV leaking	
	yes	no	yes	no	yes	no	yes	no	yes	no	yes	no
Overall Missed Care	1.9	1.8	2.05*	1.79	2.19*	1.79	2.29*	1.77	2.13*	1.73	2.05*	1.75
Communication	1.92	1.66	1.96*	1.64	1.84	1.65	2.20*	1.62	1.95*	1.6	1.91*	1.61
Time to Respond	1.61	1.5	1.80*	1.48	1.99	1.48	1.93*	1.48	1.69*	1.47	1.68*	1.46
Basic Care	2.23	2.29	2.46	2.27	2.84*	2.27	2.81*	2.25	2.83*	2.16	2.67*	2.19

TABLE 8.2.   **Nursing staff sample characteristics (n = 1495).**

Variable	Label	n	%
Education	LPN Diploma	7	0.5
	RN Diploma	67	4.5
	Associate degree in nursing	437	29.2
	Bachelor degree	643	43.0
	Master degree	44	3.0
Gender	Male	147	9.8
	Female	1309	87.6
Age	Under 25 years old	234	15.7
	26 to 34 years old	474	31.7
	35 to 44 years old	406	27.2
	45 to 54 years old	276	18.5
	55 years and older	99	6.6
Job	RN/LPN	1187	79.4
	Nursing assistant	308	20.6
Shift Type	8-hour shift	309	20.7
	10-hour shift	11	0.7
	12-hour shift	1064	71.2
	8-hour and 12-hour rotating shift	101	6.8
	Other	9	0.6
Work Hours	Days (8- or 12-hour shift)	628	42.6
	Evenings (8- or 12-hour shift)	120	8.0
	Nights (8- or 12-hours shift)	487	32.6
	Rotation	256	17.1

breakdown/pressure ulcers, medication errors, new infections, IV running dry, IV infiltrating, and other problems reported significantly more overall missed nursing care as well as missed communication and timeliness. Patients reported more missed basic care if they experienced the adverse events of medication errors, new infection, IV running dry, IV leaking (infiltrating), and other problems. The "other problems" included lack of pain management, problems with their food, fluid overload, and complaints of noise. The sample size was too small to conduct tests of significance on these responses.

Comparison of Patients, RNs, and NAs

We also surveyed nursing staff (i.e., RNs, NAs) on the units where the patients were hospitalized to allow us to compare the reports of the type and amount of missed nursing care between patients and nursing

TABLE 8.3.   **Comparison of reports of missed nursing care: RNs versus patients (n = 1937).**

Variable	RNs (Mean ± SD) (n = 1187)	Patients (Mean ± SD) (n = 750)	Z-value	p-value
Overall	1.82 ± 0.47	1.82 ± 0.58	−1.300	0.193
Ambulation	2.26 ± 0.77	2.17 ± 1.09	−2.588	0.010*
Turning	1.85 ± 0.69	2.17 ± 1.12	−3.825	0.000**
Feeding	1.99 ± 0.76	2.09 ± 1.16	−0.344	0.731
Education	1.85 ± 0.73	1.91 ± 1.06	−1.481	0.139
Emotional support	1.73 ± 0.76	1.35 ± 0.69	−12.142	0.000**
Bathing/Skin care	1.64 ± 0.66	1.88 ± 1.04	−2.653	0.008**
Mouth care	2.13 ± 0.83	2.53 ± 1.25	−6.599	0.000**
IV/Other line monitoring	1.55 ± 0.66	1.55 ± 0.84	−2.361	0.018*
Call-light response	1.84 ± 0.75	1.44 ± 0.69	−12.160	0.000**
PRN medication	1.54 ± 0.65	1.82 ± 0.89	−5.287	0.000**
Toileting	1.76 ± 0.71	1.54 ± 0.73	−5.938	0.000**

Note: $*p < .05, **p < .01$

staff members. The aim was to determine the extent to which patient and nursing staff reports of missed nursing care were congruent.

Sample

A total of 1,480 nursing staff in the same two hospitals where patient data (n = 729) was collected participated in this study. They completed the *MISSCARE Survey*, which was utilized to collect the nursing staff reports. The predominant gender was female (87.6%) and 52% were 34 years or older. The respondents included 79.2% RNs and 20.8% NAs. Nursing staff education level, shift type, and work hours are contained in Table 8.2.

Comparisons

RNs versus patients

As can be seen in Table 8.3, there was not a significant difference in the overall ratings of missed nursing care between RNs and patients. There were, however, significant differences for the individual elements of nursing care. Nurses reported more missed ambulation, emotional support, call-light responses, and toileting assistance than did patients. Patients, on the other hand, reported more missed turning, bathing, mouth care, and PRN medication. Patients and nurses were similar

TABLE 8.4.   **Comparison of reports of missed nursing care by NAs versus patients (n = 2245).**

Variable	Nursing assistants (Mean ± SD) (n = 1495)	Patients (Mean ± SD) (n = 750)	Z-value	p-value
Overall	1.62 ± 0.56	1.82 ± 0.58	−5.636	0.000**
Ambulation	1.94 ± 0.82	2.17 ± 1.09	−2.368	0.018*
Turning	1.62 ± 0.78	2.17 ± 1.12	−6.061	0.000**
Feeding	1.64 ± 0.79	2.09 ± 1.16	−3.081	0.002**
Education	1.58 ± 0.74	1.91 ± 1.06	−3.241	0.001**
Emotional support	1.49 ± 0.76	1.35 ± 0.69	−3.373	0.001**
Bathing/Skin care	1.48 ± 0.76	1.88 ± 1.04	−5.585	0.000**
Mouth care	1.80 ± 0.87	2.53 ± 1.25	−8.382	0.000**
IV/Other line monitoring	1.36 ± 0.66	1.55 ± 0.84	−2.536	0.011*
Call-light response	1.68 ± 0.80	1.44 ± 0.69	−4.858	0.000**
PRN medication	1.72 ± 0.83	1.82 ± 0.89	−1.240	0.215
Toileting	1.48 ± 0.71	1.54 ± 0.73	−1.289	0.197

Note: * $p < .05$, ** $p < .01$

(i.e., no statistical difference) in the amount of missed feeding assistance and patient education.

NAs versus patients
NAs reported less missed nursing care than patients and RNs. NAs did not differ from patients in their assessments of missed PRN medications and toileting. Patients reported more missed ambulation, turning, feeding, education, bathing, mouth care, and IV site care than NAs did (Table 8.4). Emotional support and response to call lights was reported to be missed more by NAs than patients.

RNs versus NAs
Overall, RNs reported more missed care than NAs. The specific elements of nursing care for which RNs reported higher levels of missed care were: ambulation, turning, feeding, education, emotional support, bathing, mouth care, IV and other line monitoring, call-light response, and toileting. On the other hand, NAs reported more missed PRN medications than RNs (Table 8.5).

This study uncovered differences and similarities in the amount and type of missed nursing care as reported by RNs, NAs, and patients. Patients reported less missed emotional support and timely response

TABLE 8.5. **Comparison of reports of missed nursing care by RNs versus NAs (n = 1495).**

Variable	Nurses (Mean ± SD) (n = 1187)	Nurse assistants (Mean ± SD) (n = 308)	Z-value	p-value
Overall	1.82 ± 0.47	1.62 ± 0.56	−7.425	0.000**
Ambulation	2.26 ± 0.77	1.94 ± 0.82	−6.169	0.000**
Turning	1.85 ± 0.69	1.62 ± 0.78	−5.806	0.000**
Feeding	1.99 ± 0.76	1.64 ± 0.79	−6.931	0.000**
Education	1.85 ± 0.73	1.58 ± 0.74	−5.318	0.000**
Emotional support	1.73 ± 0.76	1.49 ± 0.76	−5.483	0.000**
Bathing/Skin care	1.64 ± 0.66	1.48 ± 0.76	−5.057	0.000**
Mouth care	2.13 ± 0.83	1.80 ± 0.87	−6.363	0.000**
IV/Other line monitoring	1.55 ± 0.66	1.36 ± 0.66	−4.587	0.000**
Call-light response	1.84 ± 0.75	1.68 ± 0.80	−3.698	0.000**
PRN medication	1.54 ± 0.65	1.72 ± 0.83	−2.325	0.020*
Toileting	1.76 ± 0.71	1.48 ± 0.71	−6.983	0.000**

Note: * $p < .05$, ** $p < .01$

to call lights than did RNs and NAs. This suggests that nursing staff may feel the patient needs more emotional support and quicker responses to call lights than patients see the need for. It may be that patients do not recognize their own requirements for emotional support or do not see that it is the role of the nursing staff to provide that care. Nurses may overestimate what the patients need or patients do not perceive they had unmet needs. The other explanation could be that patients do not feel that the nurses could provide this psychological support because they had other work to do. In regard to the timely response to call lights, patients may not recognize the danger (e.g., falls) of nurses not responding to call lights in a timely fashion. Patients may overestimate their own ability to walk and stand and proceed to the bathroom, or they may refuse to believe that they are dependent on the nursing staff in this way.

On the other hand, patients report more missed turning, mouth care, and bathing than RNs and NAs. RNs reported more missed ambulation and toileting than did patients and NAs. Studies have consistently pointed to the lack of patient ambulation in acute care hospitals and other studies have demonstrated the impact of that lack on patients in these settings. As such, there is a need to educate NAs and for that matter, patients, as to the importance of mobility. There are also instances where patients resist ambulation, and this may account for some of the differences between patients and staff.

Providing PRN medications was an area that patients and NAs felt was missed, but RNs did not agree. Perhaps RNs are sometimes unaware of patients' needs for medications, such as for pain. It is possible that they may place it lower on the priority scale than patients who want the relief. Additionally, NAs, who may be face-to-face with the patient more often than RNs, may be more knowledgeable about the patient's needs. On another note, RNs and patients reported the same level of missed feedings and patient education while NAs said it was missed less.

RNs and patients are similar in their rating of the overall amount of missed care as well as ambulation, feeding assistance, patient education, and monitoring IV lines. The differences found between RNs and NAs substantiates an earlier study which found that NAs reported less missed ambulation, mouth care, feeding, turning, toileting, bathing, timely response to call lights, and emotional support than RNs (Kalisch, 2009).

NAs, however, report significantly less missed nursing care. This finding substantiates the earlier study of the difference between nurses' and NAs' ratings of the amounts and types of missed nursing care. The possible reason for the lower ratings by NAs is that they may not be as aware of the patients' needs as nurses. On the other hand, their assessments may be more accurate since they may spend more actual time in the patients' rooms.

Implications of Studies
Patient Ability to Report
The results of these studies show that it is possible for patients and/ or family members to report some aspects of missed nursing care but not all errors of omission. This information from patients potentially has high-level value for the improvement of quality and patient satisfaction. For example, we learned that mouth care is a very important contributor to patient satisfaction. We also determined that both quantitative and qualitative data is valuable. Quantitative data provides us with the extent of the problem of missed nursing care and qualitative data gives us insights into patient and family reactions, concerns, and values.

A Measurement Tool
Using missed nursing care as a process measurement of the quality of nursing care makes sense and could offer nursing staff the data they

need to improve care. Both nurses and patients could be surveyed. A comparison between hospitals showed that while there was no significant difference in the overall missed nursing care score between the two hospitals, Hospital 1 missed more basic nursing care and the nursing staff members in Hospital 2 were less timely in their responses, especially with assisting patients to the bathroom. This suggests that the *MISSCARE Survey—Patient* might be used to compare hospitals regarding their completion of nursing care and offer a benchmark measurement of care.

In the case of wanting to measure the impact of an intervention, such as using activity lists or increasing teamwork, potential Hawthorne effect could be minimized. The Hawthorne effect refers to people improving or altering their behavior because they are aware they are being observed. Since nursing staff would be aware of any intervention being tested to reduce missed nursing care, surveying patients would be a way to avoid this problem.

Adverse Events and Quality

This study uncovered substantial areas of missed nursing care. We found that adverse events are significantly associated with the amount of missed nursing care, which gives evidence to the fact that not completing nursing care is a serious problem that needs to be addressed. These omissions have potential for serious negative patient outcomes, which is the subject of the next chapter.

A previous study of the agreement between patients' and physicians' reports of adverse events found agreement in 72.2% of the cases. Patients demonstrated the ability to recognize and report on many inpatient adverse events, yielding their reports valuable and complementary to other incident-detection methods (Zhu et al., 2011).

In addition to these adverse events, the quality of care is seriously impacted by missed nursing care. Not having mouth care, for example is the most frequent element of missed nursing care identified by patients in this study (50.3%) and also by nursing staff (25.5%) in other studies (Kalisch, Tschannen, Lee, & Friese, 2011). This could contribute to serious problems, including chest infection, pneumonia, poor nutrition intake, decreased self-esteem, and increased hospitalized days, especially when patients have physical or cognitive problems that require them to rely on others for their personal care (Blevins, 2011; Dickinson, 2012; Sona et al., 2009). Mouth care is supposed to be a part of the daily nursing routine in most hospitals (Kuramoto et al., 2011). Although the majority of nurses feel responsible to ensure that patients receive mouth care, Pettit, McCann, Schneiderman, Farren, and Campbell and other investigators have noted that they do not usually consider mouth care as a priority in the acute setting and are somewhat ill-prepared to provide adequate mouth care (Dickinson, 2012; Pettit et al., 2012; Soh, Soh, Japar, Raman, & Davidson, 2011).

Missed ambulation is an even more important issue reported by both nursing staff and patients. This finding, along with the results of other studies that have asked nursing staff to report on the extent to which this care is provided, indicates that most patients are confined to bed or a chair and experience a lack of mobility during their hospitalization. Previous studies reveal that inpatient mobilization has a vital positive impact on patients' physical function as well as emotional and social well-being (Kalisch, Lee, & Dabney, 2014). Moreover, patient ambulation potentially could yield important organizational benefits, including cost reduction, decreased length of stays, and lower mortality rates (Kalisch, Xie, & Dabney, 2013). Effective interventions and policies that increase mobilization need to be developed and integrated into nursing practice in the acute care setting. In order to decrease the amount of missed care, system improvements (such as adequate staffing, reminders, check lists, mid-shift debriefings, etc.) are needed.

This study also uncovers inadequate communication between patients and nursing staff. Patients reported that the tests and treatment were not discussed with them (missed 27% and 26.5% of time, respectively), and their opinions were not considered (missed 20.4%). Effective communication between patients and healthcare providers is critical to ensure the delivery of quality patient care, patient satisfaction, and patient safety (McCabe, 2004; Rao, 2011). Failure to communicate effectively with patients and their family members can contribute to problems such as errors, inadequate pain relief, extended hospital stays, increased costs, and patient anguish and disorientation (Rao, 2011). Essential training and other interventions, as well as organizational improvements, should be provided to facilitate patient-centered communication. More information on the impact of missed nursing care is the subject of the next chapter.

Patient Engagement

A substantial body of evidence demonstrates that patients who are more actively involved in their healthcare experience have better health outcomes at lower costs (Hibbard & Greene, 2013). With more patient education about the care they should be receiving, they could be even more engaged in monitoring and contributing to the quality and safety of their own care. Moreover, the greater involvement of patients and their family members could better prepare them for care after discharge and potentially lead to a decrease in readmissions and complications. Although this probably would require more time on the part of staff members while the patient is hospitalized, the result could be a higher quality of care and even potential reduction in the overall costs of health care. Studies are needed to demonstrate the effect of engaging patients and families more extensively in their nursing care. The patient's ability to work with the staff to reduce errors depends on them being well informed.

Summary

Contained in this chapter are summaries of several studies of patient-reported missed nursing care. First, the results of a qualitative study with the aim to determine what elements of missed nursing care can be reported by patients showed that there are fully reportable, partially reportable, and not reportable elements of nursing care. In this study we also collected data on elements of missed nursing care that showed that mouth care, ambulation, discharge planning, patient education, listening to patients, and keeping them informed were frequently missed. A quantitative study of patient reports of missed nursing care using the *MISSCARE Survey—Patient* revealed the most missed nursing care in the subscale of basic care (2.29 ± 1.06) followed by communication (1.69 ± 0.71) and time to respond (1.52 ± 0.64). Finally, a comparison of reports of missed nursing care identified by RNs, NAs, and patients revealed that patients reported less missed emotional support and timely response to call lights than did RNs and NAs. Patients also reported more missed turning, mouth care, and bathing than RNs and NAs. RNs reported more missed ambulation and toileting than did patients and NAs.

References

Adamsen, L., & Tewes, M. (2000). Discrepancy between patients' perspectives, staff's documentation and reflections on basic nursing care. *Scandanavian Journal of Caring Sciences, 14*(2), 120–129.

Blevins, J. Y. (2011). Oral health care for hospitalized children. *Pediatric Nursing, 37*(5), 229–235; quiz 236.

Bush, H. (2012). Patient safety congress. How important is patient satisfaction? *Hosptials & Health Networks, 86*(7), 17.

Centers for Disease Control and Prevention (2013). FastStats: Michigan facts. Retrieved from http://www.cdc.gov/nchs/fastats/popup_mi.htm

Corbin, J., & Strauss, A. (2008). *Basics of qualitative research: Techniques and procedures for developing grounded theory* (3rd ed.). Los Angeles, CA: Sage Publications.

Dickinson, H. (2012). Maintaining oral health after stroke. *Nursing Standard, 26*(49), 35–39.

Englebright, J., Aldrich, K., & Taylor, C. R. (2014). Defining and incorporating basic nursing care actions into the electronic health record. *Journal of Nursing Scholarship, 46*(1), 50–57.

Heidegger, M. (1962). *Being and time.* New York, NY: Harper and Row.

Hibbard, J. H., & Greene, J. (2013). What the evidence shows about patient activation: Better health outcomes and care experiences; fewer data on costs. *Health Affairs, 32*(2), 207–214.

Kalisch, B. J. (2009). Nurse and nurse assistant perceptions of missed nursing care: What does it tell us about teamwork? *The Journal of Nursing Administration, 39*(11), 485–493.

Kalisch, B. J., Lee, S., & Dabney, B. W. (2014). Outcomes of inpatient mobilizaiton: A literature review. *Journal of Clinical Nursing, 23*(11–12), 1486–1501.

Kalisch, B. J., McLaughlin, M., & Dabney, B. W. (2012). Patient perceptions of missed nursing care. *The Joint Commission Journal on Quality and Patient Safety, 38*(4), 161–167.

Kalisch, B. J., Tschannen, D., Lee, H., & Friese, C. R. (2011). Hospital variation in missed nursing care. *American Journal of Medical Quality, 26*(4), 291–299.

Kalisch, B. J., Xie, B., & Dabney, B. W. (2013). Patient-reported missed nursing care correlated with adverse events. *American Journal of Medical Quality, 29*(5), 415–422.

Kuramoto, C., Watanabe, Y., Tonogi, M., Hirata, S. Sugihara, N., Ishii, T., & Yamane, G. Y. (2011). Factor analysis on oral health care for acute hospitalized patients in Japan. *Geriatrics & Gerontology International, 11*(4), 460–466.

McCabe, C. (2004). Nurse-patient communication: An exploration of patients' experiences. *Journal of Clinical Nursing, 13*(1), 41–49.

Pettit, S. L., McCann, A. L., Schneiderman, E. D., Farren, E. A., & Campbell, P. R. (2012). Dimensions of oral care management in Texas hospitals. *Journal of Dental Hygiene, 86*(2), 91–103.

Pipe, T. B., Connolly, T., Sparhr, N., Lendzion, N., Buchda, V., Jury, R., & Cisar, N. (2012). Bringing back the basics of nursing: Defining patient care essentials. *Nursing Administration Quarterly, 36*(3), 225–233.

Rao, P. R. (2011). From the president: Our role in effective patient-provider communication. *The ASHA Leader, 16*(13), 17.

Soh, K. L., Soh, K. G., Japar, S., Raman, R. A., & Davidson, P. M. (2011). A cross-sectional study on nurses' oral care practice for mechanically ventilated patients in Malaysia. *Journal of Clinical Nursing, 20*(5–6), 733–742.

Sona, C. S., Zack, J. E., Schallom, M. E., McSweeney, M., McMullen, K., Thomas, J., ... Schuerer, D. J. (2009). The impact of a simple, low-cost oral care protocol on ventilator-associated pneumonia rates in a surgical intensive care unit. *Journal of Intensive Care Medicine, 24*(1), 54–62.

Williams, A. M. (1998). The delivery of quality nursing care: A grounded theory study of the nurse's perspective. *Journal of Advanced Nursing, 27*(4), 808–816.

Zhu, J., Stuver, S. O., Epstein, A. M., Schneider, E. C., Weissman, J. S., & Weingart, S. N. (2011). Can we rely on patients' reports of adverse events? *Medical Care, 49*(10), 948–955.

— 9 —

Patient Outcomes of Missed Nursing Care

During hospitalization, patients are commonly deprived of sleep, experience disruption of normal circadian rhythms, are nourished poorly, have pain and discomfort, confront a baffling array of mentally challenging situations, receive medications that can alter cognition and physical function, and become deconditioned by bed rest or inactivity. Each of these perturbations can adversely affect health and contribute to substantial impairments during the early recovery period, an inability to fend off disease, and susceptibility to mental error. (Krumholz, 2013)

Krumholz is referring to what he terms the post-hospital syndrome (i.e., an acquired, transient period of vulnerability) where patients experience susceptibility to a range of adverse events. He suggests that the risks in the 30-day period after discharge might derive as much from the allostatic load (the physiologic consequences of adapting to repeated or chronic stress). Another way to put it is the wear and tear on the body, which accumulates over time when the individual is exposed to the repeated stress that patients experience while hospitalized. For example, if a dehydrated individual does not reinstate normal body function, the body systems will wear out. The human body is adaptable, but it cannot maintain allostatic overload for very long without consequences (Sadatsafavi, Lynd, & FitzGerald, 2013). A great proportion of these problems can be traced to missed nursing care.

The impact of hospitalization in and of itself may be more harmful than the lingering effects of the original acute illness which led to the hospitalization in the first place. At the time of discharge, Krumholz writes, the "physiological systems are impaired, reserves are depleted, and the body cannot effectively defend against health threats" (2013, p. 100). In older patients, acute medical illness that requires hospitalization is a sentinel event that often precipitates disability. This results in the subsequent inability to live independently and complete basic activities of daily living (ADLs). This hospitalization-associated disability occurs in approximately one-third of patients older than 70 years of age and may be triggered even when the illness that necessitated the hospitalization is successfully treated.

Former Secretary of State and presidential candidate Hillary Clinton's health problems illustrate how a seemingly minor health issue can snowball and lead to more severe problems. Clinton first suffered a gastrointestinal illness, which left her dehydrated and weak. That led her to fall, where she hit her head and suffered a concussion. Trauma to the head then led to a blood clot in her head, causing her to be hospitalized.

Snowballing is a common occurrence in hospitalized or recently hospitalized patients. For example, the 70-year-old patient's call light is not answered promptly and he decides to get up on his own to go to the bathroom. He falls and sustains a fracture which leads to a need for surgery and a longer length of stay. When the patient is discharged from the hospital, he is in a deconditioned state and cannot return home to live on his own. He is discharged to a rehabilitation long-term care facility for 4 to 6 weeks. When he is finally discharged from the rehabilitation facility, he has to undergo additional physical therapy. A seemingly minor omission in nursing care results in a major and costly illness.

About 20% of Medicare patients are readmitted to the hospital within the first month after discharge. It has been referred to as the revolving door syndrome, and is estimated to cost $26 billion annually. More than $17 billion of it pays for unnecessary return hospitalizations that would not have happened if patients got appropriate care. The Affordable Care Act of 2010 required the government to establish a readmission reduction program designed to provide incentives for hospitals to implement strategies to reduce the number of costly and unnecessary hospital readmissions (American College of Emergency Physicians, 2013). The incentives are escalating penalties that decrease the amount of payments that hospitals receive for all of their Medicare cases. The payment penalty was as much as 1% of all Medicare payments for a hospital in 2012 that was deemed to have excessive readmissions for acute myocardial infarction or congestive health failure, and pneumonia. In 2013, the penalty went up to 2% and increased to 3% in 2014. In 2015, additional conditions and measures for the initial inpatient admission will be added to the current list of three. In addition to the loss of revenue for hospitals, missed nursing care has a definite negative impact on patients. In this chapter, we review the available research that demonstrates the impact of missed nursing care overall, as well as specific elements of nursing care (e.g., ambulation, turning, nourishment, etc.).

The Consequences of Not Providing Nursing Care
Overall Missed Nursing Care
The studies evaluating the impact of missed care on patient outcomes have been limited. We identified three studies which tested the impact of missed nursing care on patient outcomes. These are summarized below.

In the first study, missed nursing care and patient falls were studied. Up to 12% of hospitalized patients experience at least one fall during their hospital stay (Coussement et al., 2008). A fall is defined as any event in which patients are found on the floor (observed or unobserved) or an unplanned lowering of the patient to the floor by staff or visitors (Rutledge, Donaldson, & Pravikoff, 1998). In 2010 and 2012, falls were identified as one of the top 10 sentinel event categories by the Joint Commission (2014). Fall rates in hospitals range from 2 to 14 falls per 1,000 patient days (Oliver, Hopper, & Seed, 2000). With the adoption of the Centers of Medicare and Medicaid rule in 2008—which no longer reimburses hospitals at the higher diagnosis-related group for the care and treatment associated with patient falls that occur during hospitalization—a clearer understanding of what factors influence fall rates among hospitalized patients has been highlighted (Centers for Medicare and Medicaid Services, 2008). The causes of patient falls and interventions to prevent them have received considerable attention (Ferrari, Harrison, Campbell, Maddens, & Whall, 2010; Yauk et al., 2005; Fick, Waller, & Inouye, 2013). Yauk and colleagues

(2005) identified ambulation assistance, disorientation, bowel control problems, and fall history as predictors of falls among hospitalized medical–surgical patients. Ferrari and colleagues (2010) also found inattention and lack of mobility contributed to falls.

Falls have adverse consequences for patients (e.g., mortality, fractures, functional dependence, and fear of reoccurrence) and staff who provide direct patient care (e.g., feelings of guilt, apprehension). Although several national and professional organizations have developed evidence-based guidelines that set forth strategies for reducing falls, consistency in implementation of these strategies has been limited (Degelau et al., 2012; Gray-Micelli, 2008). Findings from 188 medical–surgical units in 48 hospitals across the United States found that risk-specific interventions (such as ambulation and medication management) are not being implemented consistently (Titler, 2008).

To determine if missed nursing care mediated patient falls, we utilized data from 124 patient units in 11 acute care hospitals. The term mediated tells us how or why the level of staffing (in this case) predicts patient falls (the outcome criteria in this case). In fact, a number of studies have shown that the level of staffing predicts patient falls. By using the mediator approach, we were able to identify and explicate the process that underlies the relationship between staffing levels and patient falls. The study questions were: (1) Do nurse staffing levels (hours per patient day) predict patient falls? and (2) Does missed nursing care mediate the effect of staffing levels on patient falls?

The level of staffing (hours per patient day), the case mix index (as an indication of patient acuity), the number of patient falls, and the nursing staff reports of missed nursing care using the *MISSCARE Survey* (n = 4412) were collected for these units. Since patient falls are reported at the patient unit level, we examined falls and staffing at that level. Unit inclusion criteria were (1) an average patient length of stay of 2 days or more and (2) a patient population older than 18 years. Exclusion criteria were (1) short stay units (≤ 23 hours) and (2) pediatric, women's health, perioperative, and psychiatric units (Kalisch, Tschannen, & Lee, 2012).

Correlations were calculated to examine the relationships among the variables and showed that (Table 9.1) hours per patient day (HPPD) was negatively associated with patient falls ($r = -0.36$, $p < .01$). The higher the overall missed nursing care score, the higher the patient fall rates ($r = 0.30$, $p < .01$). More patient falls were significantly related to the following specific elements of missed nursing care: ambulation ($r = 0.22$, $p < .05$), shift patient assessment ($r = 0.19$, $p < .05$), call-light response ($r = 0.22$, $p < .05$), and toilet assistance ($r = 0.30$, $p < .01$).

TABLE 9.1. **Staffing, missed nursing care, and patient falls: Correlation matrix.**

Variables	1	2	3	4	5	6	7	8	9
1. Square root of fall rate	–								
2. HPPD	–.36†	–							
3. CMI	–.19	.64†	–						
4. Overall missed nursing care	.30†	–.26†	–.13	–					
5. Ambulation	.22*	.00	–.00	.66†	–				
6. Each shift pt assessments	.19*	–.01	.05	.63†	.11	–			
7. Focused reassessment	.16	–.15	–.13	.70†	.13	.71†	–		
8. Call-light response	.22*	–.38†	–.23*	.76†	.40†	.22*	.41†	–	
9. Toilet assistance	.30†	–.41†	–.17	.86†	.50†	.45†	.50†	.65†	–

Note: $*p < .05$. $†p < .01$

As noted in the Figure 9.1, results indicated that HPPD was significantly associated with missed nursing care ($F\,1,120 = 8.46$, $p = .004$). Hours per patient day explained 6.7% of the variance in missed nursing care. In the second equation, patient falls, the outcome variable, was regressed on the predictor variable, HPPD. Hour per patient day was significantly associated with patient falls ($F\,1,115 = 17.20$, $p < .001$). Hour per patient day explained 13.0% of the variance in patient falls. In the final equation, patient falls, the outcome variable, was regressed on both the predictor variable (HPPD) and the mediator variable (missed nursing care). Missed nursing care negatively affected patient falls ($t = 2.49$, $p = .014$), explaining 9.2% of variance in patient falls. With missed nursing care present, the proportion of variance of patient falls accounted for by HPPD was reduced from 13.0% (second equation) to 8.3% (third equation), and the standardized regression coefficient was decreased from –.36 to –.30 from the second to third equation. Thus, the reduced direct association between HPPD and patient falls when missed nursing care was in the model supported the hypothesis that missed nursing care acts as a mediator in the relationship between HPPD and patient falls.

In another study, patient reports of missed nursing care were predictive of patient reported adverse events during the current hospitalization (Kalisch & Xie, 2014). The aim of this study, reported in Chapter 8, was to determine the extent and type of missed nursing care as reported by patients and the association with patient-reported

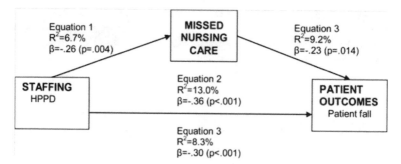

FIGURE 9.1. **Missed nursing care as mediator of patient falls (n = 4412).**

adverse outcomes. A total of 729 inpatients on 20 units in two acute care hospitals were surveyed. The *MISSCARE Survey—Patient* was used to collect patient reports of missed care. As noted in the previous chapter, patients reported more missed nursing care in the domain of basic care (2.29 ± 1.06) than in communication (1.69 ± 0.71) and in time to respond (1.52 ± 0.64). The five most frequently reported elements of missed nursing care were the following:

1. mouth care (50.3%)
2. ambulation (41.3%)
3. getting out of bed into a chair (38.8%)
4. providing information about tests/procedures (27%)
5. bathing (26.4%).

Patients who reported skin breakdown, pressure ulcers, medication errors, new infections, IVs running dry, IVs infiltrating, and other problems during the current hospitalization reported significantly more overall missed nursing care.

Finally, Schubert and colleagues' (2008) investigation showed that even though specific elements of missed nursing care (which they termed rationed care) were low in incidence, they still resulted in adverse outcomes, namely medication errors, patient falls, infections, and pressure ulcers.

Specific Elements of Nursing Care

Research studies which have examined the impact of not providing specific elements of nursing care (i.e., ambulation, turning/positioning, medication administration, hand washing and other infection control procedures, mouth care, emotional support, promoting sleep, discharge planning, patient teaching, nourishment, bathing and skin care, and interdisciplinary rounds) are summarized below.

Ambulation
The fact that ambulation of hospitalized adults is regularly missed indicates that many patients are confined to a bed or a chair and are mostly immobile throughout their hospital stay (Callen, Mahoney, Grieves, Wells, & Enloe (2004). Studies exploring inpatient immobility have uncovered many negative consequences of not ambulating that affect the cardiovascular, respiratory, gastrointestinal, integumentary, musculoskeletal, renal, endocrine, and nervous systems (Convertino, 1997; Convertino, Bloomfield, & Greenleaf, 1997; Creditor, 1993; Graf, 2006).

Patients begin to experience a decline in walking ability within two days of being hospitalized (Hirsch, Sommers, Olsen, Mullen, & Winograd, 1990). Lack of inpatient mobility can be especially devastating to the older person where the aging process contributes to more rapid functional decline (Graf, 2006). This new walking dependence among the older population may lead to discharge to a nursing home and has been found to result in continued walking dependence three months after discharge in 27% of older patients (Mahoney, Sager, & Jalaluddin, 1998). It may also lead to rehospitalization within 30 days of discharge resulting in higher costs for the hospital (Morandi et al., 2013).

Failure to ambulate patients has been linked to new onset delirium, pneumonia, delayed wound healing, pressure ulcers, increased length of stay and delayed discharge, increased pain and discomfort, muscle wasting, fatigue, and physical disability (Bansal, Scott, Stewart, & Cockerell, 2005; Kamel, Iqbal, Mogallapu, Maas, & Hoffmann, 2003; Mundy, Leet, Darst, Schnitzler, & Dunagan, 2003; Munin, Rudy, Glynn, Crossett, & Rubash, 1998; Price & Fowlow, 1994; Pasero & Belden, 2006; Whitney & Parkman, 2004; Yohannes & Connolly, 2003). Any patient with impaired mobility can also be at risk of pressure ulcers, which are typically caused by "periods of uninterrupted pressure on the skin, soft tissue, muscle, and bone" (Darling, Shea, & Linscott, 2008).

In a review of the research that has been completed on the outcomes of mobility conducted with patients in acute care hospitals, we uncovered 36 studies which met the criteria for inclusion in the review (Kalisch, Lee, & Dabney, 2013). Four areas (study design, sample size, measurement, and statistical analysis) were evaluated for methodological quality. A synthesis of the findings generated four themes of the effects of inpatient mobilization:

1. Physical outcomes including pain, deep vein thrombosis, fatigue, etc.
2. Psychological outcomes including anxiety, depressive mood, distress, discomfort, and dissatisfaction.
3. Social outcomes including quality of life and independence.
4. Organizational outcomes including length of stay, mortality, and cost.

Mobilizing hospitalized adults is beneficial not only for physical functioning, but also their emotional and social well-being. Ambulation also yields important organizational benefits. Even though each study approached different types of patients, illnesses, and procedures, this review demonstrated the critical nature of ambulating inpatients and the negative effects of not doing so.

Turning and positioning patients

For the past century, turning or repositioning patients every 2 hours has been the standard and required nursing care for patients who are not mobile (Makic, Rauen, Watson, & Poteet, 2014). The idea of repositioning is to remove pressure from the surface the patient is lying on to prevent skin breakdown, but also to mobilize the body to prevent venous stasis, improve muscle strength, pulmonary function, and cardiovascular tone. The negative outcomes of not turning patients include pressure ulcers, pneumonia, venous stasis, thrombosis, embolism, stone formation, urinary tract infection (kidney and bladder), muscle wasting, bone demineralization, and atelectasis (Krishnagopalan, Johnson, Low, & Kaufman, 2002).

To avoid pressure ulcer development, the mechanical load needs to be decreased in patients who spend a large amount of time in bed or sitting and for patients who cannot adequately turn or reposition themselves. The incidence of pressure ulcers varies by clinical setting: 0.4% to 38.0% for hospitals, 2.2% to 23.9% for long-term care, and 0% to 17% for home care (Lyder, 2003). A Healthcare Cost and Utilization Project study reported an average cost of $37,800 to treat pressure ulcers (Russo & Elixhauser, 2006). Cost data vary greatly, depending on what factors are included or excluded from the economic models (e.g., nursing time, support surfaces). It has been estimated that the cost of treating pressure ulcers is 2.5 times the cost of preventing them (Oot-Giromini et al., 1989).

Only a few studies have been published relating to optimal turning schedules. Norton, McLaren, and Exton-Smith (1975) conducted an observational study where they divided older adults into three turning treatment groups (every 2 to 3 hours [n = 32], every 4 hours [n = 27], or turned two to four times/day [n = 41]) (Norton et al., 1975). Those patients turned every 2 to 3 hours had fewer ulcers. A more recent study by DeFloor, De Bacquer, and Grypdonck (2005) suggests that, depending on the support surface used, less-frequent turning may be acceptable to prevent pressure ulcers in a long-term care facility. Four different turning frequencies (every 2 hours on a standard mattress, every 3 hours on a standard mattress, every 4 hours on a viscoelastic foam mattress, and every 6 hours on a viscoelastic foam mattress) were compared. The incidence of early pressure ulcers (Stage I) did not differ in the four groups. However, patients being turned every 4 hours on a viscoelastic foam mattress developed significantly less severe pressure ulcers (Stage II and greater) than the three other groups. Reddy, Gill, and Rochon (2006) questioned the methodology in the DeFloor study, suggesting that the every 2 hour turning standard should not be abandoned before more research is conducted. Thus, there is emerging research to support the continued turning of patients at least every 2 hours (Reddy et al., 2006). Some patients may actually need to be turned more often (Salcido, 2004).

The current national practice guidelines recommend that the patient's skin be assessed for injury and that they are turned or repositioned every two hours. Pressure ulcers can develop within 2 to 6 hours (Kosiak, 1959; Kosiak, Kubicek, Olsen, Danz, & Kottke, 1958). Special mattresses or specialty bed support surfaces are beneficial to patients but do not replace turning. Although pressure ulcers do not typically cause death, mortality has been associated with pressure ulcers. Several studies noted mortality rates as high as 60% for older persons with pressure ulcers within one year of hospital discharge (Allman, Goode, Patrick, Burst, & Bartolucci, 1995; Thomas, Goode, Tarquine, & Allman, 1996). These studies further suggest that the development of skin breakdown post-surgery can lead to major functional impairment.

Medication administration

Inappropriate medication omissions can clearly lead to harm from lack of therapeutic effect. Green, Du-Pre, Elahi, Dunckley, and McIntyre (2009) and Barker, Flynn, Pepper, Bates, & Mikeal (2002) studied the impact of omitted medications. They note that nurses administering medicines may decide that omission of a dose is appropriate in certain circumstances (e.g., when patients show signs of a possible adverse drug reaction [ADR]) (Warne et al., 2010; Kanaan et al., 2013). Other examples include omission of a laxative in an admission with a fall risk and omission of amlodipine for hypertension in a patient with a urinary tract infection. However, they found that in 7% of cases, the omission was evaluated to be potentially detrimental and adversely affected outcome and length of stay. For example, they found that a patient with Clostridium difficile (C. difficile) missed the first two doses of Vancomycin, another patient with diarrhea missed three doses of metronidazole for C. difficile treatment, and two patients with acute coronary syndrome missed Enoxaparin. These medications are first-line treatments and they should not be omitted. In addition, time spent by the healthcare team tracking missed doses can have an effect on time available for direct patient care (Sagnga et al., 2014).

In another study, researchers reviewed missing medication reports that nurses are required to complete if the medication they are seeking to administer is not available. This can occur if an incorrect medication was delivered by the pharmacy for that patient, a specific medication for a patient cannot be located, or a new medication order has not been delivered by the pharmacy within an allotted time period. Missing medication reports in this organization were reported to be consistently high, with approximately 650 reports filed per week, representing 2.83% of all orders. Consequences of not having medications available include increased processing times for the pharmacy as they rework orders, and decreased availability of the nursing staff for patient care as they search for medications and follow up on reports. The high level of frustration this creates for nurses is illustrated in the following direct quotes from RN focus group participants:

> Today I have had late medications on both of my patients and that is because the pharmacy first got me the wrong med, and then they had to get the new med from [another part of the hospital] and I had to wait. It was 3 hours late. And I was 2 hours late on a magnesium that was ordered just because it wasn't here. I don't know the reasoning why it wasn't here, but that puts off my Zosyn that I was going to hang at noon because now the mag is hanging for two hours and I can't hang the Zosyn until the mag is done.

> It got to the point with me that I would check all of my medications for the day the second I got to work so that I could call the pharmacy to remind them to bring some of my nine o' clock medications. I knew if I did not do it in advance, I would not have the medications at the right time.

> I think the biggest [problem] we have with our resources is the pharmacy stocking our medications. It is very frustrating when

it's not there. And then you call and they say, "Oh it's on the run right now." Well they just dropped the run off and it's not here. "Well, we sent it twice." "Well, the bottom line is it's not here so I need you to make it again. I'll just come and get it." We usually have what we need, thankfully, and if we don't, we know where to find it.

We have to spend time tracking down the pharmacy, calling them. That's time away from doing the tasks that we need to do.

Hand washing

Effective hand hygiene practices have long been recognized as the most important way to reduce the transmission of potentially deadly bacteria in healthcare settings. Healthcare-associated infections (HAIs) are a major, yet often preventable, threat to patient safety (Centers for Disease Control and Prevention, 2015). HAIs include central line-associated bloodstream infections (CLABSIs), catheter-associated urinary tract infections (CAUDIs), and ventilator-associated pneumonia (VAPs). Infections may also occur at surgery sites, known as surgical site infections.

Based on a large sample of U.S. acute care hospitals, a survey conducted by the CDC found that on any given day, about 1 in 25 hospital patients has at least one HAI. There were an estimated 722,000 HAIs in U.S. acute care hospitals in 2011. About 75,000 hospital patients with HAIs died during their hospitalizations and more than half of all HAIs occurred outside of the intensive care unit (Centers for Disease Control and Prevention, 2014; Caplan, Williams, Daly, & Abraham, 2004). Tables 9.2 and 9.3 show detailed estimates.

CLABSIs (central line infections) result in thousands of deaths each year and billions of dollars in added costs to the U.S. healthcare

TABLE 9.2. **Estimates of healthcare-associated infections occurring in acute care hospitals in the United States, 2011.**

Major Site of Infection	Estimated No.
Pneumonia	157,500
Gastrointestinal illness	123,100
Urinary tract infections	93,300
Primary bloodstream infections	71,900
Surgical site infections from any inpatient surgery	157,500
Other types of infections	118,500
Estimated total number of infections in hospitals	**721,800**

TABLE 9.3. **Estimates of selected* healthcare-associated infections occurring in acute care hospitals, 2011± or 2012†.**

Type of Healthcare-Associated Infection	Estimated No.
Catheter-associated urinary tract infections (wards and critical care units)	54,500†
Central line-associated bloodstream infections (medical–surgical and critical care units)	30,100†
Surgical-site infections associated with 10 surgical procedures	53,700†
Hospital-onset Clostridium difficile infections (all hospital locations)	107,700±

Note: * Infections closely tied to performance measures reported as part of the CMS Hospital Quality Reporting Program

system, yet these infections are preventable. CAUTIs (urinary tract infections) are the most common type of healthcare-associated infection reported to the National Healthcare Safety Network (Centers for Disease Control and Prevention, 2012a). Among UTIs acquired in the hospital, approximately 75% are associated with a urinary catheter and between 15% and 25% of hospitalized patients receive urinary catheters during their hospital stays. Prolonged use of the urinary catheters is the most important risk factor for developing a CAUTI (Institute for Healthcare Improvement, 2014a). Urinary catheters should only be used for appropriate indications and should be removed as soon as they are no longer needed.

A surgical site infection is an infection that occurs after surgery in the part of the body where the surgery took place. Surgical site infections can sometimes be superficial infections involving the skin only. Other surgical site infections are more serious and can involve tissues under the skin, organs, or implanted material.

Besides hand hygiene, studies have shown that other preventive measures for CLABSIs and CAUTIs are to use them only if necessary, remove them as soon as possible, and use maximal sterile barrier precautions (Centers for Disease Control and Prevention, 2012b; Institute for Healthcare Improvement, 2014a). For CLABSIs, the best site to minimize infections and mechanical complications should be selected, and the site should be covered with sterile gauze or sterile, transparent, semipermeable dressings (Centers for Disease Control and Prevention, 2012b). For the prevention of VAP, besides hygiene, elevating the head of the bed, providing mouth care, maintaining cuff pressure, changing the respiratory circuit only when necessary, continuous suctioning and other interventions, need to be consistently completed (Institute for Healthcare Improvement, 2014b).

Mouth care
(by Elizabeth Hetrick and Laura Sinko, University of Michigan)
The importance of proper oral hygiene on patients' clinical outcomes and overall well-being is well documented. The absence of proper mouth care in an inpatient setting has the potential to cause hospital-acquired infections, particularly respiratory disease, as well as a decline in nutritional status and a decrease in overall quality of life (Hanne, Ingelise, Linda, & Ulrich, 2012; Paulsson, Wardh, Andersson, & Ohrn, 2008; Miller & Rubenstein, 1987; Ohrn, Sjoden, Wahlin, & Elf, 2001). For those patients undergoing chemotherapy or oral intubation, a lack of oral care may increase risk for oral mucositis or ventilator-associated pneumonia (VAP), lead to discomfort, cause a delay or discontinuation of treatment, and lead to increased length of stay (Koenig & Truwit, 2006; Miller & Rubenstein,1987; Ohrn et al., 2001; Richards, Edwards, Culver, & Gaynes, 2000; Scannapieco, Bush, & Paju, 2003; Sona, Zack, & Schallom, 2009; Sousa, Silva Filho, Mendes, Moita Neto, & Prado, Jr., 2014). These consequences can be costly, uncomfortable, and even life-threatening.

Sousa and colleagues (2014) investigated dental plaque build-up among patients on non-critical care units. The researchers found that even short periods of hospitalization in non-intensive care units impact oral health. Without proper oral hygiene practices, dental plaque biofilm can accumulate among non-ICU patients, leading to an onset of or an increase in gingival inflammation. Researchers note that it is important to control dental biofilm to prevent oral and respiratory diseases (Seneviratne, Zhang, & Samaranayake, 2011; Sousa et al., 2014). Accumulations of biofilm can exacerbate preexisting oral conditions or cause new conditions, such as pulmonary infections, to occur (Sousa et al., 2014).

Among oncology patients, a different concern arises. Oral mucositis can develop as a result of chemotherapeutic or radiotherapeutic agents used in the treatment of cancer. These treatments affect rapidly dividing cells, causing lesions to develop in the mouth (Miller & Rubenstein, 1987). The lesions occur in 20% to 40% of patients receiving conventional chemotherapy and approximately 80% of patients receiving high-dose chemotherapy (Lalla, Saunders, & Peterson, 2014). The lesions of mucositis can be incredibly painful (Miller & Rubenstein, 1987). The pain can become so severe that it negatively impacts oral intake of both nutrients and medications, and decreases patient reports of overall quality of life (Saunders et al., 2013). Saito and colleagues (2014) report that approximately half of the patients developing severe oral mucositis require changing, postponing, or discontinuing their oncology treatments. Delaying or discontinuing therapy may in turn contribute to increased morbidity, length of stay, and cost.

Sona and colleagues (2009) conducted a study of 53 hematopoietic stem-cell transplant patients to evaluate the effectiveness of oral care strategies in preventing oral mucositis. After dividing the oral care program into two periods, the "examination and trial period" (2003 and 2004) and "intensive oral care period" (2005 and 2006), the researchers concluded that oral care practices did indeed reduce oral mucositis rates from 76% of patients in 2003 to only 20% in 2006 (Sona et al., 2009). More recently, McGuire and colleagues (2013) undertook a systematic review of available literature and concluded that the use of proper oral care protocol is appropriate for both the prevention and the treatment of oral mucositis.

Pneumonia is the second most common nosocomial infection in critically ill patients, affecting 27% of these patients at some point during their stay (Koenig & Truwit, 2006). Of all these pneumonia cases, 86% are associated with mechanical ventilation (Richards et al., 2000). VAP is usually caused by aspirated bacteria that settle in the oropharynx (Pettit, McCann, Schneiderman, Farren, & Campbell, 2012). It causes fever, low blood pressure, hypoxemia, or even death. The mortality rates of VAP range from 24% to 50%, making it a leading cause of death in the intensive care unit. In addition, VAP not only puts the patient at risk, but also has an economic cost. The diagnosis of VAP leads to an increase of 4 to 13 days in the intensive care unit for the patient (Richards et al., 2000). Costs associated with VAP have been estimated between $5,000 and $20,000 per case (Richards et al., 2000). To determine the factor that oral hygiene plays in VAP, Scannapieco and colleagues (2003) conducted a systematic review of 36 empirical studies. These researchers found that mechanical and/or topical chemical disinfection interventions in the oral cavity reduced the incidence of nosocomial pneumonia by an average of 40% (Scannapieco et al., 2003). This greatly reduced the prevalence of VAP and increased the chances of patient survival.

Emotional support

Patient psychosocial distress may significantly interfere with their health outcomes and quality of life. Nurses are typically in the best position to screen for and provide timely intervention. Hospitalization, along with ongoing treatment and the need to make critical decisions, can lead to stress, anxiety, and depression. Most patients need individualized support, listening, and encouragement when hospitalized. They need the opportunity to verbalize their feelings and be listened to as they work through their concerns and make important care decisions.

Cancer patients often need to deal with difficult and physically demanding treatments (chemotherapy, radiation, etc.) and permanent impairment can occur. These treatments increase emotional distress, can cause psychological problems, and can lead to social problems (e.g., patients may not be able to work and will have reduced income as a result) (Adler & Page, 2008).

In a study of ICU patients, Hupcey (2001) found that feeling safe was an overwhelming need for them while they were in the ICU and that nurses play a major role in this. Impacting the experience of feeling safe were the need to know information, regain control, hope, and trust. When these needs were not met, patients did not feel safe and their experiences ranged from being upset or frustrated to being distressed, paranoid, or in some cases, violent (Hupcey, 2001).

Besides safety, patients in or out of the ICU need hope in order to effectively battle their illness. Nurses are responsible for assessing progress toward the development and maintenance of hope. Its presence can be powerful in the healing and coping process and the nurse has a key role in helping patients with this task (Johnson, Dahlen, & Roberts, 1997).

Positive feelings about the ICU were found to be influenced by supportive behaviors of the nursing staff (Geary, Tringali, & George, 1997). The critically ill adults had positive feelings when they felt supported by the nursing staff and negative feelings when they did not receive that care (Geary et al., 1997).

Promoting sleep
Although patients may appear to sleep in the hospital, it may not be refreshing or restorative. The reasons for this can be categorized into three groups: environmental, physiological, and psychological. These factors can work concomitantly, making sleep virtually impossible for some patients. Nurses can help their patients by understanding what influences sleep patterns and acting on this knowledge. This may include a variety of interventions, from allowing patients to carry out their own bedtime routine to explaining to elderly people how their sleeping patterns change with age.

Insomnia can lead to an increase in accidents including falls, illness, impaired cognitive functioning, problems with remembering, hospitalization, and referrals to nursing homes (Isaia et al., 2011; Reznik et al., 2011; Hilton, 1976). Patients who do not get adequate sleep scored significantly lower on the Medical Outcomes Study Cognitive Scale than controls, thereby reflecting problems with concentration, memory, reasoning, and problem-solving (Zammit, Weiner, Damato, Sillup, & McMillan, 1992). In a study by Breslau, Roth, Rosenthal, and Andreski (1996), patients with insomnia were nearly four times more likely to suffer major depression than those without insomnia.

Nursing actions designed to promote sleep include: reducing the noise, keeping interruptions to only those that are required, being sure the patient is clean and dry, administering pain medication close to time of sleep, keeping lights off or dimmed and blinds down, and maintaining diurnal rhythm (sleep and awake times) of the patients (i.e., not waking patients early if not necessary).

Discharge planning

The period following hospital discharge is a vulnerable time for patients and families, not only because they are recovering from an acute illness and consequently have to adjust to new medications, treatments, and other interventions, but also because they must recover from the hospitalization itself (as described in the beginning of this chapter) (Burke, Whitfield, & Prochazka, 2013; Jencks, Williams, & Coleman, 2009). The role of the hospital discharge planning process is to bridge the gap between the care provided in the hospital and the care needed at home. Nurses are uniquely positioned to provide discharge planning since they are present with patients in the hospital and knowledgeable about the care that will be needed post-hospitalization as well as the resources the patient has available to them. However, this care is often missed. Studies have shown that discharge planning is not completed in a quality and timely manner. Patients report that there is a significant decline in the level of care they receive after discharge. They suffer a whole host of problems which often leads to readmission to the hospital and/or adverse events. For Medicare patients, 20% are readmitted within 30 days after discharge. In another study, reports on the experiences of family members of the hospital discharge planning process indicated that the needs of family members were often not addressed in the hospital discharge process and that discharge planning and execution is in need of improvement (Bauer, Fitzgerald, Koch, & King, 2011).

Discharge planning has many different meanings to nurses. For some, discharge planning is confined to reviewing and printing a plan for the patient and then going over it with the patient (or their family) when they are ready to leave the hospital. For other nurses, it is a comprehensive analysis of patient and family needs they will have after they return home or to the community and the implementation of a plan to ensure the patient receives the care they need after they leave the hospital. In other words, it has been noted that some believe that nurses involved in discharge planning should take more of an administrative role, whereas others see the roles of nurses to be teaching patients and families complex post-discharge treatments, such as breathing treatments, decubitus and skin care, feeding tubes, and home injections (Holliman, Dziegielewski, & Teare, 2003).

Studies have shown the positive influence of discharge planning (Psotka & Teerlink, 2013). Higher overall patient satisfaction and satisfaction with discharge planning were found to be associated with lower 30-day risk-standardized hospital readmission rates after adjusting for clinical quality (Boulding, Glickman, Manary, Schulman, & Staelin, 2011). There have been a number of trials conducted which study the impact of discharge planning. In a Cochran review of 24 trials, discharge planning is shown to result in shorter lengths of hospital stay (mean difference length of stay –0.91, 95% CI –1.55 to –0.27, 10 trials) and fewer readmissions, at least for medical patients (mean difference length of stay –0.91, 95% CI –1.55 to –0.27, 10 trials) (Shepperd et al., 2013). The impact of discharge planning on mortality, health outcomes and cost, however, remains uncertain.

Patient teaching

Hospitalized patients and their care givers have major needs for information and skill. The nurse is in a key position to provide that education or ensure that it is provided by others.

Many studies have been conducted to show the outcome of education and training for patients. A sample of these studies will be reviewed here but it is by no means comprehensive.

In one study, patients were surveyed to determine awareness and knowledge regarding risks and consequences of and prevention of surgical site infection (SSI), and found that 26% of respondents thought that education for SSI prevention could be improved and that 16% could not recall discussing SSI risks and prevention with a healthcare worker at all. Only 60% of patients recalled receiving an informational flyer in the hospital (Anderson et al., 2013). In another study,

40% of patients surveyed thought that education regarding CLABSI could be improved, 22% could not recall discussing risks of infection of a central line with a healthcare worker, and only 46% of patients recalled receiving an informational flyer in the hospital regarding CLABSI (Anderson, Ottum, Zerbel, Sethi, & Safdar, 2013).

Nourishment

The outcomes of poor nutritional status in hospitalized patients include increased length of stay, readmissions, susceptibility to other illnesses, poor quality of life, increased risk of unsuccessful outcomes of treatment, and higher costs. Mortality may also be increased in hospitalized malnourished older people (Friedmann, Jense, Smiciklas-Wright, & McCamish, 1997; Rasmussen et al., & Wengler, 2004; Tappenden et al., 2013).

Covinsky and colleagues (1999) found that malnutrition leads to adverse outcomes including greater mortality, delayed functional recovery, and higher rates of nursing home use. These adverse outcomes were not explained by greater acute illness severity, comorbidity, or functional dependence in malnourished patients on hospital admission (Covinsky et al., 1999). Söderström, Rosenblad, Adolfsson, Saletti, and Bergkvist (2014) found that nutritional status independently predicted preterm death in people aged 65 years and older. In another study, Lim and colleagues (2012) discovered that malnourished patients (29%) had longer hospital stays (6.9 ± 7.3 days vs. 4.6 ± 5.6 days, $p < 0.001$) and were more likely to be readmitted within 15 days (adjusted relative risk = 1.9, 95% CI 1.1–3.2, $p = 0.025$). Mortality was higher in malnourished patients at 1 year (34% vs. 4.1%), 2 years (42.6% vs. 6.7%), and 3 years (48.5% vs. 9.9%); $p < 0.001$ for all. Overall, malnutrition was a significant predictor of mortality (adjusted hazard ratio = 4.4, 95% CI 3.3–6.0, $p < 0.001$). Increased length of hospital stay has also been found by other researchers (Chima et al., 1997; Heersink, Brown, Diamaria-Ghalili, & Locher, 2010; Ordóñez, Madalozzo Schieferdecker, Cestonaro, Cardoso Neto, & Ligocki Campos, 2013).

Higher costs are associated with malnourished patients. The compromised health status increases costs by extending length of stay in the hospital, promoting the development of comorbidities, and requiring more intensive care. The most costly complication associated with poor nutrition status is acute respiratory infections ($13,350 to $19,530 per hospitalization), while institutional long-term care is the greatest chronic cost contributor across many diseases ($77,000 per year of care) (Cangelosi, Rodday, Saunders, & Cohen, 2013; Heersink et al., 2010; Ordóñez et al., 2013; Pasquini, Neder, Araujo-Junqueira, & De-Souza, 2012).

Factors associated with inadequate food intake were poor appetite, higher BMI, diagnosis of infection or cancer, delirium, and need for assistance with feeding (Mudge et al., 2011a). Ross, Mudge, Young, and Banks (2011b) conducted a qualitative study with staff members to determine what the barriers were to maintaining an adequate nutritional level by inpatients. Study participants identified patient-level barriers to nutrition care, such as not following nutrition plans, and hospital-level barriers including lack of enough nursing staff, lack of multidisciplinary collaboration and communication, lack of a coordinated approach, and a lack of a sense of shared responsibility for nutrition care. All staff talked about competing activities at meal times and felt disempowered to prioritize nutrition in the acute hospital setting. In another study, the intervention of mealtime assistance significantly improved nutritional status of hospitalized patients and increased the achievement of adequate energy intake (Young, Mudge, Banks, Ross, & Daniels, 2013).

Bathing and skin care
A daily shower or bath is a deeply ingrained American habit. For many people, the bath is very important psychologically to ensure they smell and look good. Taking a bath is important for hygiene, but it is also a great tool for creating relaxation and sense of well-being.

As far as the use of bathing to decrease infection, there have been a series of studies using daily chlorhexidine-impregnated washcloths. In a multicenter, cluster-randomized, non-blinded crossover trial evaluating the effect of chlorhexidine on the acquisition of multidrug-resistant organisms (MDROs) and the incidence of CLABSIs, the overall rate of MDRO acquisition was 5.10 cases per 1,000 patient-days with chlorhexidine bathing versus 6.60 cases with nonantimicrobial washcloths ($p < 0.03$), the equivalent of a 23% lower rate with chlorhexidine bathing (Climo et al., 2013). The overall rate of hospital-acquired bloodstream infections was 4.78 cases per 1,000 patient-days with chlorhexidine bathing versus 6.60 cases per 1,000 patient-days with nonantimicrobial washcloths ($p < 0.007$), a 28% lower rate with chlorhexidine-impregnated washcloths.

In another study, 7,102 and 7,699 adult medical patients were admitted to control and intervention groups, respectively. The control group received daily bathing with soap and water while the intervention patients were bathed daily with chlorhexidine-impregnated cloths (Kassakian, Mermel, Jefferson, Parenteau, & Machan, 2011). The intervention group had a 64% reduced risk of developing the composite incidence of methicillin-resistant Staphylococcus aureus (MRSA) and Vancomycin-resistant Enteroccocus HAIs (hazard ratio, 0.36 [95% CI, 0.2–0.8] $p > .01$). We have not been able to find studies which investigated patients who received no bath at all.

Although expert opinion maintains that there is a relationship between skin care and pressure ulcer development, there is a paucity of research to support this assumption. How and the frequency with which the skin is cleansed may make a difference. One study found that the incidence of Stages I and II pressure ulcers could be reduced by educating the staff and using body wash and skin protection products (Thompson, Langemo, Anderson, Hanson, & Hunter, 2005).

Interdisciplinary rounds
In 2000, the Joint Commission added a standard to their accrediting process which states that patient care, treatment, and rehabilitation should be planned, evaluated, and revised by an interdisciplinary collaborative team. This is a team made up of individuals from various healthcare disciplines that plan together for the care of the patient. According to the standard, conferences or rounds should take place from three times a week to every day.

Care by a multidisciplinary group of providers has been shown to have many benefits (i.e., improvement in the health outcome of elderly inpatients after discharge, reduced readmissions, increased resection rate of lung cancers, reduced medication variance, better treatments, increased survival rates, and hypertension control) (Adorian, Silverberg, Tomer, & Wamosher, 1990; Davison et al., 2004; Junor, Hole, & Gillis, 1994; Rubenstein et al., 1984; Sim & Joyner, 2002; Townsend-Gervis, Cornell, & Vardaman, 2014). Decisions from a multidisciplinary discussion have been found to be more accurate and effective than the sum of individual opinions (no one of us is as smart as all of us). Other benefits include consistency in the standard of patient management (Ruhstaller, Roe, Thurlimann, & Nicoll, 2006). The multidisciplinary decision-making process has been shown to greatly reduce the wide variations in decisions made by professionals acting independently (Adorian et al., 1990; Caplan et al., 2004; Chang et al., 2001).

Interdisciplinary rounds held on medical units resulted in fewer adverse events. The rate of adverse events was 3.9 per 100 patient days for the intervention unit compared with 7.2 per 100 patient-days, respectively, for the control (O'Leary et al., 2011a). In another study, a combination of the Situation Background Assessment Recommendation (SBAR) protocol, a readmissions risk assessment and daily interdisciplinary rounds on medical–surgical units resulted in an improvement in timely removal of urinary catheters from 78% to 94%, and a decrease in readmissions from 14.5% to 2.1% (Townsend et al., 2014). Physicians and nurses valued the pharmacists' services and reported that this collaboration improved patients' therapy. Instituting multidisciplinary rounds resulted in a drop in LOS by one day and an increase in patient satisfaction (Katz, 2008). Daily rounds by a multidisciplinary team were associated with lower mortality among medical ICU patients (Kim, Barnato, Angus, Fleisher, & Kahn, 2010).

O'Leary and colleagues (2010) conducted a study where they assigned hospitalists to specific units. They interviewed nurses and physicians pre- and post-localization. After localization, a higher percentage of patients' nurses and physicians were able to correctly identify one another (93% vs. 71%; $p < 0.001$ and 58% vs. 36%; $p < 0.001$, respectively). Nurses and physicians reported more frequent communication after localization (68% vs. 50%; $p < 0.001$ and 74% vs. 61%; $p < 0.001$, respectively). Nurse–physician agreement was significantly improved for two aspects of the plan of care: planned tests and anticipated length of stay. O'Leary and colleagues (2011b) also completed a study of the impact of interdisciplinary rounds on a hospitalist unit. They found that nurses rated communication and teamwork higher than on the control unit that did not conduct these rounds.

Summary

In this chapter, research on the consequences of not providing nursing care are summarized. Overall missed nursing care has been shown to result in an increase in patient falls and the adverse events of skin breakdown and pressure ulcers, medication errors, new infections, IVs running dry, and IVs infiltrating. The impact of missing specific elements of nursing care—that is ambulation, turning, medication administration, hand washing and other infection control procedures, mouth care, promoting sleep, emotional support, discharge planning, patient teaching, nourishment, bathing and skin care, and interdisciplinary rounds—are summarized.

References

Adler, N. E., & Page, A. E. K. (Eds.). (2008). *Cancer care for the whole patient: Meeting psychosocial needs.* Washington, DC: National Academies Press.

Adorian, D., Silverberg, D. S., Tomer, D., & Wamosher, Z. (1990). Group discussions with the health care team – a method of improving care of hypertension in general practice. *Journal of Human Hypertension, 4*(3), 265–268.

Allman, R. M., Goode, P. S., Patrick, M. M., Burst, N., & Bartolucci, A. A. (1995). Pressure ulcer risk factors among hospitalized patients with activity limitation. *The Journal of the American Medical Association, 273*(11), 865–870.

American College of Emergency Physicians. (2013). Medicare's hospital readmission reduction program FAQ. Retrieved from https://www.acep.org/Physician-Resources/Practice-Resources/Administration/Financial-Issues-/-Reimbursement/Medicare-s-Hospital-Read

Anderson, M., Ottum, A., Zerbel, S., Sethi, A., Gaines, M. E., & Safdar, N. (2013). A survey to examine patient awareness, knowledge, and perceptions regarding the risks and consequences of surgical site infections. *American Journal of Infection Control, 41*(12), 1293–1295.

Anderson, M., Ottum, A., Zerbel, S., Sethi, A., & Safdar, N. (2013). Are hospitalized patients aware of the risks and consequences of central line-associated bloodstream infections? *American Journal of Infection Control, 41*(12), 1275–1277.

Bansal, C., Scott, R., Stewart, D., & Cockerell, C. J. (2005). Decubitus ulcers: A review of the literature. *International Journal of Dermatology, 44*(10), 805–810.

Barker, K. N., Flynn, E. A., Pepper, G. A., Bates, D. W., & Mikeal, R. L. (2002). Medication errors observed in 36 health care facilities. *Archives of Internal Medicine, 162*(16), 1897–1903.

Bauer, M., Fitzgerald, L., Koch, S., & King, S. (2011). How family carers view hospital discharge planning for the older person with a dementia. *Dementia, 10*(3), 3317–3323.

Boulding, W., Glickman, S. W., Manary, M. P., Schulman, K. A., & Staelin, R. (2011). Relationship between patient satisfaction with inpatient care and hospital readmission within 30 days. *The American Journal of Managed Care, 17*(1), 41–48.

Breslau, N., Roth, T., Rosenthal, L., & Andreski, P. (1996). Sleep disturbance and psychiatric disorders: a longitudinal epidemiological study of young adults. *Biological Psychiatry, 39*(6), 411–418.

Burke, R. E., Whitfield, E., & Prochazka, A. V. (2013). Effect of a hospital-run postdischarge clinic on outcomes. *Journal of Hospital Medicine, 9*(1), 7–12.

Callen, B. L., Mahoney, J. E., Grieves, C. B., Wells, T. J., & Enloe, M. (2004). Frequency of hallway ambulation by hospitalized older adults on medical units of an academic hospital. *Geriatric Nursing, 25*(4), 212–217.

Cangelosi, M. J., Rodday, A. M., Saunders, T., & Cohen, J. T. (2013). Evaluation of the economic burden of diseases associated with poor nutrition status. *Journal of Parenteral and Enteral Nutrition.* Advance online publication. doi: 10.1177/0148607113514612

Caplan, G. A., Williams, A. J., Daly, B., & Abraham, K. (2004). A randomized, controlled trial of comprehensive geriatric assessment and multidisciplinary intervention after discharge of elderly patients in an emergency department – the DEED ll study. *Journal of the American Geriatrics Society, 52*(9), 1417–1423.

Centers for Disease Control and Prevention. (2012a). Catheter-associated urinary tract infections (CAUTI). Retrieved from http://www.cdc.gov/HAI/ca_uti/uti.html

Centers for Disease Control and Prevention. (2012b). Central line-associated bloodstream infection (CLABSI). Retrieved from http://www.cdc.gov/HAI/bsi/bsi.html

Centers for Disease Control and Prevention. (2014). Healthcare-associated infections (HAIs): Data and statistics. Retrieved from http://www.cdc.gov/HAI/surveillance/index.html

Centers for Disease Control and Prevention. (2015). *National and state healthcare-associated infections (HAI) progress report.* Retrieved from http://www.cdc.gov/HAI/pdfs/progress-report/hai-progress-report.pdf

Centers for Medicare and Medicaid Services. (2008). Medicare and Medicaid move aggressively to encourage greater patient safety in hospitals and reduce never events. Retrieved from http://www.cms.gov/Newsroom/MediaReleaseDatabase/Press-releases/2008-Press-releases-items/2008-07-313.html

Chang, J. H., Vines, E., Bertsch, H., Fraker, D. L., Czerniecki, B. J., Rosato, E. F., ... Solin, L. J. (2001). The impact of a multidisciplinary breast cancer center on recommendations for patient management: The University of Pennsylvania experience. *Cancer, 91*(7), 1231–1237.

Chima, C. S., Barco, K., Dewitt, M. L., Maeda, M., Teran, J. C., & Mullen, K. D. (1997). Relationship of nutritional status to length of stay, hospital costs, and discharge status of patients hospitalized in the medicine service. *Journal of the American Dietetic Association, 97*(9), 975–978.

Climo, M. W., Yokoe, D. S., Warren, D. K., Perl, T. M., Bolon, M., Herwaldt, L. A., ... Wong, E. S. (2013). Effect of daily chlorhexidine bathing on hospital-acquired infection. *The New England Journal of Medicine, 368*(6), 533–542.

Convertino, V. A. (1997). Cardiovascular consequences of bed rest: effect on maximal oxygen uptake. *Medicine and Science in Sports and Exercise, 29*(2), 191–196.

Convertino, V. A., Bloomfield, S. A., & Greenleaf, J. E. (1997). An overview of the issues: Physiological effects of bed rest and restricted physical activity. *Medicine and Science in Sports and Exercise, 29*(2), 187–190.

Coussement, J., De Paepe, L., Schwendimann, R., Denhaerynck, K., Dejaeger, E., & Milisen, K. (2008). Interventions for preventing falls in acute- and chronic-care hospitals: A systematic review and meta-analysis. *Journal of the American Geriatrics Society, 56*(1), 29–36.

Covinsky, K. E., Martin, G. E., Beyth, R. J., Justice, A. C., Sehgal, A. R., & Landefeld, C. S. (1999). The relationship between clinical assessments of nutritional status and adverse outcomes in older hospitalized medical patients. *Journal of the American Geriatrics Society, 47*(5), 532–538.

Creditor, M. C. (1993). Hazards of hospitalization of the elderly. *Annals of Internal Medicine, 118*(3), 219–223.

Darling, H., Shea, G., & Linscott, K. (2008). Serious adverse events working group. Report presented at the National Quality Forum, National Priorities Partners Meeting 2008, Washington, D.C.

Davison, A. G., Eraut, C. D., Haque, A. S., Doffman, S., Tanqueray, A., Trask, C. W., ... Sharma, A. (2004). Telemedicine for multidisciplinary lung cancer meetings. *Journal of Telemedicine and Telecare, 10*(3), 140–143.

DeFloor, T., De Bacquer, D., & Grypdonck, M. (2005). The effect of various combinations of turning and pressure reducing devices on the incidence of pressure ulcers. *International Journal of Nursing Studies, 42*(1), 37–46.

Degelau, J., Belz, M., Bungum, L., Flavin, P. L., Harper, C., Leys, K., ... Webb, B. (2012). *Prevention of falls (acute care). Institute for Clinical Systems Improvement.* Retrieved from https://www.icsi.org/_asset/dcn15z/Falls-Interactive0412.pdf

Ferrari, M. A., Harrison, B. E., Campbell, C., Maddens, M., & Whall, A. L. (2010). Contributing factors associated with impulsivity-related falls in hospitalized, older adults. *Journal of Nursing Care Quality, 25*(4), 320–326.

Fick, D. M., Steis, M. R., Waller, J. L., & Inouye, S. K. (2013). Delirium superimposed on dementia is associated with prolonged length of stay and poor outcomes in hospitalized older adults. *Journal of Hospital Medicine, 8*(9), 500–505.

Friedmann, J. M., Jensen, G. L., Smiciklas-Wright, H., & McCamish, M. A. (1997). Predicting early nonelective hospital readmission in nutritionally compromised older adults. *The American Journal of Clinical Nutrition, 65*(6), 1714–1720.

Geary, P. A., Tringali, R., & George, E. (1997). Social support in critically ill adults: A replication. *Critical Care Nursing Quarterly, 20*(2), 34–41.

Graf, C. (2006). Functional decline in hospitalized older adults: It's often a consequence of hospitalization, but it doesn't have to be. *American Journal of Nursing, 106*(1), 58–67.

Gray-Micelli, D. (2008). Preventing falls in acute care. In E. Capezuti, D. Zwicker, M. Mezey, & T. Fulmer (Eds.), *Evidence based geriatric nursing protocols for best practice* (pp. 161–198). New York, NY: Springer Publishing.

Greene, C. J., Du-Pre, P., Elahi, N., Dunckley, P., & McIntyre, A. S. (2009). Omission after admission: Failure in prescribed medications being given to inpatients. *Clinical Medicine, 9*(6), 515–518.

Hanne, K., Ingelise, T., Linda, C., & Ulrich, P. P. (2012). Oral status and the need for oral health care among patients hospitalized with acute medical conditions. *The Journal of Clinical Nursing, 21*(19–20), 2851–2859.

Heersink, J. T., Brown, C. J., Dimaria-Ghalili, R. A., & Locher, J. L. (2010). Undernutrition in hospitalized older adults: Patterns and correlates, outcomes, and opportunities for intervention with a focus on processes of care. *Journal of Nutrition for the Elderly, 29*(1), 4–41.

Hilton, B. A. (1976). Quantity and quality of patients' sleep and sleep-disturbing factors in a respiratory intensive care unit. *Journal of Advanced Nursing, 1*(6), 453–468.

Hirsch, C. H., Sommers, L., Olsen, A., Mullen, L., & Winograd, C. H. (1990). The natural history of functional morbidity in hospitalized older patients. *Journal of the American Geriatrics Society, 38*(12), 1296–1303.

Holliman, D., Dziegielewski, S. F., & Teare, R. (2003). Differences and similarities between social work and nurse discharge planners. *Health and Social Work, 28*(3), 224–231.

Hupcey, J. E. (2001). The meaning of social support for the critically ill patient. *Intensive Critical Care Nursing, 17*(4), 206–212.

Institute for Healthcare Improvement. (2014a). Catheter-associated urinary tract infection. Retrieved from http://www.ihi.org/Topics/CAUTI/Pages/default.aspx

Institute for Healthcare Improvement. (2014b). Ventilator-associated pneumonia. Retrieved from http://www.ihi.org/topics/VAP/Pages/default.aspx

Isaia, G., Corsinovi, L., Bo, M., Santos-Pereira, P., Michelis, G., Aimonino, N., & Zanocchi, M. (2011). Insomnia among hospitalized elderly patients: Prevalence, clinical characteristics and risk factors. *Archives of Gerontology and Geriatrics, 52*(2), 133–137.

Jencks, S. F., Williams, M. V., & Coleman, E. A. (2009). Rehospitalizations among patients in the Medicare fee-for-service program. *New England Journal of Medicine, 360*(14), 1418–1428.

Johnson, L. H., Dahlen, R., & Roberts, S. L. (1997). Supporting hope in congestive heart failure patients. *Dimensions of Critical Care Nursing, 16*(2), 65–78.

Junor, E. J., Hole, D. J., & Gillis, C. R. (1994). Management of ovarian cancer: Referral to a multidisciplinary team matters. *British Journal of Cancer, 70*(2), 363–370.

Kalisch, B., Lee, S. H., & Dabney, B. (2013). Outcomes of inpatient mobilization: A literature review. *Journal of Clinical Nursing.* Advance online publication. doi: 10.1111/jocn.12315

Kalisch, B., Tschannen, D., & Lee, K. H. (2012). Missed nursing care, staffing, and patient falls. *Journal of Nursing Care Quality, 27*(1), 6–12.

Kalisch, B., & Xie, B. (2014). Errors of omission: Missed nursing care. *Western Journal of Nursing Research.* Advance online publication. doi: 10.1177/0193945914531859

Kamel, H. K., Iqbal, M. A., Mogallapu, R., Maas, D., & Hoffmann, R. G. (2003). Time to ambulation after hip fracture surgery: Relation to hospitalization outcomes. *The Journals of Gerontology. Series A, Biological Sciences and Medical Sciences, 58*(11), 1042–1045.

Kanaan, A. O., Donovan, J. L., Duchin, N. P., Field, T. S., Tjia, J., Cutrona, S. L., … Gurwitz, J. H. (2013). Adverse drug events after hospital discharge in older adults: Types, severity, and involvement of Beers Criteria medications. *Journal of the American Geriatrics Society, 61*(11), 1894–1899.

Kansagara, D., Englander, H., Salanitro, A., Kagen, D., Theobald, C., Freeman, M., & Kripalani, S. (2011). Risk prediction models for hospital readmission: A systematic review. *Journal of the American Medical Association, 306*(15), 1688–1698.

Kassakian, S. Z., Mermel, L. A., Jefferson, J. A., Parenteau, S. L., & Machan, J. T. (2011). Impact of chlorhexidine bathing on hospital-acquired infections among general medical patients. *Infection Control and Hospital Epidemiology, 32*(3), 238–243.

Katz, P. S. (2008, July). The push is on for multidisciplinary rounds: Are hospitalists willing to forgo some autonomy to make the concept work? *Today's Hospitalist.* Retrieved from http://www.todayshospitalist.com/index.php?b=articles_read&cnt=602

Kim, M. M., Barnato, A. E., Angus, D. C., Fleisher, L. A., & Kahn, J. M. (2010). The effect of multidisciplinary care teams on intensive care unit mortality. *Archives of Internal Medicine, 170*(4), 369–376.

Koenig, S. M., & Truwit, J. D. (2006). Ventilator-associated pneumonia: Diagnosis, treatment, and prevention. *Clinical Microbiology Reviews, 19*(4), 637–657.

Kosiak, M. (1959). Etiology and pathology of ischemic ulcers. *Archives of Physical Medicine and Rehabilitation, 40*(2), 62–69.

Kosiak, M., Kubicek, W. G., Olson, M., Danz, J. N., & Kottke, F. J. (1958). Evaluation of pressure as a factor in the production of ischial ulcers. *Archives of Physical Medicine and Rehabilitation, 39*(10), 623–629.

Krishnagopalan, S., Johnson, E. W., Low, L. L., & Kaufman, L. J. (2002). Body positioning of intensive care patients: Clinical practice versus standards. *Critical Care Medicine, 30*(11), 2588–2592.

Krumholz, H. M. (2013). Post-hospital syndrome – An acquired transient condition of generalized risk. *New England Journal of Medicine, 368*(2), 100–102.

Lim, S. L., Ong, K. C., Chan, Y. H., Loke, W. C., Ferguson, M., & Daniels, L. (2012). Malnutrition and its impact on cost of hospitalization, length of stay, readmission and 3-year mortality. *Clinical Nutrition, 31*(3), 345–350.

Lalla, R. V., Saunders, D. P., & Peterson, D. E. (2014). Chemotherapy or radiation-induced oral mucositis. *Dental Clinics of North America, 58*(2), 341–349.

Lyder, C. H. (2003). Pressure ulcer prevention and management. *The Journal of the American Medical Association, 289*(2), 223–226.

Mahoney, J. E., Sager, M. A., & Jalaluddin, M. (1998). New walking dependence associated with hospitalization for acute medical illness: Incidence and significance. *The Journals of Gerontology. Series A, Biological Sciences and Medical Sciences, 53*(4), M307–M312.

Makic, M. B. F., Rauen, C., Watson, R., & Poteet, A. W. (2014). Examining the evidence to guide practice: Challenging practice habits. *Critical Care Nurse, 34*(2). Retrieved from http://www.aacn.org/wd/Cetests/media/C1423.pdf

McGuire, D. B., Fulton, J. S., Park, J., Brown, C. G., Correa, M. E., P., Eilers, J., ... Oberle-Edwards, L. K. (2013). Systematic review of basic oral care for the management of oral mucositis in cancer patients. *Supportive Cancer Care, 21*(11), 3165–3177.

Miller, R., & Rubenstein, L. (1987). Oral health care for hospitalized patients: The nurses role. *The Journal of Nursing Education, 26*(9), 362–366.

Morandi, A., Bellelli, G., Vasileyskis, E. E., Turco, R., Guerini, F., Torpilliesi, T., ... Trabucchi, M. (2013). Predictors of rehospitalization among elderly patients admitted to a rehabilitation hospital: The role of polypharmacy, functional status, and length of stay. *Journal of the American Medical Directors Association, 14*(10), 761–767.

Mudge, A. M., Kasper, K., Clair, A., Redfern, H., Bell, J. J., Barras, M. A., ... Pachana, N. A. (2011A). Recurrent readmissions in medical patients: A prospective study. *Journal of Hospital Medicine, 6*(2), 61–67.

Mudge, A. M., Ross, L. J., Young, A. M., Isenring, E. A., & Banks, M. D. (2011B). Helping understand nutritional gaps in the elderly (HUNGER): A prospective study of patient factors associated with inadequate nutritional intake in older medical patients. *Clinical Nutrition, 30*(3), 320–325.

Mundy, L. M., Leet, T. L., Darst, K., Schnitzler, M. A., & Dunagan, W. C. (2003). Early mobilization of patients hospitalized with community-acquired pneumonia. *Chest, 124*(3), 883–889.

Munin, M. C., Rudy, T. E., Glynn, N. W., Crossett, L. S., & Rubash, H. E. (1998). Early inpatient rehabilitation after elective hip and knee arthroplasty. *Journal of the American Medical Association, 279*(11), 847–852.

Norton, D., McLaren, R., & Exton-Smith, A. (1975). *An investigation of geriatric nurse problems in hospitals.* Edinburgh, UK: Churchill Livingston.

O'Leary, K. J., Buck, R., Fligiel, H. M., Haviley, C., Slade, M. E., Landler, M. P., ... Wayne, D. B. (2011a). Structured interdisciplinary rounds in a medical teaching unit: Improving patient safety. *Archives of Internal Medicine, 171*(7), 678–684.

O'Leary, K. J., Haviley, C., Slade, M. E., Shah, H. M., Lee, J., & Williams, M. V. (2011b). Improving teamwork: Impact of structured interdisciplinary rounds on a hospitalist unit. *Journal of Hospital Medicine, 6*(2), 88–93.

O'Leary, K. J., Wayne, D. B., Haviley, C., Slade, M. E., Lee, J., & Williams, M. V. (2010). Improving teamwork: Impact of structured interdisciplinary rounds on a medical teaching unit. *Journal of General Internal Medicine, 25*(8), 826–832.

Ohrn, K. E., Sjoden, P. O., Wahlin, Y. B., & Elf, M. (2001). Oral health and quality of life among patients with head and neck cancer or haematological malignancies. *Supportive Care in Cancer, 9,* 528–538.

Oliver, D., Hopper, A., & Seed, P. (2000). Do hospital fall prevention programs work? A systematic review. *Journal of the American Geriatrics Society, 48*(12), 1679–1689.

Oot-Giromini, B., Bidwell, F. C., Heller, N. B., Parks, M. L., Prebish, E. M., Wicks, P., & Williams, P. M. (1989). Pressure ulcer prevention versus treatment, comparative product cost study. *Decubitus, 2*(3), 52–54.

Ordóñez, A. M., Madalozzo Schieferdecker, M. E., Cestonaro, T., Cardoso, N. J., & Ligocki Campos, A. C. (2013). Nutritional status influences the length of stay and clinical outcomes in hospitalized patients in internal medicine wards. *Nutricion Hospitalaria, 28*(4), 1313–1320.

Paulsson, G., Wardh, I., Andersson, P., & Ohrn, K. (2008). Comparison of oral health assessments between nursing staff and patients on medical wards. *European Journal of Cancer Care, 17*(1), 49–55.

Pasero, C., & Belden, J. (2006). Evidence-based perianesthesia care: Accelerated postoperative recovery programs. *Journal of Perianesthesia Nursing, 21*(3), 168–176.

Pasquini, T. A., Neder, H. D., Araujo-Junqueira, L., & De-Souza, D. A. (2012). Clinical outcome of protein-energy malnourished patients in a Brazilian university hospital. *Brazilian Journal of Medical and Biological Research, 45*(12), 1301–1307.

Pettit, S. L., McCann, A. L., Schneiderman, E. D., Farren, E. A., & Campbell, P. R. (2012). Dimensions of oral care practices in Texas hospitals. *Journal of Dental Hygiene, 86*(2), 91–103.

Price, P., & Fowlow, B. (1994). Research-based practice: Early ambulation for PTCA patients. *Canadian Journal of Cardiovascular Nursing, 5*(1), 23–25.

Psotka, M. A., & Teerlink, J. R. (2013). Strategies to prevent postdischarge adverse events among hospitalized patients with heart failure. *Heart Failure Clinics, 9*(3), 303–320.

Rasmussen, H. H., Kondrup, J., Staun, M., Ladefoged, K., Kristensen, H., & Wengler, A. (2004). Prevalence of patients at nutritional risk in Danish hospitals. *Clinical Nutrition, 23*(5), 1009–1015.

Reddy, M., Gill, S. S., & Rochon, P. A. (2006). Preventing pressure ulcers: A systematic review. *Journal of the American Medical Association, 296*(8), 974–84.

Reznik, R., Mehta, B., Thirumala, R., Lessnau, K., Difabrizio, L., Rogers, M., & Posner, D. (2011, May). Sleep quality in hospitalized patients – A prospective study safety and outcomes. Presented at the American Thoracic Society International Conference, Denver, CO.

Richards, M. J., Edwards, J. R., Culver, D. H., & Gaynes, R. P. (2000). Nosocomial infections in medical intensive care units in the United States. *Infection Control and Hospital Epidemiology, 21*, 510–515.

Ross, L. J., Mudge, A. M., Young, A. M., & Banks, M. (2011). Everyone's problem but nobody's job: Staff perceptions and explanations for poor nutritional intake in older medical patients. *Nutrition & Dietetics, 68*(1), 41–46.

Rubenstein, L. Z., Josephson, K. R., Wieland, G. D., English, P. A., Sayre, R. L., & Kane, R. L. (1984). Effectiveness of a geriatric evaluation unit: A randomized clinical trial. *The New England Journal of Medicine, 311*(26), 1664–1670.

Ruhstaller, T., Roe, H., Thurlimann, B., & Nicoll, J. J. (2006). The multidisciplinary meeting: An indispensible aid to communication between different specialties. *European Journal of Cancer, 42*(15), 2459–2462.

Russo, C. A., & Elixhauser, A. (2006). Hospitalizations related to pressure sores, 2003. *Agency for Healthcare Research and Quality: Healthcare Cost and Utilization Project, Statistical brief #3.* Retrieved from http://www.hcup-us.ahrq.gov/reports/statbriefs/sb3.pdf

Rutledge, D. N., Donaldson, N. E., & Pravikoff, D. S. (1998). Fall risk assessment and prevention in healthcare facilities. *Online Journal of Clinical Innovations, 1*(9), 1–33.

Sadatsafavi, M., Lynd, L. D., & FitzGerald, M. (2013). Post-hospital syndrome in adults with asthma: A case-crossover study. *Allergy, Asthma & Clinical Immunology, 9*(1), 49.

Sagnga, F., Landi, F., Ruggiero, C., Corsonello, A., Vetrano, D. L., Lattanzio, F., ... Onder, G. (2014). Polypharmacy and health outcomes among older adults discharged from hospital: Results from the CRIME study. *Geriatrics & Gerontology International.* Advance online publication. doi: 10.1111/ggi.12241

Saito, H., Watanabe, Y., Sato, K., Ikawa, H., Yoshida, Y., Katakura, A., ... Sato, M. (2014). Effects of professional oral health care on reducing the risk of chemotherapy-induced oral mucositis. *Supportive Care in Cancer, 22*(11), 2935–2940.

Salcido, S. (2004). Patient turning schedules: Why and how often? *Advances in Skin and Wound Care, 17*(4 Pt 1), 156.

Saunders, D. P., Epstein, J. B., Elad, S., Allemano, J., Bossi, P., van de Wetering, M. D., ... Lalla, R. V. (2013). Systematic review of antimicrobials, mucosal coating agents, anesthetics, and analgesics for the management of oral mucositis in cancer patients. *Supportive Care in Cancer, 21*(11), 3191–3207.

Scannapieco, F. A., Bush, R. B., & Paju, S. (2003). Associations between periodontal disease and risk for atherosclerosis, cardiovascular disease, and stroke. A systematic review. *Annals of Periodontology, 8*(1), 38–53.

Schubert, M., Glass, T. R., Clarke, S. P., Aiken, L. H., Schaffert-Witvliet, B., Sloane, D. M., & De Geest, S. (2008). Rationing of nursing care and its relationship to patient outcomes: the Swiss extension of the International Hospital Outcomes Study. *International Journal for Quality in Health Care, 20*(4), 227–237.

Seneviratne, C. J., Zhang, C. F., & Samaranayake, L. P. (2011). Dental plaque biofilm in oral health and disease. *The Chinese Journal of Dental Research, 14*(2), 87–94.

Shepperd, S., Lannin, N. A., Clemson, L. M., McCluskey, A., Cameron, I. D., & Barras, S. L. (2013). Discharge planning from hospital to home. *The Cochrane Database of Systematic Reviews,* 1. doi:10.1002/14651858.CD000313.pub4

Sim, T. A., & Joyner, J. (2002). A multidisciplinary team approach to reducing medication variance. *The Joint Commission Journal on Quality Improvement, 28*(7), 403–409.

Söderström, L., Rosenblad, A., Adolfsson, E. T., Saletti, A., & Bergkvist, L. (2014). Nutritional status predicts preterm death in older people: A prospective cohort study. *Clinical Nutrition, 33*(2), 354–359.

Sona, C. S., Zack, J. E., & Schallom, M. E. (2009). The impact of a simple, low cost oral care protocol on ventilator associated pneumonia rates in a surgical intensive care unit. *Journal of Intensive Care Medicine, 24*(1), 54–62.

Sousa, L. L. A., Silva Filho, W., Mendes, R. F., Moita Neto, J. M., & Prado, Jr., R. R. (2014). Oral health of patients under short hospitalization period: Observational study. *Journal of Clinical Periodontology, 41*(6), 558–563.

Tappenden, K. A., Quatrara, B., Parkhurst, M., Malone, A. M., Fanjiang, G., & Ziegler, T. R. (2013). Critical role of nutrition in improving quality of care: An interdisciplinary call to action to address adult hospital malnutrition. *Journal of the Academy of Nutrition and Dietetics, 1131*(9), 1219–1237.

The Joint Commission. (2014). Summary data of sentinel events reviewed by The Joint Commission. Retrieved from http://www.jointcommission.org/assets/1/18/2004_to_2Q_2013_SE_Stats_-_Summary.pdf

Thomas, D. R., Goode, P. S., Tarquine, P. H., & Allman, R. M. (1996). Hospital-acquired pressure ulcers and risk of death. *Journal of the American Geriatrics Society,44*(12), 1435–1440.

Thompson, P., Langemo, D., Anderson, J., Hanson, D., & Hunter, S. (2005). Skin care protcols for pressure ulcers and incontinence in long-term care: A quasi-experimental study. *Advances in Skin & Wound Care, 18*(8), 422–429.

Titler, M. (2008, July 16–17). Impact of system-centered factors, and processes of nursing care on fall prevalence and injuries from falls. Presented at the third annual meeting of Robert Wood Johnson Foundation's Interdisciplinary Nursing Quality Research Initiative, Princeton, NJ.

Townsend-Gervis, M., Cornell, P., & Vardaman, J. M. (2014). Interdisciplinary rounds and structured communication reduce re-admissions and improve some patient outcomes. *Western Journal of Nursing Research.* Advance online publication. doi: 10.1177/0193945914527521

Warne, S., Endacott, R., Ryan, H., Chamberlain, W., Hendry, J., Boulanger, C., & Donlin, N. (2010). Non-therapeutic omission of medications in acutely ill patients. *Nursing in Critical Care, 15*(3), 112–117

Whitney, J. D., & Parkman, S. (2004). The effect of early postoperative physical activity on tissue oxygen and wound healing. *Biological Research for Nursing, 6*(2), 79–89.

Yauk, S., Hopkins, B. A., Phillips, C. D., Terrell, S., Bennion, J., & Riggs, M. (2005). Predicting in-hospital falls: Development of the Scott and White Falls Risk Screener. *Journal of Nursing Care Quality, 20*(2), 128–133.

Yohannes, A. M., & Connolly, M. J. (2003). Early mobilization with walking aids following hospital admission with acute exacerbation of chronic obstructive pulmonary disease. *Clinical Rehabilitation, 17*(5), 465–471.

Young, A. M., Mudge, A. M., Banks, M. D., Ross, L. J., & Daniels, L. (2013). Encouraging, assisting and time to EAT: Improved nutritional intake for older medical patients receiving protected mealtimes and/or additional nursing feeding assistance. *Clinical Nutrition, 32*(4), 543–549.

Zammit, G. K., Weiner, J., Damato, N., Sillup, G. P., & McMillan, C. A. (1992). Quality of life in people with insomnia. *Sleep, 22*(Suppl 2), S379–S385.

Nursing Staff Outcomes of Missed Nursing Care

In the previous chapter, we reviewed the impact of missed nursing care on patient outcomes. Nursing staff are also influenced when they miss their patients' care. Dissatisfaction with job and occupation, intent to leave, turnover, moral distress, compassion fatigue, and burnout are outcomes that may result when nursing care is missed. These issues will be examined in this chapter.

RN Shortages

The ability to attract and retain nursing staff is obviously critical for maintaining and enhancing the quality of patient care. There have been nursing shortages on and off for the past 70 years. The first shortages occurred during World War II when there were not enough nurses to care for both the wounded soldiers and the civilian population. The government established the U.S. Cadet Nurse Corps at that time to address this issue (Kalisch & Kalisch, 1976). This large and widespread program conducted a high-level advertising campaign to attract young people to the profession, provided funds to hospitals to increase the quality of the programs and the number of enrollees, and distributed financial assistance to students (as well as uniforms, which made them part of the war effort) (Kalisch & Kalisch, 1974). After the war, nurses left the workforce in droves and stayed at home as house-wives and mothers. The average U.S. birth rate at the time exceeded that of India. Since then, there have been shortages created by such factors as fewer women entering the traditional female professions, an increase in demand for nursing care as the population ages, the decrease in federal funds for nursing education, the negative media image of nurses (Kalisch & Kalisch, 1987), and poor working condi-tions (e.g., hours, pay, autonomy, level of staffing, etc.).

Although there is not currently an acute shortage of nurses, the U.S. Bureau of Labor Statistics (BLS) predicts that there will be a need for more than one million new and replacement registered nurses (RNs) by 2016 (Dohm & Shniper, 2007). Furthermore, it is estimated that by 2020 there will be a 36% shortfall of RNs (U.S. Department of Health and Humans Services, 2006). Close to 600,000 new positions in nursing will be created through 2016 (a 23.5% increase), making nursing the nation's top profession in terms of projected job growth (Dohm & Shniper, 2007). In addition, the cost of RN turnover is very high, ranging from $21,514 to $67,100 per nurse turnover (Jones, 2005; O'Brien-Pallas et al., 2006).

The need for nursing assistive personnel is also projected to grow tremendously (U.S. Department of Health and Human Services, 2003). Employment of nursing assistants and orderlies is projected to grow 21% from 2012 to 2022, faster than the average for all occupations. Because of the growing elderly population, many nursing assistants and orderlies will be needed in long-term care facilities and homes as well as in hospitals. Therefore, efforts are needed to retain nursing staff in light of the projected shortages, growing demand, and the cost of nurse turnover.

Previous Studies
Job and Occupation Satisfaction
The job satisfaction of RNs and NAs has been the focus of many studies. Work environment has been identified as a major cause of RN dissatisfaction and turnover (Aiken, Clarke, Sloane, Lake, & Cheney, 2008; Ejaz, Noelker, Menne, & Bagaka, 2008; Friese, 2005; Toh, Ang, & Devi, 2012) as well as the level and type of nurse staffing (Aiken, Clarke, Sloane, Sochalski, & Silber, 2002; Newman, Maylor, & Chansarkar, 2008; Shaver & Lacey, 2003; Tovey & Adams, 1999). Aiken and colleagues (2008), for example, found that the likelihood of a nurse reporting dissatisfaction increased by one-tenth each time another patient was added to his or her workload.

In a meta-analysis of research, Blegen identified seven characteristics that correlate with job satisfaction: recognition, autonomy, stress, organizational commitment, communication with supervisor and peers, and routinization of the work. In a subsequent meta-analysis by Irvine and Evens (1995), compensation, job characteristics (e.g., autonomy, feedback, etc.), and work environment (e.g., management, leadership, stress, participation in decision-making) were found to be moderately correlated with RN job satisfaction. In a more recent study by Best and Thurston (2004), RNs identified autonomy, status, relationships, task requirements, organizational policies, and pay to be factors which contributed to job satisfaction or dissatisfaction.

For NAs, pay, teamwork, management, being appreciated, listened to, and treated with respect have been found to be important (Ejaz et al., 2008; Kemper et al., 2008). In another study, NA satisfaction has also been positively linked with manager support and negatively associated with job stress (McGilton, Hall, Wodchis, & Petroz, 2007). Empowerment has also been significantly associated with greater job satisfaction (Kuo, Yin, & Li, 2008).

Very few studies of nursing staff job satisfaction have looked at the correlation between job satisfaction and the quality of patient care being provided. One research team determined that a primary reason for satisfaction was interacting with and caring for patients (Newman, Maylor, & Chansarkar, 2002). Best and Thurston (2004) found that nurses overwhelmingly felt that satisfaction was associated with "patient care, patient response, making a difference, and quality of the patient care" (p. 287). A study of nurses who had been terminated or changed their position revealed that 46% of nurses were frustrated with the quality of care they could deliver, many of whom provided descriptions of incidents of substandard care and concern about patient errors (Strachota, Normandin, O'Brien, Clary, & Krukow, 2003). There were no studies found linking the quality and completeness of nursing care and NA job satisfaction. There was one study that linked physician satisfaction with practice quality and involvement in quality-improvement activities (Quinn, 2000). They found that physicians reporting more quality problems had lower satisfaction, higher levels of stress, and more feelings of isolation.

Turnover and Intent to Leave

Turnover among nursing staff results in significant organizational cost as well as potential ramifications for the quality of care delivered at the bedside. Evidence shows that high turnover rates lead to negative patient outcomes. Zimmerman, Gruber-Baldini, Hebel, Sloane,

& Magaziner (2002), while examining how nursing home care affects patient infection rates, found that each loss of an RN proportionately increased the risk of infection almost 30% and the risk of hospitalization more than 80%. In another study, organizations with low turnover (4% to 12%) had lower risk adjusted mortality and shorter patient length of stay than organizations with moderate (12% to 22%) or high (22% to 44%) turnover rates (Gelinas & Loh, 2004).

Job satisfaction has been directly associated with nurse retention and turnover (Coomber & Barribal, 2007; Ingersoll, Olsan, Drew-Cates, DeVinney, & Davies 2002; Ulrich, Buerhaus, Donelan, Norman, & Dittus, 2005; Yin & Yang, 2002). Ingersoll and colleagues (2002) found that dissatisfied nurses had a 65% lower probability of staying in their jobs than satisfied nurses. Due to the link between nurse satisfaction and turnover, it is important to take predictors of nurse satisfaction into consideration.

Although several studies have identified predictors of intent to leave and turnover, only a few, like studies of job satisfaction, have considered the impact of the quality of nursing care provided at the bedside on subsequent turnover (Gelinas & Loh, 2004; Zimmerman et al., 2002). For example, a study by Strachota and colleagues (2003) reported that 46% of nurses who had voluntarily terminated or changed their position were unhappy with the quality of care they were providing. A few studies have identified a link between intention to leave and turnover with the nursing care provided to patients. Nurses who were satisfied with the nursing care they provided, who were able to meet clinical challenges, and had the opportunity to be of service and do research were 2.4 times more likely than other RNs to indicate no intention to leave (Larrabee et al., 2003). One research team found caregivers were more satisfied when they were able to provide what they perceived as high-quality care (Castle, Degenholtz, & Rosen, 2006). This includes being able to complete all the necessary nursing care required for the patient.

In this chapter, the results of the studies we conducted on satisfaction, intent to leave, turnover, and missed nursing care will be reported for 11 study hospitals. Our previous publications in this area used 10 hospitals (Kalisch, Tschannen, & Lee, 2011). The research questions were:

- Does missed nursing care predict satisfaction with current position and occupation and teamwork and intent to leave after controlling for staff characteristics?

- Does missed nursing care predict staff turnover while controlling for unit staff characteristics?

Study Method

The sample population for this study included the nursing staff employed on 124 adult units (medical–surgical, rehabilitation, intermediate, and intensive care units) in 11 hospitals. This secondary analysis was completed on the sample described in Chapter 2. A total of 3,341 RNs and 976 NAs participated in the study with response rates ranging from 29.1% to 100% across the 124 participating patient care units. By job title, response rates were 61.8% for RNs, 53.4% for NAs, and 60% overall. Licensed practical nurses (LPNs) were excluded from the analysis due to a small sample size and unequal distribution across hospitals. As has been previously noted in the reported studies in earlier chapters, the *MISSCARE Survey* was used to collect nursing staff perceptions of the type and extent of missed nursing care. Also contained in this survey are questions for nursing staff on intent to leave their current position, satisfaction with their current job, occupation (RN or NA), and with teamwork. Additionally, there were questions about overtime in the past three months, absenteeism in the last three months, and perceptions of staffing adequacy. Administrative records at each hospital were used to gather the staffing, unit level case mix index (CMI) and turnover data. Turnover, CMI and staffing CMI data were collected for two months (during and one month prior to distribution of the *MISSCARE Survey*). Two months were utilized to account for any possible unusual events on the unit in a given month. Researchers computed the variables of interest (using the raw data) to ensure consistency in calculation across institutions.

Data Analysis

In this study, the unit of analysis was the individual and patient care unit. The research questions about how missed nursing care predicts job satisfaction with current position, occupation, teamwork, and intent to leave were analyzed using individual level data but when controlling for unit characteristics (staffing levels, CMI), the unit was the level of analysis. Turnover required the unit level of analysis since that is the way it is collected and reported. We estimated regression models using the robust cluster estimation commands for all analyses in order to control for the cluster effect by patient care units. Using correlation analysis, missed nursing care and other independent variables (age, gender, job title, education, staffing adequacy, work hours per week, overtime, years of experience, type of shift, and type of unit) were tested separately for their potential predictive ability on the dependent variables (Bliese, 2000). The overall mean score of missed nursing care (continuous variable) was the average amount of missed care identified for each of the elements of nursing care (e.g., ambulation, interdisciplinary rounds, etc.) for each participant. Finally, multivariate analyses were conducted with significant independent variables based on the preliminary analysis results.

For unit-level analyses, characteristics of the sample, although collected at the individual level (n = 4317), were aggregated to the unit level in order to test the relationships between turnover, intent to leave, missed care, and other unit characteristics. To do this, each of the unit variables was computed into the proportion of staff above a referent point (i.e., median). For example, education values represented the proportion of nursing staff who had a baccalaureate degree (BSN) or higher within each unit. The experience value for each unit represented the proportion of nursing staff that had experience of more than five years (in their occupation) on a given unit. The referent value for intent to leave was assessed with staff members who had plans to leave (either in six months or a year) and absenteeism was determined by calculating who had missed work for one or more days. For missed care, a unit-level missed care score was calculated as the average amount of missed care identified for each of the elements of nursing care by staff on each unit.

Study Findings

As noted in Table 10.1, both RNs and NAs were predominantly female, under 34 years of age, and worked full time. The majority of RNs held a baccalaureate degree (51.9%) while the NAs held a high school diploma (27.7%). A high percentage of RNs had greater than ten years of experience (35.2%), whereas the majority of NAs sampled had between six months to less than five years of experience (63.7%). Approximately half of the RNs and NAs worked the day shift. Both RNs and NAs worked primarily full time (82.8% and 75.5%, respectively).

Current Job Satisfaction

The correlation matrix of the job satisfaction variables of missed nursing care and staff characteristics revealed that missed nursing care, age, absenteeism, staffing adequacy, and type of unit were significantly associated with satisfaction with current position (Table 10.2). In order to control for different hospitals where the nursing staff worked, the hospital variable was also entered in the regression models as a control factor in this study. Except age, the three independent variables (missed nursing care, staffing adequacy, and unit

TABLE 10.1. Sample characteristics (n = 4317).

		RN (n = 3341)	NA (n = 976)
Gender	Male	254 (7.8)	152 (15.8)
	Female	3014 (92.2)	813 (84.2)
Age	Under 25	380 (11.4)	281 (28.9)
	26 to 34	1088 (32.6)	285 (29.4)
	35 to 44	890 (26.7)	205 (21.1)
	45 to 54	678 (20.3)	144 (14.8)
	55+	298 (8.9)	56 (5.8)
Highest degree	High School or GED	235 (7.1)	13 (27.7)
	Associate Degree	1367 (41)	8 (17)
	Baccalaureate Degree or greater	1731 (51.9)	26 (55.3)
Experience in the role	≤6 months	151 (4.5)	59 (6.1)
	>6 months to ≤2 yrs	722 (21.8)	273 (28.2)
	>2 yrs to ≤5 yrs	653 (19.7)	252 (26)
	>5 yrs to ≤10 yrs	626 (18.9)	188 (19.4)
	≥10 yrs	1167 (35.2)	197 (20.3)
Experience on current unit	≤6 months	243 (7.3)	114 (11.8)
	>6 months to ≤2 yrs	960 (29)	376 (38.9)
	>2 yrs to ≤5 yrs	826 (24.9)	240 (24.8)
	>5 yrs to ≤10 yrs	661 (19.9)	141 (14.6)
	≥10 yrs	625 (18.9)	96 (9.9)
Work hours per week	≤30 hrs/week (part time)	574 (17.2)	238 (24.5)
	>30 hrs/week (full time)	2760 (82.8)	735(75.5)
Shift worked	Days	1614 (48.5)	486 (50)
	Evenings	217 (6.5)	142 (14.7)
	Nights	1235 (37.1)	285 (29.3)
	Rotates	265 (8)	58 (6)
Overtime	None	897 (26.9)	398 (40.9)
	Yes	2432 (73.1)	574 (59.1)
Absenteeism	None	1447 (43.6)	400 (41.4)
	Yes	1873 (56.4)	567 (58.6)

(Continued)

TABLE 10.1. **Sample characteristics (n = 4317) (continued).**

		RN (n = 3341)	NA (n = 976)
Type of unit	ICU	893 (26.7)	128 (13.1)
	Intermediate	586 (17.5)	204 (20.9)
	Med–Surg	1732 (51.8)	596 (61.1)
	Rehab	130 (3.9)	48 (4.9)
Perceived Staffing Adequacy	100% of the time	472 (14.2)	109 (11.3)
	75% of the time	1874 (56.5)	503 (52.2)
	50% of the time	648 (19.5)	233 (24.2)
	25% of the time	270 (8.1)	102 (10.6)
	0% of the time	55 (1.7)	17 (1.8)
Missed nursing care (mean ± S.D.)*		1.60 ± .39	1.31 ± 42
Satisfaction with current position (mean ± S.D.)		3.93 ± .83	3.88 ± .89
Occupation satisfaction (mean ± S.D.)		4.30 ± .76	4.05 ± .86
Teamwork satisfaction (mean ± S.D.)		4.06 ± .90	3.71 ± 1.05

Note: ( ) indicates percent; valid percentages used. * Means and standard deviations are presented for missed nursing care and the two satisfaction variables

type) were significant predictors of job satisfaction (Table 10.3). The lower the level of missed nursing care, the higher the job satisfaction level ($p < 0.001$). Compared to the staff on intensive care units, those working on medical–surgical areas reported lower levels of job satisfaction ($p = .013$), while those on rehabilitation units reported the lowest levels of job satisfaction ($p < .001$).

Occupation Satisfaction
The model testing occupation satisfaction included eight independent variables: missed nursing care, age, gender, job title, education, absenteeism, staffing adequacy, and hospital (Table 10.2). All of the eight predictors, except age and hospital, were significantly associated with levels of occupation satisfaction. The logistic regression (Table 10.4) verified that staff who reported less missed care were more satisfied with their occupation, while those who reported more missed care were less satisfied (OR = 0.49, 95% CI = 0.37–0.64). Females were more satisfied compared to males (OR = 1.79, 95% CI = 1.29–2.47) and NAs were less satisfied compared to RNs (OR = 0.42, 95% CI = 0.21–0.81).

TABLE 10.2. **Satisfaction with current job, occupation, teamwork, missed nursing care, and staff and unit characteristics at the individual level: Correlation matrix (n = 4317).**

	1	2	3	4	5	6	7	8	9	10	11	12	13	14	15	16
1. Satisfaction with current position	1.00															
2. Occupation satisfaction	.52**	1.00														
3. Teamwork satisfaction	.44**	.30**	1.00													
4. Missed nursing care	-.31**	-.14**	-.24**	1.00												
5. Education	-.01	-.04*	.03	.01	1.00											
6. Gender	-.01	.06**	-.01	.05**	.01	1.00										
7. Age	.038*	.08**	-.04*	.07**	-.22**	.03	1.00									
8. Job title	-.02	-.13**	-.14**	-.23**	-.02	-.11**	-.16**	1.00								
9. Full-time equivalency	-.01	.02	-.01	-.01	-.01	-.04*	-.01	-.08**	1.00							
10. Shifts	-.01	-.02	.05**	-.02	.07**	-.05**	-.13**	-.05**	.05**	1.00						
11. Experience in role	-.01	.01	-.07**	.11**	-.07**	.08**	.63**	-.13**	-.10**	-.21**	1.00					
12. Experience on current unit	.01	.03	-.05**	.10**	-.10**	.08**	.49**	-.14**	-.09**	-.24**	.73**	1.00				
13. Overtime	-.01	.03	-.01	.05**	-.03	-.03	.06**	-.13**	.17**	-.01	-.01	.02	1.00			
14. Absenteeism	-.08**	-.05**	-.05**	.07**	.01	.01	-.09**	.01	.06**	.04**	-.05**	-.05**	.05**	1.00		
15. Staffing adequacy	-.38**	-.20**	-.26**	.24**	-.04*	.05**	.01	.07**	.02	-.02	-.02	.01	.08**	.07**	1.00	
16. Unit type	-.08**	.01	-.08**	.06**	-.11**	.07**	.02	.11**	-.05**	-.04**	-.06**	-.01	.02	.02	.07**	1.00

Note: * p < .05; ** p < .01

TABLE 10.3. **Summary of logistic regression analysis for variables predicting satisfaction with current position: RNs and NAs (n = 4317).**

Independent Variables	Odds Ratio	Robust Std. Err	p	95% CI	
Missed nursing care	0.35	0.05	<.001**	0.26	0.46
Age	1.06	0.04	0.121	0.98	1.14
Staffing adequacy	0.45	0.02	<.001**	0.4	0.5
Absenteeism	0.81	0.07	0.020*	0.68	0.97
Unit type					
ICU(R)					
Intermediate	0.89	0.12	0.406	0.67	1.18
Med–Surg	0.71	0.1	0.013*	0.54	0.93
Rehabilitation	0.51	0.08	<.001**	0.38	0.68
Hospital			0.396		

Note: $\chi 2$= 466.05, $p < .001$. * $p < .05$; **$p < .01$. (R) is the reference variable. Analysis included a dummy variable for study hospitals to control for its effect, but coefficients were not included in the table for the privacy of data (output suppressed)

Satisfaction with Teamwork

The model testing satisfaction with teamwork included these independent variables: missed nursing care, age, experience in role, experience on current unit, staffing adequacy, job title, shifts, absenteeism, unit types, and hospital (Table 10.2 and 10.5). The level of missed nursing care, experience in role, staffing adequacy, job title, night shift, and unit type were the significant predictors of satisfaction with teamwork. The nursing staff who reported less missed nursing care were happier with the teamwork on their unit (OR = 0.37, 95% CI = 0.23–0.59). Nursing staff members with more experience in their role reported less satisfaction with teamwork. Compared to RNs, NAs reported less satisfaction with teamwork. Nurses working on night shifts reported higher levels of satisfaction with teamwork compared with those on day shifts.

Intent to Leave

Intent to leave was significantly correlated with eight variables in the bivariate analyses: turnover, missed care, skill mix, education, age, experience, overtime, and absenteeism (Table 10.6). Turnover and intent to leave were positively correlated with one another ($r = .26$, $p < .05$). Greater amounts of missed care were associated with higher intention to leave ($r = 53$, $p < .01$). The higher the skill mix ($r = .34$,

TABLE 10.4.   Summary of logistic regression analysis for variables predicting occupation satisfaction in RNs and NAs (n = 4317).

Independent Variables	Odds Ratio	Robust Std. Err	p	95% CI	
Missed nursing care	0.49	0.07	<.001**	0.37	0.64
Age	1.02	0.05	0.690	0.932	1.11
Staffing adequacy	0.68	0.04	<.001**	0.6	0.77
Education					
Grade school or lower (R)					
Associate degree of nursing	2	0.37	<.001**	1.39	2.89
BSN or greater	1.58	0.3	0.017*	1.08	2.29
Gender					
Male (R)					
Female	1.79	0.3	<.001**	1.29	2.47
Job title					
RN (R)					
NA	0.42	0.15	0.013*	0.21	0.83
Absenteeism	0.72	0.09	0.009**	0.56	0.92
Hospital			0.507		

Note: $\chi 2$ = 168.11, p < .001. * p < .05; **p < .01. (R) is the reference variable. Analysis included a dummy variable for study hospitals to control for its effect, but coefficients were not included in the table for the privacy of data (output suppressed)

$p < .01$), the greater the intention to leave. Education and perceived absenteeism were also significantly related to intent to leave. Specifically, greater absenteeism ($r = .48$, $p < .01$) and higher education ($r = .34$, $p < .01$) were associated with greater intent to leave. In contrast, age ($r = -.30$, $p < .01$), experience ($r = -.35$, $p < .01$), and overtime ($r = -.26$, $p < .01$) were negatively associated with intent to leave. In other words, units with nursing staff who were older, had greater years of experience, and worked more overtime were less likely to report intention to leave.

Findings from the preliminary analysis were used to determine the variables to include in the multivariate regression analyses, which would demonstrate whether missed nursing care and unit characteristics predict intent to leave. A multiple regression model was computed with the following independent variables (Table 10.7): missed care, skill mix, education (BSN or higher), age (above 35 years), experience (greater than 5 years), overtime, and absenteeism. The overall model accounted for 41.2% of the variation in intent to leave ($p < .0001$).

TABLE 10.5.   **Summary of logistic regression analysis for variables predicting teamwork satisfaction in RNs and NAs (n = 4317).**

Independent Variables	Odds Ratio	Robust Std. Err	p	95% CI	
Missed nursing care	0.37	0.09	<.001	0.23	0.59
Age	1.01	0.05	0.74	0.92	1.12
Experience in role	0.85	0.05	0.00	0.76	0.94
Experience on current unit	1.01	0.06	0.29	0.95	1.17
Staffing adequacy	0.61	0.32	<.001	0.55	0.67
Job title					
RN(R)					
NA	0.35	0.05	<.001	0.27	0.46
Shifts					
Days (R)					
Evenings	0.96	0.13	0.768	0.74	1.25
Nights	1.38	0.16	0.005	1.11	1.73
Rotates	0.8	0.13	0.185	0.57	1.11
Absenteeism	0.88	0.07	0.09	0.76	1.02
Unit type					
ICU (R)					
Intermediate	0.67	0.17	0.105	0.41	1.09
Med–Surg	0.75	0.17	0.201	0.49	1.16
Rehabilitation	0.47	0.11	0.002	0.29	0.75
Hospital			0.99		

Note: χ^2 = 378.91, $p < .001$. * $p < .05$; ** $p < .01$. (R) is the reference variable. Analysis included a dummy variable for study hospitals to control for its effect, but coefficients were not included in the table for the privacy of data (output suppressed)

Missed nursing care, skill mix, and absenteeism were significantly associated with intent to leave. Units with higher missed care ($\beta = .34$, $p < .0001$) and greater absenteeism rates ($\beta = .29$, $p = .008$) had more staff with plans to leave. A higher level of skill mix (or more RNs as a proportion of the staff) predicted less intention to leave ($\beta = 0.25$, $p = .002$). Other variables in the model were not significant predictors of the intent to leave.

Turnover

At the bivariate level, six variables were significantly related to nurse turnover: intention to leave, missed care, skill mix, gender, percentage of time working, and absenteeism (Table 10.6). Greater amounts

TABLE 10.6. Intent to leave, RN turnover, missed care, and unit characteristics at the unit level: Correlation matrix.

Variables	1	2	3	4	5	6	7	8	9	10	11	12	13	14	15
1. Intent to leave	1														
2. RN turnover	.26*	1													
3. Missed care	.53**	.37**	1												
4. HPPD	-.13	-.19	-.16	1											
5. CMI	.23	-.04	-.08	.56**	1										
6. Skill mix	.42**	.43**	.35**	-.15	.17	1									
7. Education (above BSN)	.34**	-.23	.175	.246	.34**	.34**	1								
8. Gender (Female)	.06	-.28*	.07	.01	-.29*	-.28*	.10	1							
9. Age (above 35 yrs)	-.30*	.16	-.02	.131	-.09	-.04	-.51**	-.09	1						
10. Experience (more than 5 yrs)	-.35**	-.10	-.31*	.32*	.12	-.04	-.28*	-.06	.71**	1					
11. Shift (12 hours)	-.24	-.01	-.10	.39**	.26*	-.36**	.01	.01	-.09	.01	1				
12. Work hours (Full time)	-.15	.26*	.12	.10	.01	-.11	-.44**	-.17	.47**	.253	.28*	1			
13. Work hours (day or rotate)	.27*	.10	.31*	-.13	-.18	.14	.09	.22	-.15	-.09	.01	.19	1		
14. Overtime	-.26*	.14	.03	-.06	-.09	.06	-.04	-.10	.16	.10	-.14	.09	-.09	1	
15. Absenteeism	.48**	.39**	.48**	-.24	-.01	.67**	.21	-.06	.05	-.06	-.24	.04	.26*	-.03	

Note: *$p < .05$; **$p < .01$

TABLE 10.7. **The predictors of intention to leave.**

Variable	B	SE B	β	t	p
Missed care	0.21	0.05	0.34	4.47	0.000**
Skill mix	0.25	0.08	0.35	3.10	0.002 **
Education (BSN or above)	0.00	0.06	0.01	0.07	0.945
Age (>35 yrs)	−0.09	0.07	−0.16	−1.31	0.192
Experience (>5 yrs)	−0.09	0.07	−0.14	−1.20	0.233
Shift (Day and rotate)	0.03	0.08	0.03	0.40	0.692
Overtime	−0.10	0.05	−0.14	−1.86	0.066
Absenteeism	0.19	0.07	0.29	2.72	0.008**
R^2			$R^2 = .412$		
F (p)			8.727 (.000)		

Note: ** $p < .01$. Analysis included ten dummy variables for study hospitals to control for their effects, but coefficients were not included in the table for the privacy for data

of missed care were associated with higher turnover rates ($r = .37$, $p < .01$) (Tschannen, Kalisch, & Lee, 2010). Positive correlations were also identified with skillmix ($r = .43$, $p < .01$) and absenteeism ($r = .39$, $p < .01$). Furthermore, units with higher percentages of females had lower turnover rates. However, in a multiple linear regression model with independent variables of missed care, skill mix, gender, absenteeism, working full time, intent to leave, and hospital type, none of these variables were significant predictors of turnover.

Summary of Findings

The research on the job satisfaction and turnover rates of RNs and NAs has largely examined how these factors are impacted by work environment characteristics, actual staffing levels, recognition, management, and emotional exhaustion. Very little research has dealt with the relationship between nursing care that is provided at the point of care and staff members' job satisfaction, intent to leave, and turnover. The findings of these studies point to a predictive relationship between missed nursing care and satisfaction and intent to leave. Nursing staff reporting less missed nursing care had greater satisfaction with their current position, occupation, and teamwork, and they were found to be less intent on leaving their job. Missed nursing care and perceptions of staffing adequacy, however, did not predict turnover. This may have been due to the timing of the study during an economic downturn where even retirements were delayed.

In the satisfaction models (job, occupation, and teamwork satisfaction), missed nursing care and perceptions of the adequacy of staffing were predictors. Age, hours worked per week, overtime, years of experience, and type of shift were not significant predictors for the models of satisfaction.

In terms of occupation, RNs were more satisfied with their occupation than were NAs. The reason NAs are less satisfied with their occupation may be explained by findings in other studies that have uncovered NA dissatisfaction due to excessive workload (Crickmer, 2005; Mather & Bakas, 2002; Pennington, Scott, & Magilvy, 2003) and not being recognized for their contributions (Counsell & Rivers, 2002; Crickmer, 2005; Mather & Bakas, 2002; Spilsbury & Meyer, 2004). In addition, some NAs may be working towards other educational degrees, thus satisfaction with being a NA may be lower since they do not see it as their permanent occupation.

Nursing staff working on intensive care units were more satisfied, while those on rehabilitation units were the least satisfied. Perhaps this is due to the nature of the work and the number of assigned patients.

In examining the link between missed nursing care, nurse turnover, and intention to leave, the variables in the model (missed care, skill mix, overtime, gender, absenteeism, and intention to leave) failed to show significance. In addition, several indicators identified as predictors of turnover in the literature review (i.e., workload and work schedules) failed to show an association with turnover, even in the preliminary analysis. This may be partly due to (1) the low turnover rate for this study (1%), and (2) economic conditions at the time of data collection where the unemployment rate was exceptionally high (Bureau of Labor Statistics, 2010). Research has shown that the importance of a nurse's income to the family significantly reduces intention to leave (and potentially turnover) (Zeytinoglu et al., 2006). Due to the high unemployment rate in the country at the time of this study, the reliance on a nurse's income for financial wellbeing was high. Estryn-Béhar and colleagues (2007) found that having children still living at home resulted in lower rates of intention to leave. This may partly explain why intention to leave was not a significant predictor of turnover in the present study. Staff with children to support may be more willing to remain in their current position even though they are unhappy with clinical practice and environmental conditions.

There are several theories as to why we find that missed nursing care predicts satisfaction and intent to leave. They are relational job design theory, moral distress, compassion fatigue, and burnout.

Explanatory Theories
Relational Job Design
Findings of this study support the relational job design theory where employees are more motivated when they witness a positive impact of their actions on their beneficiaries (Grant et al., 2007). When nursing staff see that their patients are receiving good nursing care, and that the required elements of care are completed, satisfaction increases. Conversely, when they see that elements of nursing care are missed, their satisfaction decreases. In the case of nursing, unlike some other occupations, the providers have direct, and many times, immediate knowledge about the impact of the quality of their work on their patients. In fact, they cannot avoid it (unless they are in denial). Thus, they are fully cognizant of the impact of missing care on their patients, and when it is negative, their satisfaction diminishes.

Although there are rare exceptions, the vast majority of nursing staff want to have a positive influence in their patients' lives. Thompson and Bunderson (2003) refer to the phrase "making a difference" that is often mentioned in the mission statements of organizations, including those in health care. People in service work often describe their work as protecting the welfare of others (Colby, Sippola, & Phelps, 2001). It is logical that nurses, like other service professionals, choose the field because they have altruistic values and are concerned with impacting their patients and families positively (Meglino & Korsgaard, 2004; Penner, Midili, & Kegelmeyer, 1997; Rioux & Penner, 2001). Some researchers refer to these individuals as "benevolent employees" who are motivated to give more to others than they get back (Grant et al., 2007; Huseman, Hatfield, & Miles, 1987). Nursing staff want to do the best job they can (Cameron & Caza, 2004; Wooten & Crane, 2004). Given that nursing staff value an orientation to service, they are highly motivated to make a positive difference in their patients' lives (Ulrich et al., & Grady, 2007). Thus, when they cannot or do not provide acceptable care, they are more dissatisfied with their jobs than employees who do not have these values and service orientation.

Findings from this study point to the need to develop systems and approaches that result in less missed care. Like the general patient safety movement, missed care needs to first be measured and acknowledged. It should be tracked by units, but, as in the overall safety movement, it cannot be done in a punitive way. Staff members themselves need to be engaged in evaluating missed care (along with other indicators) and developing action plans to improve care. Only by understanding the elements of care being missed can targeted interventions aimed at minimizing missed nursing care be implemented, which in turn should lead to greater job satisfaction and occupation satisfaction, as well as less intent to leave and improved patient outcomes.

Moral Distress

Jameton (1984) defined moral distress as occurring "when one knows the right thing to do, but institutional constraints make it nearly impossible to pursue the right course of action" (p. 6). People feel powerless to take what they believe is the correct action. Corley extended the definition as follows: "The painful psychological disequilibrium that results from recognizing the ethically appropriate action, yet not taking it, because of such obstacles as lack of time, supervisory reluctance, an inhibiting medical power structure, institution policy, or legal considerations" (Corley, Elswick, Gorman, & Clor, 2001, pp. 250–251).

Moral distress is a significant problem for nurses (Riahl, 2011; Hooper, Craig, Janvrin, Wetsel, & Reimels, 2010; Meltzer & Huckabay, 2004). Research has identified many varied sources of moral distress experienced by nurses. Moral distress results in such feelings as anger, guilt, sadness, and hopelessness. It has also been demonstrated that the experience of moral distress leads some nurses to leave their jobs or the profession. It has physical, emotional, and psychological outcomes and a negative impact on the quality, quantity, and cost of patient care. A strong correlation between moral distress and burnout in nurses has been identified (Espeland, 2006; Fenton, 1988; Jameton, 1992; Maslach, Schaufeli, & Leiter, 2001; Vahey, Aiken, Sloane, Clarke, & Vargas, 2004).

Moral distress occurs with other healthcare professionals, including pharmacists (Sporrong, Hoglund, Hansson, Westerholm, & Arnetz, 2005), respiratory therapists (Schwenzer & Wang, 2006), psychologists (Austin, Rankel, Kagan, Bergum, & Lemermeyer, 2005), physicians (Austin, Kagan, Rankel, & Bergum, 2008; Chen, 2009; Forde & Aasland, 2008; Hamric & Blackhall, 2007; Lee & Dupree, 2008; Lomis, Carpenter, & Miller, 2009), chaplains, social workers, and nutritionists (Chen, 2009). There are some differences in what causes moral distress and in how it is manifested among the professions, but it is basically the same phenomena (Austin et al., 2008; Austin, Lemermeyer, Goldberg,

Bergum, & Johnson, 2005; Forde & Aasland, 2008; Hamric, Davis, & Childress, 2006; Hamric & Blackhall, 2007; Lee & Dupree, 2008; Lomis et al., 2009; Schwenzer & Wang, 2006; Sporrong et al., 2005).

DeTienne, Agle, Phillips, and Ingerson (2012) conducted a study comparing the impact of moral distress with other job stressors on three important employee variables—fatigue, job satisfaction, and turnover intentions—by utilizing survey data from 305 customer-contact employees of a financial institution's call center. Statistical analysis of the interaction of moral stress and the three employee variables was performed while controlling for other types of job stress as well as demographic variables. The results revealed that, even after including the control variables in the statistical models, moral stress remains a statistically significant predictor of increased employee fatigue, decreased job satisfaction, and increased turnover intentions. In another study of nurses and social workers, respondents reported feeling powerless (32.5%) and overwhelmed (34.7%) with ethical issues in the workplace, and frustrated (52.8%) and fatigued (40%) when they could not resolve these issues (Edwards, McClement, & Read, 2013).

In an editorial in *Bioethical Inquiry*, Rich and Ashby (2013) wrote that, for many nurses, the channels to express these concerns are poorly developed or nonexistent. Much of this goes underground and is internalized by nurses, and this in itself, presumably, has largely unquantified negative impacts on professionals, potentially leading to compassion exhaustion, burnout, and job dissatisfaction (Argentero, Dell'Olivo, & Ferretti, 2008; Back, Deignan, & Potter, 2014).

Moral Residue and the Crescendo Effect
In addition to moral distress, there is moral residue, which is caused by unresolved moral distress. Webster and Bayliss (2000) explain that moral residue is "that which each of us carries with us from those times in our lives when in the face of moral distress we have seriously compromised ourselves or allowed ourselves to be compromised" (p. 208). In situations of moral distress, one's moral values have been violated due to constraints beyond one's control. After these distressing situations, the moral wound of having to act against one's values remains. Moral residue is long-lasting and powerfully integrated into one's thoughts and views of the self. It is this aspect of moral distress—the residue that remains—that can be damaging to the self and to one's career, particularly when morally distressing episodes are repeated over time (Epstein & Hamric, 2009).

The crescendo effect refers to the fact that over time, with repeated experiences of moral distress, moral residue increases gradually. A steady increase in baseline moral distress can create increasingly higher crescendos. Each time that new situations occur, they evoke stronger reactions as the nurse is reminded of previous instances.

Burnout
Burnout is a state of physical, emotional, or mental exhaustion combined with self-doubts about one's competence (Freudenberger, 1974). Freudenberger and North (Price, 2012) have theorized that the burnout process can be divided into phases, which are not necessarily followed sequentially. It starts with an urge to prove oneself and this desire can turn into a compulsion. The person works harder and harder, showing that they are a good nurse. They begin to have little time and energy for friends and family. They may see that what they are doing is not right but they cannot identify the source (Maslach, 1993; Maslach, Jackson, & Leiter, 1996). Physical symptoms can occur at this point. Sometimes the individual experiencing burnout becomes isolated and denies their physical and emotional needs. The person becomes increasingly intolerant, cynical, and irritable with others. They begin to have trouble going to work and getting started on the shift when they get there. Outsiders tend to see more aggression and sarcasm. This is when they often begin to feel they are not valuable or competent. Sometimes these feelings evolve into depression (Ribeiro et al., 2014).

Burnout overlaps with other disorders, such as chronic fatigue syndrome (Leone, Wessely, Huibers, Knottnerus, & Kant, 2011), post-traumatic stress disorder (PTSD) (Mitani, Fujita, Nakata, & Shirakawa, 2006) and depression (Ahola et al., 2005; Iacovides, Fountoulakis, Kaprinis, & Kaprinis, 2003), all of which have been associated with objectively assessed cognitive deficits. Burnout causes cognitive weariness in the form of slow thinking processes and reduced mental agility (Shirom, Nirel, & Vinokur, 2006). Individuals with burnout often complain of concentration and memory lapses in everyday tasks (Schaufeli, Leiter, & Maslach, 2009; Weber & Jaekel-Reinhard, 2000).

In a systematic review of the relationships between burnout and cognitive functioning (Deligkaris, Panagopoulou, Montgomery, & Masoura, 2014), 13 of 15 studies reviewed (Diestel, Cosmar, & Schmidt, 2013; Jonsdottir et al., 2013; Morgan et al., 2011; Ohman, Nordin, Bergdahl, Birgander, & Neely, 2007; Oosterholt, Van der Linden,

Maes, Verbraak, & Kompier, 2012; Orena, Caldiroli, & Cortellazzi, 2013; Osterberg, Karlson, & Hansen, 2009; Sandström, Rhodin, Lundberg, Olsson, & Nyberg, 2005; Sandström et al., 2011; Van Dam, Keijsers, Eling, & Becker, 2011; Van Dam, Keijsers, Verbraak, Eling, & Becker, 2012; Van der Linden, Keijsers, Eling, & Van Schaijk, 2005) found burnout to be associated with selective cognitive deficits, whereas only one study (Castaneda et al., 2011) found higher burnout scores to be associated with better performance on neuropsychological tests. In only one study was there no significant relationship between neuro-cognitive performance and burnout (McInerney, Rowan, & Lawlor, 2012).

Burnout results from, among many factors, a lack of control. The inability of a nurse to influence the care he or she can or cannot provide contributes to the development of burnout. Another cause of burnout is a mismatch in values between the nurse and the team he or she works with or the organization he or she works for. Burnout has long-lasting consequences that influence an individual's ability to work, and also impacts their health and personal relationships.

Compassion Fatigue

Compassion fatigue, also known as secondary traumatic stress (STS), is a condition characterized by a gradual decrease in compassion over time. It was first recognized in nurses in the 1950s and is common among individuals working in health care. Between 16% and 85% of healthcare workers in various fields develop compassion fatigue. In one study, 85% of emergency nurses met the criteria for compassion fatigue, and in another, more than 25% of ambulance paramedics were identified as having severe ranges of post-traumatic symptoms (Beck, 2011). In addition, 34% of hospice nurses met the criteria for secondary traumatic stress/compassion fatigue in the same study by Beck.

People caring for dependent people can also experience compassion fatigue; this can become a cause of abusive behavior in caring professions. It results from the challenge of showing compassion for someone whose suffering is continuous and unresolvable. One may still care for the person as required by policy; however, the natural human desire to help them is significantly diminished. A study on mental health professionals that were caring for Katrina victims found that rates of negative psychological symptoms increased in the group. Of those interviewed, 72% reported experiencing anxiety, 62% had increased suspiciousness about the world around them, and 42%

admitted feeling increasingly vulnerable after treating the Katrina victims (Culver, McKinney, & Paradise, 2011).

Symptoms included hopelessness, a decrease in experiences of pleasure, constant stress and anxiety, sleeplessness or nightmares, and a pervasive negative attitude. This can have detrimental effects on individuals, both professionally and personally, including a decrease in productivity, the inability to focus, and the development of new feelings of incompetency and self-doubt. It is aggravated by organizational cultures where stressful events, such as deaths in an ICU, are not discussed afterwards (Meadors & Lamson, 2008). Lack of awareness of symptoms and poor training regarding the risks associated with high-stress jobs can also contribute to high rates of compassion fatigue.

Creating and sustaining a cultural emphasis on quality is a difficult task but is worthwhile for patients, nursing staff members, and healthcare organizations. Having nursing staff that are satisfied and not burned out or stressed contributes substantially to the delivery of quality care.

Summary

Missed nursing care predicts nursing staff satisfaction and intent to leave. The more nursing care that is missed, the lower the rates of satisfaction with their current position and with their occupation and the higher their intent to leave. Potential theories (i.e., relational job design theory, moral distress, compassion fatigue, and burnout) that explain dissatisfaction and turnover are discussed.

References

Ahola, K., Honkonen, T., Isometsä, E., Kalimo, R., Nykyri, E., Aromaa, A., & Lönnqvist, J. (2005). The relationship between job-related burnout and depressive disorders—results from the Finnish health 2000 study. *Journal of Affective Disorders, 88,* 55–62.

Aiken, L., Clarke, S., Sloane, D., Lake, E., & Cheney, T. (2008) Effects of Hospital Care Environment on Patient Mortality and Nurse Outcomes. *Journal of Nursing Administration, 38*(5), 223–229.

Aiken, L., Clarke, S., Sloane, D., Sochalski, J., & Silber, J. (2002). Hospital nurse staffing and patient mortality, nurse burnout, and job dissatisfaction. *Journal of the American Medical Association, 288*(16), 1987–1993.

Argentero, P., Dell'Olivo, B., & Ferretti, M. S. (2008). Staff burnout and patient satisfaction with the quality of dialysis care. *American Journal of Kidney Diseases, 51*(1), 80–92.

Austin, W. J., Kagan, L., Rankel, M., & Bergum, V. (2008). The balancing act: Psychiatrists' experience of moral distress. *Medicine, Health Care & Philosophy, 11*(1), 89–97.

Austin, W., Lemermeyer, G., Goldberg, L., Bergum, V., & Johnson, M. S. (2005). Moral distress in healthcare practice: The situation of nurses. *HEC Forum, 17*(1), 33–48.

Austin, W., Rankel, M., Kagan, L., Bergum, V., & Lemermeyer, G. (2005). To stay or to go, to speak or stay silent, to act or not to act: Moral distress as experienced by psychologists. *Ethics & Behavior, 15*(3), 197–212.

Back, A. L., Deignan, P. F., & Potter, P. A. (2014). Compassion, compassion fatigue, and burnout: Key insights for oncology professionals. *American Society of Clinical Oncology Educational Book*. Advance online publication. doi: 10.14694/EdBook_AM.2014.34.e454

Beck, C. (2011). Secondary traumatic stress in nurses: A systematic review. *Archives of Psychiatric Nursing, 25*(1), 1–10.

Best, M., & Thurston, N. (2004). Measuring nurse job satisfaction. *Journal of Nursing Administration, 34*(6), 283–290.

Blegen, M. A. (1993). Nurses' job satisfaction: A meta-analysis of related variables. *Nursing Research, 42*(1), 36–41.

Bliese, P. D. (2000). Within-group agreement, non-independence, and reliability: Implications for data aggregation and analysis. In K. J. Klein and S. W. Kozlowski (Eds.), *Multilevel theory, research and methods in organizations* (pp. 349–381). San Francisco, CA: Jossey-Bass.

Bollen, K., & Lennox, R. (1991). Conventional wisdom on measurement: A structural equation perspective. *Psychological Bulletin, 110*(2), 305–314.

Bureau of Labor Statistics. (2010). *Regional and state employment and unemployment summary*. Retrieved from http://www.bls.gov/schedule/archives/laus_nr.htm#2010

Cameron, K., & Caza, A. (2004). Contributions to the discipline of organizational scholarship. *American Behavioral Scientist, 47*(6), 1–9.

Castle, N. G., Degenholtz, H., & Rosen, J. (2006). Determinants of staff job satisfaction of caregivers in two nursing homes in Pennsylvania. *BMC Health Services Research, 6*, 60.

Chen, P. W. (2009). When nurses and doctors can't do the right thing. *New York Times*. Retrieved from http://www.nytimes.com/2009/02/06/health/05chen.html?_r=0

Colby, A., Sippola, L., & Phelps, E. (2001). Social responsibility and paid work in contemporary American life. In A. Rossi (Ed.), *Caring and doing for others: Social responsibility in the domains of family, work, and community* (pp. 463–502). Chicago, IL: University of Chicago Press.

Coomber, B., & Barribal, K. (2007). Impact of job satisfaction components on intent to leave and turnover for hospital-based nurses: A review of the literature. *International Journal of Nursing Studies, 44*(2), 297–314.

Corley, M. C., Elswick, R. K., Gorman, M., & Clor, T. (2001). Development and evaluation of a moral distress scale. *Journal of Advanced Nursing, 33*(2), 250–256.

Counsell, C. M., & Rivers, R. (2002). Inspiring support staff employees. *Journal of Nursing Administration, 32*(3), 120–121.

Crickmer, A. (2005). Who wants to be a CNA? *Journal of Nursing Administration, 35*(9), 380–381.

Culver, L., McKinney, B., & Paradise, L. (2011). Mental health professionals' experiences of vicarious traumatization in post-Hurricane Katrina New Orleans. *Journal of Loss and Trauma,* 16(1), 33–42.

Deligkaris, P., Panagopoulou, E., Montgomery, A. J., & Masoura, E. (2014). Job burnout and cognitive functioning: A systematic review. *Work & Stress, 28*(2), 107–123.

DeTienne, K. B., Agle, B. R., Phillips, J. C., & Ingerson, M. C. (2012). The impact of moral stress compared to other stressors on employee fatigue, job satisfaction, and turnover: An empirical investigation. *Journal of Business Ethics, 110*(3), 377–391.

Diestel, S., Cosmar, M., & Schmidt, K. H. (2013). Burnout and impaired cognitive functioning: The role of executive control in the performance of cognitive tasks. *Work & Stress, 27,* 164–180.

Dohm, A., & Shniper, L. (2007). Employment outlook: 2006–16. Occupational employment projections to 2016. *Monthly Labor Review,* (November), 86–125. Retrieved from http://www.bls.gov/opub/mlr/2007/11/art5full.pdf

Edwards, M. P., McClement, S. E., & Read, L. R. (2013). Nurses' responses to initial moral distress in long-term care. *Journal of Bioethical Inquiry, 10*(3), 325–336.

Ejaz, F. K., Noelker, L. S., Menne, H. L., & Bagakas, J. G. (2008). The impact of stress and support on direct care workers' job satisfaction. *The Gerontologist, 48*(SI1), 60–70.

Epstein, E. G., & Hamric, A. B. (2009). A moral distress, moral residue, and the crescendo effect. *The Journal of Clinical Ethics, 20*(4), 330–342.

Espeland, K.E. (2006). Overcoming burnout: How to revitalize your career. *Journal of Continuing Education in Nursing, 37*(4),178–184.

Estryn-Béhar, M., Le Nezet, O., Van der Heijden, B., Oginska, H., Camerino, D., Conway, P. M., ... Hasselhorn, H. M. (2007). Inadequate teamwork and burnout as predictors of intent to leave nursing according to seniority. Stability of associations in a one-year interval in the European NEXT study. *Ergonomia, 29*(3-4), 225–233.

Fenton, M. (1988). Moral distress in clinical practice: Implications for the nurse administrator. *Canadian Journal of Nursing Administration, 1*(3), 8–11.

Forde, R., & Aasland, O. G. (2008). Moral distress among Norwegian doctors. *Journal of Medical Ethics, 34*(7), 521–525.

Freudenberger, H. J. (1974). Staff burnout. *Journal of Social Issues, 30*(1), 159–165.

Friese, C. R. (2005). Nurse practice environments and outcomes: Implications for oncology nursing. *Oncology Nursing Forum, 32*(4), 765–772.

Gelinas, L., & Loh, D. Y. (2004). The effect of workforce issues on patient safety. *Nursing Economics, 22*(5), 266–279.

Grant, A. M. (2007). Relational job design and the motivation to make a prosocial difference. *Academy of Management Review, 32*(1), 393–417.

Grant, A. M., Campbell, E. M., Chen, G., Cottone, K., Lapedis, D., & Lee, K. (2007). Impact and the art of motivation maintenance: The effects of contact with beneficiaries on persistence behavior. *Organizational Behavior and Human Decision Processes, 103*(1), 53–67.

Hamric, A. B., & Blackhall, L. J. (2007). Nurse-physician perspectives on the care of dying patients in intensive care units: Collaboration, moral distress, and ethical climate. *Critical Care Medicine, 35*(2), 422–429.

Hamric, A. B., Davis, W. S., & Childress, M. D. (2006). Moral distress in health care professionals. *Pharos, 69*(1), 16–23.

Hooper, C., Craig, J., Janvrin, D. R., Wetsel, M. A., & Reimels, E. (2010). Compassion satisfaction, burnout, and compassion fatigue among emergency nurses compared with nurses in other selected inpatient specialties. *Journal of Emergency Nursing, 36*(5), 420–427.

Huseman, R. C., Hatfield, J. D., & Miles, E. W. (1987). A new perspective on equity theory: The equity sensitivity construct. *The Academy of Management Review 12*(2), 222–234.

Iacovides, A., Fountoulakis, K. N., Kaprinis, S., & Kaprinis, G. (2003). The relationship between job stress, burnout and clinical depression. *Journal of Affective Disorders, 75*(3), 209–221.

Ingersoll, G. L., Olsan, T., Drew-Cates, J., DeVinney, B. C., & Davies, J. (2002). Nurses' job satisfaction, organizational commitment, and career intent. *Journal of Nursing Administration, 32*(5), 250–263.

Irvine, D. M., & Evans, M. G. (1995). Job satisfaction and turnover among nurses: Integrating research findings across studies. *Nursing Research, 44*(4), 246–253.

Jameton, A. (1984). *Nursing practice: The ethical issues.* Englewood Cliffs, NJ: Prentice-Hall.

Jameton, A. (1992). *Nursing ethics and the moral situation of the nurse.* Chicago, IL: American Hospital Association.

Jones, C. B. (2005). The cost of nurse turnover, part 2: Application of the nursing turnover cost calculation methodology. *Journal of Nursing Administration, 35*(1), 41–49.

Jonsdottir, I. H., Nordlund, A., Ellbin, S., Ljung, T., Glise, K., Wahrborg, P., & Wallin, A. (2013). Cognitive impairment in patients with stress-related exhaustion. *Stress, 16*, 181–190.

Kalisch, B. J. (2006). Missed nursing care: A qualitative study. *Journal of Nursing Care Quality, 21*(4), 306–313.

Kalisch, B., Tschannen, D., & Lee, H. (2011). Does missed nursing care predict job satisfaction? *Journal of Healthcare Management, 56*(2), 117–134

Kalisch, B. J., & Kalisch, P. (1974). *From training to education: The impact of federal aid on schools of nursing in the United States in the 1940's.* Final Report of NU00443 Research Grant, Division of Nursing, U.S. Public Health Service.

Kalisch, B. J., & Kalisch, P. (1976). The U.S. cadet nurse corps in World War II. *American Journal of Nursing, 76*, 240–242.

Kalisch, B. J., Landstrom, G., & Williams, R. (2009). Missed nursing care: Errors of omission. *Nursing Outlook, 57*(1), 3–9.

Kalisch, B. J., Tschannen, D., & Lee, H. (2011a). Does missed nursing care predict job satisfaction? *Journal of Healthcare Management, 56*(2), 117–134.

Kalisch, P., & Kalisch, B. J. (1987). *The changing image of the nurse.* Menlo Park: Addison-Wesley.

Kemper, P., Heier, B., Barry, T., Brannon, D., Angelelli, J., Vasey, J., & Anderson-Knott, M. (2008). What do direct care workers say would improve their jobs? Differences across settings. *Gerontologist, 48*(S1), 17–25.

Kuo, H. T., Yin, T. J., & Li, I. C. (2008). Relationship between organizational empowerment and job satisfaction perceived by nursing assistants at long-term care facilities. *Journal of Clinical Nursing, 17*(22), 3059–3066.

Larrabee, J. H., Janney, M. A., Ostrow, C. L., Withrow, M. L., Hobbs, G. R., & Burant, C. (2003). Predicting registered nurse job satisfaction and intent to leave. *Journal of Nursing Administration, 33*(5), 271–283.

Lee, K. J., & Dupree, C. Y. (2008). Staff experiences with end-of-life care in the pediatric intensive care unit. *Journal of Palliative Medicine, 11*(7), 986–990.

Leone, S. S., Wessely, S., Huibers, M. J., Knottnerus, J. A., & Kant, I. (2011). Two sides of the same coin? On the history and phenomenology of chronic fatigue and burnout. *Psychology & Health, 26*(4), 449–464.

Lomis, K. D., Carpenter, R. O., & Miller, B. M. (2009). Moral distress in the third year of medical school; a descriptive review of student case reflections. *American Journal of Surgery, 197*(1), 107–112.

Maslach, C. (1993). Burnout: A multidimensional perspective. In W. B. Schaufeli, C. Maslach, & T. Marek (Eds.), *Professional burnout: Recent developments in theory and research* (pp. 19–32). Philadelphia, PA: Taylor & Francis.

Maslach, C., Jackson, S. E., & Leiter, M. P. (1996). *MBI: The Maslach Burnout Inventory: Manual.* Palo Alto, CA: Consulting Psychologists Press.

Maslach, C., Schaufeli, W. B., & Leiter, M. P. (2001). Job burnout. *Annual Review of Psychology 52*, 397–422.

Mather, K. F., & Bakas, T. (2002). Nursing assistants' perceptions of their ability to provide continence care. *Geriatric Nursing, 23*(2), 76–81.

McGilton, K. S., Hall, L. M., Wodchis, W. P., & Petroz, U. (2007). Supervisory support, job stress, and job satisfaction among long-term care nursing staff. *Journal of Nursing Administration, 37*(7–8), 366–372.

McInerney, S., Rowan, M., & Lawlor, B. (2012). Burnout and its effect on neurocognitive performance. *Irish Journal of Psychological Medicine, 29*, 176–179.

Meadors, P., & Lamson, A. (2008). Compassion fatigue and secondaty traumatization: Provider self care on intensive care units for children. *Journal of Pediatric Health, 22*(1), 24–34.

Meglino, B. M., & Korsgaard, A. (2004). Considering rational self-interest as a disposition: Organizational implications of other orientation. *The Journal of Applied Psychology, 89*(6), 946–959.

Meltzer, L. S., & Huckabay, L. M. (2004). Critical care nurses' perceptions of futile care and its effect on burnout. *American Journal of Critical Care, 13*(3), 202–208.

Mitani, S., Fujita, M., Nakata, K., & Shirakawa, T. (2006). Impact of post-traumatic stress disorder and job-related stress on burnout: A study of fire service workers. *The Journal of Emergency Medicine, 31*(1), 7–11.

Morgan, C. A., Russell, B., McNeil, J., Maxwell, J., Snyder, P. J., Southwick, S. M., & Pietrzak, R. H. (2011). Baseline burnout symptoms predict visuospatial executive function during survival school training in special operations military personnel. *Journal of the International Neuropsychological Society, 17*(3), 1–8.

Newman, K., Maylor, U., & Chansarkar, B. (2002). "The nurse satisfaction, service quality and nurse retention chain": Implications for management of recruitment and retention. *Journal of Management in Medicine, 16*(4), 271–291.

O'Brien-Pallas, L., Griffin, P., Shamian, J., Buchan, J., Duffield, C., Hughes, F., … Stone, P. W. (2006). The impact of nurse turnover on patient, nurse, and system outcomes: A pilot study and focus for a multicenter international study. *Policy, Politics, & Nursing Practice, 7*(3), 169–179.

Ohman, L., Nordin, S., Bergdahl, J., Slunga Birgander, L., & Stigsdotter Neely, A. (2007). Cognitive function in outpatients with perceived chronic stress. *Scandinavian Journal of Work, Environment & Health, 33*, 223–232.

Oosterholt, B. G., Van der Linden, D., Maes, J. H., Verbraak, M. J., & Kompier, M. A. (2012). Burned out cognition—cognitive functioning of burnout patients before and after a period with psychological treatment. *Scandinavian Journal of Work, Environment & Health, 38*, 358–369.

Orena, E. F., Caldiroli, D., & Cortellazzi, P. (2013). Does the Maslach Burnout Inventory correlate with cognitive performance in anesthesia practitioners? A pilot study. *Saudi Journal of Anaesthesia, 7*, 277–282.

Osterberg, K., Karlson, B., & Hansen, A. M. (2009). Cognitive performance in patients with burnout, in relation to diurnal salivary cortisol. *Stress, 12*(1), 70–81

Penner, L. A., Midili, A. R., & Kegelmeyer, J. (1997). Beyond job attitudes: A personality and social psychology perspective on the causes of organizational citizenship behavior. *Human Performance, 10*(2), 111–131.

Pennington, K., Scott, J., & Magilvy, K. (2003). The role of certified nursing assistants in nursing homes. *Journal of Nursing Administration, 33*(11), 578–584.

Price, J. V. (2012). The 12 symptoms and stages of burnout that you can't ignore. *HR News You Can Use*. Retrieved from http://jumpstart-hr.com/the-12-symptoms-and-stages-of-burnout-that-you-cant-ignore/

Quinn, R. E. (2000). *Change the world: How ordinary people can achieve extraordinary results*. San Francisco: Jossey-Bass.

Riahl, S. (2011). Role stress amongst nurses at the workplace: Concept analysis. *The Journal of Nursing Management, 19*(6), 721–731.

Ribeiro, V. F., Filho, C. F., Valenti, V. E., Ferreira, M., de Abreu, L. C., de Carvalho, T. D., ... Ferreira, C. (2014). Prevalence of burnout syndrome in clinical nurses at a hospital of excellence. *Internal Archives of Medicine, 7,* 22.

Rich, L. E., & Ashby, M. A. (2013). "Speak what we feel, not what we ought to say": Moral distress and bioethics. *Journal of Bioethical Inquiry, 10*(3), 277–281.

Rioux, S. M., & Penner, L. A. (2001). The causes of organizational citizenship behavior: A motivational analysis. *Journal of Applied Psychology, 86*(6), 1306–1314.

Sandström, A., Peterson, J., Sandström, E., Lundberg, M., Nystrom, I. L., Nyberg, L., & Olsson, T. (2011). Cognitive deficits in relation to personality type and hypothalamic-pituitary-adrenal (HPA) axis dysfunction in women with stress-related exhaustion. *Scandinavian Journal of Psychology, 52*(1), 71–82.

Sandström, A., Rhodin, I. N., Lundberg, M., Olsson, T., & Nyberg, L. (2005). Impaired cognitive performance in patients with chronic burnout syndrome. *Biological Psychology, 69,* 271–279.

Schaufeli, W. B., Leiter, M. P., & Maslach, C. (2009). Burnout: 35 years of research and practice. *Career Development International, 14,* 204–220.

Schwenzer, K. J., & Wang, L. (2006). Assessing moral distress in respiratory care practitioners. *Critical Care Medicine, 34*(12), 2967–2973.

Shaver, K., & Lacey, L. (2003) Job and career satisfaction among staff nurses: Effects of job setting and environment. *Journal of Nursing Administration, 33*(3), 166–172.

Shirom, A., Nirel, N., & Vinokur, A. D. (2006). Overload, autonomy, and burnout as predictors of physicians' quality of care. *Journal of Occupational Health Psychology, 11*(4), 328–342.

Spilsbury, K., & Meyer, K. (2004). Use, misuse and non-use of health care assistants: Understanding the work of health care assistants in a hospital setting. *Journal of Nursing Management, 12*(6), 411–418.

Sporrong, S. K., Hoglund, A. T., Hansson, M. G., Westerholm, P., & Arnetz, B. (2005). "We are white coats whirling round"—Moral distress in Swedish pharmacies. *Pharmacy World & Science, 27*(3), 223–229.

Strachota, E., Normandin, P., O'Brien, N., Clary, M., & Krukow, B. (2003). Reasons registered nurses leave or change employment status. *The Journal of Nursing Administration, 33*(2), 111–117.

Tschannen, D., Kalisch, B., & Lee, K. (2010). Missed nursing care: The impact on intention to leave and turnover. *Canadian Journal of Nursing Research, 42*(4), 22–39.

Thompson, J. A., & Bunderson, J. S. (2003). Violations of principle: Ideological currency in the psychological contract. *Academy of Management Review, 28*(4), 571–586.

Toh, S. G., Ang, E., & Devi, M. K. (2012). Systematic review on the relationship between the nursing shortage and job satisfaction, stress and burnout levels among nurses in oncology/haematology settings. *International Journal of Evidence-Based Healthcare, 10*(2), 126–141.

Tovey, E., & Adams, A. (1999). The changing nature of nurses' job satisfaction: An exploration of sources of satisfaction in the 1990s. *Journal of Advanced Nursing, 30*(1), 150–158.

Ulrich, A., O'Donnell, P., Taylor, C., Farrar, A., Danis, M., & Grady, C. (2007). Ethical climate, ethics stress, and the job satisfaction of nurses and social workers in the United States. *Social Science and Medicine, 65*(8), 1708–1719.

Ulrich, B. T., Buerhaus, P. I., Donelan, K., Norman, L., & Dittus, R. (2005). How RNs view the work environment: Results of a national survey of registered nurses. *Journal of Nursing Administration, 35*(9), 389–396.

U.S. Department of Health and Human Services (U.S. DDHS). (2003). *The future supply of long-term care workers in relation to the aging baby boom generation: Report to Congress.* Retrieved from http://aspe.hhs.gov/daltcp/reports/ltcwork.pdf

U.S. Department of Health and Human Services (U.S. DHHS). (2006). What is behind HRSA's projected supply, demand, and shortage of registered nurses? Washington, D.C.: U.S. DHHS, HRSA.

Vahey, D., Aiken, L., Sloane, D., Clarke, S., & Vargas, D. (2004). Nurse burnout and patient satisfaction. *Medical Care, 42*(2), 1157–1166.

Van Dam, A., Keijsers, G. P. J., Eling, P. A. T. M., & Becker, E. S. (2011). Testing whether reduced cognitive performance in burnout can be reversed by a motivational intervention. *Work & Stress, 25,* 257–271.

Van Dam, A., Keijsers, G. P. J., Verbraak, M. J. P. M., Eling, P. A. T. M., & Becker, E. S. (2012). Burnout patients primed with success did not perform better on a cognitive task than burnout patients primed with failure. *Psychology, 3,* 583–589.

Van der Linden, D., Keijsers, G. P. J., Eling, P., & Van Schaijk, R. (2005). Work stress and attentional difficulties: An initial study on burnout and cognitive failures. *Work & Stress 19,* 23–36.

Weber, A., & Jaekel-Reinhard, A. (2000). Burnout syndrome: A disease of modern societies? *Occupational Medicine, 50*(7), 512–517.

Webster, G. C., & Bayliss, F. (2000). Moral residue. In S. B. Rubin & L. Zoloth (Eds.), *Margin of error: The ethics of mistakes in the practice of medicine* (pp. 217–230). Hagerstown, MD: University Publishing Group.

Williams, C. L. (1995). Hidden advantages for men in nursing. *Nursing Administration Quarterly, 19*(2), 63–70.

Wooten, L., & Crane, P. (2004). Generating dynamic capabilities through a humanistic work ideology: The case of a certified-nurse midwife practice in a professional bureaucracy. *American Behavioral Scientist, 47*(6), *848–866.*

Yin, J., & Yang, K. (2002). Nursing turnover in Taiwan: A meta-analysis of related factors. *International Journal of Nursing Studies, 39*(6), 573–581.

Zeytinoglu, I. U., Denton, M., Davies, S. Baumannc, A., Blythe, J., & Boos, L. (2006). Retaining nurses in their employing hospitals and in the profession: Effects of job preference, unpaid overtime, importance of earnings and stress. *Health Policy, 79*(1), 57–72.

Zimmerman, S., Gruber-Baldini, A. L., Hebel, J. R., Sloane, P. D., & Magaziner, J. (2002). Nursing home facility risk factors for infection and hospitalization: Importance of registered nurse turnover, administration, and social factors. *Journal of the American Geriatrics Society, 50*(12), 1987–1995.

— 11 —

Staffing and Missed Nursing Care

Staffing and Patient Outcomes

Numerous studies have demonstrated the impact of nurse staffing on patient outcomes. Increased nurse staffing levels have been linked to a reduction in several patient outcomes including mortality rates (Aiken, Clarke, Cheung, Sloane, & Silber, 2003; Needleman, Buerhaus, Mattke, Stewart, & Zelevinsky, 2002), infection rates (Cimiotti, Haas, Saiman, & Larson, 2006; Hugonnet, Chevrolet, & Pittet, 2007; Stone et al., 2007), pressure ulcers (Unruh, 2003), and falls (Kane, Shamliyan, Mueller, Duval, & Wilt, 2007). These complications, in many instances, lead to longer hospital stays and increased costs (Cho, Ketefian, Barkauskas, & Smith, 2003; Dorr, Horn, & Smout, 2005).

Kane and associates (2007) conducted a review of over 100 studies of the association of nurse staffing and patient outcomes. The findings from this meta-analysis of 96 studies showed that staffing levels were associated with hospital-related mortality. Greater RN staffing was consistently associated with a reduction in the adjusted odds ratio of hospital-related mortality. An increase by 1 RN FTE (full-time equivalent) per patient day was associated with a 9% reduction in odds of death in ICUs, 16% in surgical, and 6% in medical patients. The authors estimated that "if the association was causal, an increase of 1 RN FTE per patient day would save 5 lives per 1,000 hospitalized patients in ICUs, 5 lives per 1,000 medical patients, and 6 per 1,000 surgical patients" (Kane et al., 2007, p. 1197). They also reported that better RN staffing was associated with lower odds of hospital-acquired pneumonia (19% less likely) and respiratory failure (60% lower odds per RN FTE). Each additional RN FTE per patient day in the ICU resulted in 51% less unplanned extubation and 28% fewer cardiac arrests. In surgical patients, odds of failure to rescue and of nosocomial bloodstream infection were reduced by 16% and 36%, respectively. On the other hand, they found that staffing was not associated with urinary tract infections, surgical bleeding, falls, or pressure ulcers.

Although the link between staffing levels and patient outcomes has been well established, few studies have focused on the process of nursing care that results in better outcomes. In this chapter, we report the results of a study of staffing and missed nursing care, using three different measures of staffing (Kalisch, Tschannen, & Lee, 2011).

Study of Missed Nursing Care and Staffing
Research Questions
The overall aim of this study was to examine the relationship between the levels and type of nurse staffing and missed nursing care in acute care hospitals. The following are the specific research questions:

1. Does the level and type of nurse staffing (hours per patient day) predict missed nursing care?
2. Does the number of patients cared for on the previous shift predict missed nursing care?
3. Does the perceived adequacy of nurse staffing predict missed nursing care?

Setting and Sample
A total of 110 units—including medical–surgical (52%), intermediate (19%), intensive care (24%), and rehabilitation (5%)—in 10 acute care hospitals and 4,288 nursing staff members participated in the study. The *MISSCARE Survey* administered to the participating staff members included questions about their perceptions of staffing adequacy and number of patients cared for on the last shift. In addition, actual unit level staffing data (HPPD, RN HPPD, and skill mix) was collected for the month during the time the surveys were administered as well a month prior to this time in order to account for any unusual monthly variation in staffing on the units. The operational definitions for these

variables (e.g., HPPD, RN HPPD, skill mix, nursing education, experience, case mix index, etc.) are contained in Chapter 5. Hospitals were asked to provide the data in raw form (i.e., numerator and denominator) in order to ensure consistency and comparability in computation. Subsequently, the research team computed the study variables.

Data Analysis
This study included both individual and unit levels data. Unit level analyses were conducted with actual staffing variables (HPPD, RN HPPD, and skill mix), while individual level data was utilized when the number of patients cared for on the previous shift and reports of staffing adequacy were being examined. For the individual analyses, a series of bivariate correlations were calculated to find the significant staff characteristics that were potential predictors of missed nursing care. To evaluate how perceived staffing adequacy and number of patients cared for on the last shift predicted the amount of missed nursing care, a linear regression model was calculated after controlling for the significant staff characteristics that were found in the bivariate correlations.

For the unit level analyses, characteristics of the sample were aggregated to the unit level in order to test the relationship between unit characteristics (HPPD, RN HPPD, and skill mix) and missed care. For these analyses, a unit-level missed care score was calculated as the average amount of missed care identified for each of the elements of nursing care by nursing staff on each unit. For aggregation to be statistically appropriate, it is necessary to demonstrate that the members of each unit reported similar scores for the unit on a given measure, and the units have significant between-unit variance for a given measure. In order to determine the degree of congruence between individual staff members' survey responses and the appropriateness of aggregating these measures to the unit level, one-way ANOVA and intraclass correlation coefficients (ICC1 and ICC2) were calculated. In this study, the ICC1 for missed care was 0.13 and the ICC2 was 0.90, which are both acceptable scores falling well within the expected ranges. The one-way ANOVA with type of unit as the independent variable and the missed care mean scores as the dependent variable was highly significant ($p < .000$). Findings from these techniques supported the creation of a unit-level missed nursing care score.

One-way ANOVA was used to test missed nursing care differences by type of units. Correlation analysis was used to address the relationship between unit characteristics and missed nursing care. A multiple regression analysis was performed to determine the predictive ability of the variables on the dependent variable, missed nursing care. In addition, accounting for hospital effect (i.e., nesting of data), nine hospital dummy variables were included in the multivariate analysis.

Findings

Of the study respondents, 15% were under 25 years of age, while 56% were 25 to 44, and another 29% were over 44 years. The majority of staff were female (90%) RNs (73.5%) who worked full time (81.7%). On average, 49.5% of the respondents worked day shifts. In terms of education, the average percentage of staff on the unit holding a BSN degree or higher was 46.7%. The majority of units sampled had staff members with greater than 5 years of experience in the profession/occupation (51.0%).

The mean missed nursing care score for the participating units was 1.55 ($SD \pm .19$), with a range of 1.09 to 2.67. HPPD values for participating units ranged from a low of 6.5 to a high of 32.0 with the mean of 11.16 ($SD \pm 4.55$). The average RN HPPD value was 8.55 ($SD \pm 4.28$), with a range of 3.5 to 20.9. The mean skill mix of staff on the units was 0.75 ($SD \pm .15$), with a range of 0.39 to 1.00 (1.00 being an all-RN staff).

Unit Characteristics Associated with Missed Care

Pearson correlations were calculated to determine unit characteristics significantly related to missed nursing care. A negative correlation was found between missed care and both HPPD and RN HPPD. The higher the HPPD ($r = -0.32$, $p < 0.01$) and RN HPPD ($r = -0.27$, $p < 0.01$), the lower the levels of missed care. Greater absenteeism was associated with higher levels of missed nursing care ($r = 0.26$, $p < 0.01$), while higher case mix index values were linked to lower amounts of missed nursing care ($r = -0.20$, $p < 0.05$). This finding is probably due to the fact that intensive care units have higher case mix indexes than other units and are staffed with more nurses, both of which may lead to less missed nursing care.

Predicting Missed Nursing Care

Multiple regression analysis was computed to determine whether unit characteristics predict missed nursing care. RN HPPD was dropped from the model due to a high correlation between HPPD and RN HPPD ($r = 0.91$, $p < 0.01$). The choice of HPPD over RN HPPD was based on the fact that the study sample included all levels of nurse staffing (RNs, LPNs, and NAs). The model (Table 11.1) considered the

TABLE 11.1. **Multiple linear regression model for missed nursing care predicting by staffing variables (n = 4288).**

Predictors	Estimate (SE)	t	p
HPPD	−0.02 (0.01)	−0.45	.002
Case mix index	0.01 (0.02)	0.04	.75
Experience (≥5 years)	0.06 (0.11)	0.06	.58
Absenteeism	0.16 (0.17)	0.15	.34
R^2 = 0.29, F = 3.03, p = .001			

Note: Analysis included nine dummy variables for study hospitals to control for hospital differences.

following indicators: HPPD, experience (greater than 5 years), absenteeism, and case mix index; all of which had significant correlations with missed nursing care.

The overall model accounted for 29.4% of the variation in missed nursing care (p < .001). HPPD was significantly associated with missed nursing care: The greater the HPPD, the lower the level of missed nursing care (β = −.45, p = .002). Other variables in the model were not significant predictors.

Staffing Adequacy and Number of Patients Cared For
A series of bivariate correlations were completed between missed nursing care and staff characteristics. The staff characteristics significantly correlated with missed nursing care included: gender, age, job title, experience in role, experience on current unit, overtime, and absenteeism (Table 11.2). After controlling these significant staff characteristics, a multiple regression model was calculated to evaluate how individual-level staffing variables—staffing adequacy and number of patients cared for on the last shift—predicted missed nursing care (Table 11.3). The results showed both staffing adequacy (β = −.103, p < .001) and number of patients cared for (β = .016, p < .001) were significant predictors for missed nursing care, and explained the 6.1% of variance in missed nursing care. In other words, those who cared for more patients had more missed care while nursing staff who perceived their staffing as adequate more often had less missed care.

Summary
Although there have been numerous studies (noted in previous chapters) which link staffing levels with patient outcomes, there has been less research that explains why these linkages exist. Findings of this study explain, at least in part, what is occurring within the process of providing nursing care. It reveals the fact that certain aspects of

TABLE 11-2. Missed nursing care, staffing adequacy, number of patients, and individual characteristics: Correlation matrix (n = 4086).

	1	2	3	4	5	6	7	8	9	10	11	12	13
1. Missed care	1												
2. Education	.012	1											
3. Gender	.057**	-.025	1										
4. Age	.058**	-.161**	.019	1									
5. Job title	-.198**	.013	-.112**	-.149**	1								
6. Full-time equivalence	-.009	-.014	-.040*	-.003	-.092**	1							
7. Shift	-.014	.057**	-.049**	-.111**	-.045**	.049**	1						
8. Experience in role	.088**	-.055**	.068**	.538**	-.114**	-.083**	-.176**	1					
9. Experience on current unit	.086**	-.091**	.065**	.408**	-.127**	-.069**	-.211**	.668**	1				
10. Overtime	.035**	-.016	-.027	.052**	-.129**	.179**	.002	-.008	.018	1			
11. Absenteeism	.061**	-.009	.006	-.076**	.023	.066**	.036*	-.044**	-.058**	.055**	1		
12. Staffing adequacy	-0.187**	.031*	-.058**	-.011	-.061**	-.011	.022	.011	-.007	-.077**	-.075**	1	
13. Number of patients cared for	-.037**	-.100**	-.015	-.073**	.578**	-.041**	-.004	-.102**	-.093**	-.047**	-.001	-.131**	1

Note: ** $p < .01$; * $p < .05$

TABLE 11.3. **Predictors of missed nursing care* (n = 4086).**

	β	St. Error	t	p
Staffing adequacy	−0.103	0.007	−14.263	<.001**
Number of patients cared for	0.016	0.003	5.584	<.001**

Note: * After controlling for age, gender, job title, experience in role, experience on current unit, overtime and absenteeism. ** $p < .01$

nursing care are not being completed, and that one reason for this is inadequate staffing.

All three staffing variables in this study—HPPD, perceived staffing adequacy, and number of patients cared for—were strong predictors of missed nursing care. When staffing is lower, nurses are unable to complete all required care. Having fewer staff leads to less care because it limits the capacity of staff members to help one another or step in whenever care is required. For example, when a nurse or nursing assistant needs to ambulate the patient, he or she is less likely to find other staff members who would have time to ambulate the patient than if staffing were adequate.

In addition, unit type was not included in the final regression model since unit type was not correlated with missed nursing care ($F[3,106] = 2.219$, $p = .10$). However, we ran the multiple regressions after including a unit type variable (i.e., ICU [reference variable] vs. non-ICU unit) to explore the effects of case mix index and unit type on missed nursing care. HPPD was a significant predictor ($\beta = 3.71$, $p < .001$). Case mix index was still negatively associated with missed care, but was not statistically significant ($\beta = -.03$, $p = .84$). As noted above, it is likely that patients who are more acutely ill get more overall attention than those who are less acute.

These findings are similar to the results of a study by Ball, Murrells, Rafferty, Morrow, and Griffiths (2014), referred to in Chapter 2. They investigated the impact of staffing levels on unfinished (missed) nursing care in English hospitals. The study used the staffing measure of nurse self-reports as to how many patients they cared for on the previous shift and if any of a list of 13 nursing actions (adequate patient surveillance, adequate documentation of nursing care, administering medication on time, comforting and talking with patients, developing or updating nursing care plans and care pathways, educating patients and family, frequent changing of patient's position, oral hygiene, pain management, planning care, preparing patients and families for discharge, skin care, and undertaking treatments and procedures) were missed. They found that the fewer patients assigned, the less care was missed ($p < 0.001$). Fewer elements of care were missed ($p < 0.01$) and the odds of missing any care were significantly lower (OR 0.343, 95% CI 0.222 to 0.53, $p < 0.001$) when RNs were caring for the fewest patients (6.13 or fewer patients per RN) compared with when caring for the highest number of patients (11.67 or more patients per RN). RN staffing level was significantly associated with missed care for 8 of the 13 care activities. The impact of staffing was strongest for patient surveillance, documentation, and comforting patients. Nurses working on shifts with 12 patients per RN were twice as likely to report inadequate patient surveillance, when compared with shifts in which there were fewer than 6.14 patients per RN. There was no relationship between number of patients cared for by the RN and repositioning, giving medications on time, managing, and discharge planning.

These studies highlight the importance of adequate nurse staffing levels to ensure that required nursing care is provided to patients on a consistent basis. As concerns for cost reduction continue, it is imperative to consider the impact of reducing staffing levels in nursing. Findings from this study also reveal insight into how we can specifically improve nursing care.

References

Aiken, L. H., Clarke, S. P., Cheung, R. B., Sloane, D. M., & Silber, J. H. (2003). Educational levels of hospital nurses and surgical patient mortality. *Journal of the American Medical Association, 290*(12), 1617–1623.

Ball, J. E., Murrells, T., Rafferty, A. M., Morrow, E., & Griffiths, P. (2014). 'Care left undone' during nursing shifts: Associations with workload and perceived quality of care. *BMJ Quality & Safety, 23*(2), 116–125.

Cho, S. H., Ketefian, S., Barkauskas, V. H., & Smith, D. G. (2003). The effects of nurse staffing on adverse events, morbidity, mortality, and medical costs. *Nursing Research, 52*(2), 71–79.

Cimiotti, J. P., Haas, J., Saiman, L., & Larson, E. L. (2006). Impact of staffing on bloodstream infections in the neonatal intensive care unit. *Archives of Pediatrics & Adolescent Medicine, 160*(8), 832–836.

Dorr, D. A., Horn, S. D., & Smout, R. J. (2005). Cost analysis of nursing home registered nurse staffing times. *Journal of the American Geriatrics Society, 53*(5), 840–845.

Hugonnet, S., Chevrolet, J. C., & Pittet, D. (2007). The effect of workload on infection risk in critically ill patients. *Critical Care Medicine, 35*(1), 76–81.

Kane, R. L., Shamliyan, T. A., Mueller, C., Duval, S., & Wilt, T. J. (2007). The association of registered nurse staffing levels and patient outcomes—Systematic review and meta-analysis. *Medical Care, 45*(12), 1195–1204.

Kalisch, B., Tschannen, D., & Lee, K. (2011). Do staffing levels predict missed nursing care? *International Journal for Quality in Health Care, 23*(3), 1–7.

Needleman, J., Buerhaus, P., Mattke, S., Stewart, M., & Zelevinsky, K. (2002). Nurse-staffing levels and the quality of care in hospitals. *New England Journal of Medicine, 346*(22), 1715–1722.

Stone, P. W., Mooney-Kane, C., Larson, E. L., Horan, T., Glance, L. G., Zwanziger, J., & Dick, A. W. (2007). Nurse working conditions and patient safety outcomes. *Medical Care, 45*(6), 571–578.

Unruh, L. (2003). Licensed nurse staffing and adverse events in hospitals. *Medical Care, 41*(1), 142–152.

— 12 —

Teamwork and Missed Nursing Care

Teamwork is essential for patient safety and quality of care. Beginning with the Institute of Medicine (IOM) study, *To Err Is Human*, administrators, regulators, and providers alike began to recognize the need for enhanced teamwork in health care to avoid patient errors (Institute of Medicine, 2000). This IOM report made recommendations to decrease errors which included enhanced teamwork.

When people work on high performing teams, they are more satisfied (Gifford, Zammuto, & Goodman, 2002; Horak, Guarino, Knight, & Kweder, 1991; Rafferty, Ball, & Aiken, 2001), they are more productive (Rondeau & Wagar, 1998) and less stressed (Carter & West, 1999), the quality of the care they deliver is higher (Liedtka & Whitten, 1997; Shortell, O'Brien, & Carman, 1995; Young et al., 1998; Schmutz & Manser, 2013), there are fewer errors (Morey et al., 2002; Sil´en-Lipponen, Tossavainen, Turunen, & Smith, 2005; Auerbach et al., 2012; Blegen et al., 2013; Chassin & Loeb, 2011; Kalisch, Tschannen, & Lee, 2011a; Weaver et al., 2010), and patients are more satisfied (Meterko, Mohr, & Young, 2004). A systematic review of 28 studies on the impact of team processes on clinical performance (e.g., fall rates, morbidity, mortality) revealed that "every study reported at least one significant relationship between team processes and performance" (Schmutz & Manser, 2013).

There are 5,723 acute care hospitals with 920,829 staffed beds in the United States alone,which have anywhere from 1 to 15 or more patient care units that operate 7 days a week, 24 hours a day. Each of these estimated 50,000 units has a team(s) of nursing staff (RNs, LPNs, NAs, and unit secretaries [USs]). Given the number of these teams, the potential magnitude of patient errors and diminished quality, caused by lack of teamwork among the members of the nursing team, is enormous (American Hospital Association, 2014).

Most definitions of teamwork contain the following three elements: two or more individuals, a common purpose, and interdependence. Team members have specific role assignments, must perform particular tasks, must make decisions, interact, and coordinate to achieve a common goal(s) or outcome(s) (Brannick, Salas, & Prince, 1997).

This chapter will review the results of several studies dealing with aspects of nursing teamwork: (1) behaviors of teamwork, (2) the dynamics of the RN–NA relationships, (3) measuring nursing teamwork, (4) characteristics of nursing teams, (5) staffing levels and teamwork, (6) job satisfaction and teamwork, (7) quality and safety and teamwork, and (8) teamwork and missed nursing care.

1. Teamwork Behaviors

Numerous theories of teamwork have been developed over the past 20 years. An extensive review of the literature uncovered 138 teamwork theories (Salas, Stagl, & Burke, 2004). Of these, we have chosen to utilize the Salas conceptual framework of teamwork in our work because it offers a real-world, behavioral, and clear-cut explanation of teamwork that can be widely understood. This theory promotes accurate diagnoses of teamwork problems and what needs to be done to correct them (Salas, Sims, & Burke, 2005).

The Salas framework (Figure 12.1) describes teamwork as five major core components, coined the "Big Five," supported by three main coordinating mechanisms. This framework has been extensively used as a foundation for studying teamwork (Baker, Day, & Salas, 2006; Eppich, Brannen, & Hunt, 2008; Nielsen & Mann, 2008). The five core components of teamwork in the Salas model are (Salas, Sims, & Burke, 2005):

1. Team leadership (i.e., coordination and support provided by the formal leader and/or other team members)
2. Collective orientation (i.e., extent to which the team needs and objectives are more important than the individual's desires)

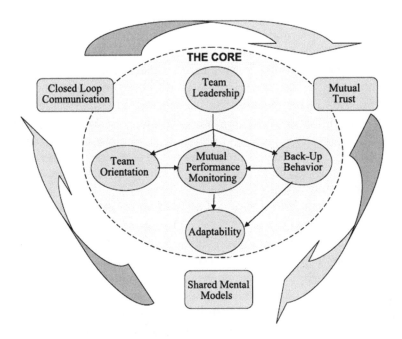

FIGURE 12.1. **The 'Big Five' framework of teamwork.**
Reprinted with permission from Ed Salas, University of Central Florida.

3. Mutual performance monitoring (i.e., team members' observation and cognizance of one another's work and issues)
4. Back-up behavior (i.e., assisting other team members with their responsibilities)
5. Adaptability (i.e., use of adjustment strategies when needed)

According to the framework, these relationships are fostered via three coordinating mechanisms:

1. Shared mental models (i.e., the extent to which team members have a shared concept of their work) (Mathieu, Heffner, Goodwin, Salas, & Cannon-Bowers, 2008)
2. Closed-loop communication (i.e., active information exchange in which receiver verifies receipt and the sender verifies whether the intended message was received) (Brown, 2004)
3. Mutual trust (i.e., shared perception that members will perform actions necessary to reach interdependent goals and act in the interest of the team)

To understand the team functioning in nursing units, we conducted a qualitative study that applied the Salas teamwork conceptual framework to nursing teams (Kalisch, Weaver, & Salas, 2009). We wanted to determine whether this concept of teamwork could be used to capture and describe teamwork in nursing teams functioning on patient care units in acute care hospitals. This study involved conducting 34 focus group interviews with RNs, LPNs, NAs, and USs from five patient care units. RNs in the focus groups were 97% female, had 18 years of experience, 10 of which were on their current unit, and had an average age of 42 years. The LPNs had a mean age of 46 years, were all women, and had an average of 25 years of experience in nursing and 23 years of practice on their current units. The NA focus group members had an average age of 25.2 years, were 94% women, and had worked 7 years as an NA, 6 of which were on their current patient care units.

To analyze the data, a grounded theory approach was used (Glaser & Strauss, 1967). Two researchers analyzed the data independently. The results showed that although differently grouped, both pulled out the same issues from the interview data. The use of the Salas model in explaining nursing teamwork was substantiated by the study. Table 12.1 provides selected data from the study, giving examples from the focus groups where the team behavior was present or not. Each behavior is further explained below.

TABLE 12.1.   **Example focus group comments illustrating the five core components of teamwork and three coordinating functions.**

	Examples of presence	Examples of absence
Team leadership	RN: The charge nurse watches over all of the staff, determining when they need assistance.	RN: We don't get our assignment for the shift until 9 o'clock. We never catch up.
Team or collective orientation	RN: According to what we hear the needs of the patients are, we divide our team. We do not go 'Ok there are eight patients so you get four and I get four.'	NA: The RNs count the patients as opposed to looking at how much demand of time everything it would take.
Mutual performance monitoring	RN: We put a board up and each person puts a green, yellow or red tag up depending on how their work is going. Red they can't take another thing, yellow is they are busy but it will probably get better soon, and green is I am on top of my work. That way the charge nurse knows who to give a new admission to and so forth. RN: We let each other know if we missed something and we don't take offense. It is the way we function.	RN: It was insane and very dangerous. There were three of us that night, and we each had eight patients. You couldn't help each other because you had eight of your own. NA: I see a little of what the other staff are doing, like if a nurse leaves a medication at the bedside, I just throw it away.

	Examples of presence	Examples of absence
Back-up behavior	RN: You ask once and everybody is there. If there is a crisis, everybody is behind you. When I had a real crisis with one patient, a nurse stayed after her shift and took care of all my other patients without me even asking.	RN: Sometimes I feel bad asking for help because I feel that if I am asking the charge nurse for help frequently, that it looks like I am just not able to handle my job, that I am not a good nurse
Adaptability	NA: Some units really watch out for their NAs and make sure they are not being given too much work.	RN: We have staff on both 8 and 12 hour shifts and instead of reassigning patients so the nurse coming on doesn't have patients on all three wings, we let her run.
Shared mental models	RN: We have a routine when a patient has to go on a road trip to have a diagnostic procedure. We know that the patient is transported on their bed, not a stretcher, that we need IV poles that roll well, that the respiratory therapist has to go on the trip if the patient is on a vent, that we need the key for the elevator so we don't have to wait, that we have to take the patient's medications with us. The charge nurse calls the respiratory therapist and transportation, and when the patient's nurse says she is ready, another nurse helps finalize the preparations.	RN: A nurse floated to our unit and did things the way they do on her floor. This created a safety problem because she thought the other staff members would give her patients their medications when she took a break. She found out several hours later that this was not the case.
Closed-loop communication	RN: I meet with the NAs I am working with as soon as I can in the shift so we know the objectives for the shift and who is going to do what.	RN: I feel angry when I have not been told the important things I need to know for my shift. It makes me look bad and the unit looks bad. I have had patients say, 'Do you talk to each other?'
Mutual trust	RN: If I work with certain people, I know a good job is being done.	RN: I would like to believe the aid when she tells me she ambulated the patient, but I am not sure.

Permission was obtained to reprint this table from Kalisch, B., Weaver, S., & Salas, E., (2009). What does nursing teamwork look like? A qualitative study. Journal of Nursing Care Quality, 24(4), 298–307.

Team Leadership

Participants identified that the overall leadership style and expectations of the nurse manager as key factors in determining whether or not they would operate as a team. There were both positive examples (e.g., "Our manager really values us working well together and expects it" [RN]) and negative ones (e.g., "The manager of our unit appears to not value teamwork since she engages in conversations with staff about other staff members, which really hurts teamwork" [RN]).

While the nurse manager oversees the unit, assistant nurse managers and/or charge nurses (appointed for each shift) are at the point of care delivery and thus in the best position to ensure teamwork on any given shift. Successful charge nurse leadership was described in the focus groups as central to unit functioning, and involved the provision of adequate resources and relationship building. A problem identified in this study was the lack of stability of the charge nurse role, which is often a rotating job (e.g., "We have a different charge nurse almost every day. You have to do things differently for each one" [RN]).

NAs were reportedly given specific tasks to do, such as ambulation, vital signs, baths and feeding, but the RN reportedly did not follow up when they delegated to determine if the delegatee performed the work. Instead of providing leadership in these instances, the RNs often assumed that the NAs were doing their job, or hoped they were (and perhaps thinking that information you don't have cannot hurt you). The leadership behaviors of the NAs were also identified (e.g., "When a patient coded, the NA, without being asked, moved a second patient out of the room" [RN]).

Team or Collective Orientation

There were many instances discussed by the focus group participants about problems with team (collective) orientation. For example, evening and night shift staff members complained about work that was not done during the day, without consideration of why this might be so. Another common area illustrating the lack of team orientation was the process of making patient assignments. In many units, RNs are said to begin the shift questioning their assignment compared to what is assigned to others on the team. In these instances, only the number of patients seems to matter, not other factors such as the acuity of the patient. Another common example of the lack of team orientation was that RNs, when asked by the patient for a bedpan or water, would search all over the unit for the NA rather than provide the care themselves (e.g., "Nurses are consistently refusing to put a patient on a bedpan when they are in the room and the patient requests it. Instead they search all over the unit for me and if I am up to my elbows cleaning a patient, it is a bad scene. The RN could have put the patient on the bedpan herself" [NA]).

Mutual Performance Monitoring

The focus group participants agreed that they need to monitor and be aware of others on the team throughout the work shift. Identified barriers to mutual performance monitoring included staffing levels, an increase in workload demands (e.g., a large number of admissions), the layout and size of the unit, the degree of comfort with asking for help, and the nature of the handoff reports. For example, one RN said, "I don't even see anyone else. I am so busy doing my work, being tied up with my patients, I don't know if anyone else is busy or what." Another RN indicated better situational awareness among unit members: "We are aware of each other. It isn't negative but if we see someone forget to wash their hands, we remind them. We do it for each other."

Back-up Behavior

Many instances of the impact of back-up behavior on the units were highlighted in the focus groups. One problem is that all team members on a nursing team did not completely understand other members' responsibilities. RNs stated that while they understand the work of the NAs and secretaries, NAs and secretaries are not always completely knowledgeable about the responsibilities of the RN. One key area that came up in all the groups was that the NAs complained about the length of time RNs spend sitting down and documenting (e.g., "She is just resting.") RNs expressed frustration that the NAs think they are goofing off, and the NAs stated that they think the RNs use documentation as an excuse to sit down and not give direct care. Other back-up problems identified were not answering one another's call lights, leaving all call lights to the NAs, and not reminding others to wash their hands if they forget. A substantial number of the focus groups participants expressed the belief that they are not responsible for what other team members do or don't do (e.g., "If she doesn't wash her hands, it is her responsibility. I won't say anything because I would provoke an attitude I don't need.") Another example of back-up problems was the it's-not-my-job syndrome, which was reported frequently. The nurses in the focus groups referred to work as "NA work" or "RN work." This is the antithesis of teamwork.

Adaptability

The adaptability of the nursing team was highlighted as very important because so many changes occur even during one shift. An RN stated, "We constantly have a change in our workload with patients getting sicker, new admissions—we can get five at a time—and we pitch in to cover the load together, rather than letting someone take on the impossible." It is essential that team members be aware of the changes in workload in order to adapt appropriately. For example, one RN said, "When an NA calls in sick at the last minute and we can't get a replacement, the one or two NAs working get assigned all of the patients instead of having the nurses take some of them. The NA can't care for 18 or 24 patients."

Shared Mental Models

Shared mental models were discussed in the focus groups. They gave examples of the positive outcome when all members of the team understood what the role of the other individuals was as well as their own. As is evident in Table 12.1, the focus group participants pointed to the presence of many task-related mental models and their impact on team effectiveness. One such example given by an RN was the following: "Everyone knows what to do when a patient codes. The charge nurse immediately pages the code team and takes the code cart to the patient's room, and everyone descends on the room."

Examples of the impact on teamwork when shared mental models were absent were also uncovered in the focus groups. One common area was the shift report, which was stated to be very different from person to person. Standard communication methods, such as Situation Background Assessment Recommendation (SBAR), were mentioned as methods for improving shared mental models. A key issue for teamwork was that RNs heard the shift report from off-going RNs, but NAs were not included in these briefings. The RNs might share information with the NA who was leaving or coming on, but there is typically no report that shares the information between the NAs and the RNs, much less a shared plan for the shift. ("We are not given any report at the beginning of the shift so we really don't know anything about the patients" [NA]).

Closed-loop Communication

Communication problems were identified as a major barrier to successful teamwork. One consistent area mentioned was the hand-offs from shift to shift and within the shift. Problems identified were the extended shift lengths, aggravated by members who came in late, a large portion of the time taken up in socialization with one another, the lack of key information, the inclusion of unnecessary information, and the use of taped reports where there were no opportunities to ask questions. When the shift report and other handoffs were inadequate, participants agreed that teamwork was adversely affected. The practice of not including the assistive personnel in the shift report, and not having a briefing with all team members early in the shift, was identified as very detrimental to teamwork.

Another communication problem was a lack of debriefings during the shift. Team members need to touch base with one another to keep informed and to monitor one another. Debriefings have not been an established practice in nursing. Each staff member has typically been focused on their own assignment. If they have to leave for an intrahospital transport or a break, for example, they are required of give another staff member a report about their patients (or they are supposed to), but these reports are not always adequate. The group of nurses working together rarely confers with one another about the whole group of patients, the overall priorities, and where they need assistance. Several contributing factors played a role in this communication disconnect: poor communication skills on the part of selected staff members, the geography of the unit where nursing staff are physically distant from one another, and the model of care. The model of care or method of assignment was identified by focus group participants to be a barrier to communication between nurses and NAs. As mentioned earlier, the NA reports to two or more RNs, assisting them in the care of their patients. No one knows the total load on the NA because the entire team does not communicate about their work.

Inability to manage conflict was another major theme. RNs and NAs reported that they were not able to manage conflict and almost always avoided it. The conflicts may be small (e.g., "I disagree with how we schedule our in-services, but the others want it that way so I go along" [RN]), or they may spiral out of control and become major (e.g., "I refuse to work when so and so works. If I see her, I walk way out of my way to avoid her" [RN]). Fear of conflict was a common thread in the discussions (e.g., "I would do anything to avoid an argument" [RN]). When questioned about this avoidance of conflict, common responses included that it would make matters worse or that the person would become defensive and take on an attitude.

The scheduling of staff with a combination of 4-, 8-, and 12-hour shifts was reported to create communication problems. This was described as a disorganized and fragmented situation in which staff come and go at all times of the day and night. The strength of the team decreased with the introduction of new staff member(s). The use of agency or per diem staff, even float staff, was also reported to create similar communication problems.

Mutual Trust

The focus group participants identified the key need for trust of their fellow team members if they were to work together effectively. Numerous examples of the lack of trust and its impact on teamwork were noted. RNs expressed distrust about the work of NAs (e.g., "I don't think the NAs do what I ask them" [RN]) and NAs pointed to a lack of trust that the RNs will do their job (e.g., "I have to watch some of the RNs—they don't give pain medication when I tell them the patient really needs it" [NA]) (Schulman-Green et al., 2005).

2. RN and NA Teamwork

The above study pointed to special issues between RNs and NAs that we wanted to investigate further. There have been several studies examining the RN–NA relationship over the past 25 years (Bernreuter & Cardonna, 1997a, 1997b; Chaboyer, McMurray, & Patterson,1998; Chaboyer et al., 2009; Chang, Lam, & Lam, 1998; Standing, Anthony, & Hertz, 2001). These studies, conducted in both acute care hospitals and nursing homes, reveal the following—the desire for more NAs to assist RNs (Huber, Belgen, & McCloskey, 1994; Keeney, Hasson, McKenna, & Gillen, 2005); the conclusion that the workload is excessive for NAs (Crickmer, 2005; Mather & Bakas, 2002; Meek, 1998); mixed opinions as to the quality of care provided by the NA (Keeney et al., 2005; Meek, 1998; Chang, Lam, & Lam, 1997); dissatisfaction with the level of training for the NA (Chase & Paul, 1995; Fisher, 1999; Huber et al., 1994; McKenna, Hasson, & Keeney, 2004); high turnover rates (Kupperschmidt, 2002); problems with RN delegation to NAs (Anthony, Standing, & Hertz, 2000; Cohen, 2004; Davis & Farrell, 1995; Huber et al., 1994; Parsons, 1999; Tourangeau, White, Scott, McAllister, & Giles, 1999;), and lack of trust by nurses in the competency level of the NA and thus a fear of delegating to them (Huber et al., 1994; Potter & Grant, 2004; Scott-Cawiezell et al., 2004).

There has been limited research specifically on teamwork between the NA and the RN. Mather and Bakas (2002) found that lack of teamwork was a barrier to continence care of nursing home patients. They point to the perception that RNs do not listen to NAs or include them in planning care. Potter and Grant (2004) completed a study of the RN and NA working relationships. They interviewed 13 RNs and 9 NAs from 22 units in one acute care hospital. They analyzed three nursing practices—assignment method, orientation and mentoring and change of shift reporting—to determine the nature of the relationships. They found that trust and respect were critical but often nonexistent in these cases. Barter, McLaughlin, and Thomas (1997), Salmond (1995a, 1995b), Scott-Cawiezell and colleagues (2004), and Potter and Grant (2004) also describe mistrust and communication problems between RNs and NAs.

In a qualitative study in three acute care hospitals, we conducted 9 focus groups with RNs (n = 81) and 12 with nursing assistants (NAs) (n = 118). Seven consistent problems emerged from the study: (1) lack of role clarity, (2) working in isolation, (3) inability to deal with conflict, (4) not engaging the NA in decision-making, (5) deficient delegation, (6) more than one boss, and (7) it's not my job syndrome (Kalisch, 2011). Table 12.2 contains a summary of these problems with examples as to how they can negatively impact the quality and safety of care.

Lack of Role Clarity

As indicated earlier, many RNs and NAs do not fully understand one another's role or they have a lack of agreement on who should complete certain tasks. The RN understands the elements of nursing care that the NA is responsible for but not necessarily the workload and barriers the NAs are experiencing in completing their work and vice versa.

- "We realize that they [RNs] have a lot of work to do. But they don't realize that we have a lot of work to do also. They have 7 patients, sometimes 10, but 7 mostly. But we have twenty. They don't seem to realize that." (NA)

- "The NAs don't understand our work and how much goes into it." (RN)

- "I don't care if you're doing charting at that moment. If my patient needs something, that comes before [documenting]. They tell us if we get a call, we have to stop our task to answer the call. Well, they should do the same thing" (NA)

It was evident from the focus group comments that RNs do not always assume their leadership role. There is a lack of acknowledgement that the RN is the leader of the RN–NA dyad. It was clear that RNs fail to consistently direct and support the NA.

246 ERRORS OF OMISSION

TABLE 12.2. **Problems in the RN–NA working relationships and resulting quality and safety problems.**

THEME	SUBTHEME	EXAMPLES OF RESULTANT NEGATIVE IMPACT ON QUALITY AND SAFETY
1. Lack of role clarity	RNs feel NAs do not understand RN responsibilities RN does not assume leadership role with accountability for all of the patients' care. NA does not see the RN as the leader of the team.	NA says she doesn't understand the need for nurse to document so much of the time. She interprets this as "not putting the patient first" and decides to not answer call lights promptly because why should she do it if the RN isn't going to. Because of this, a patient falls trying to get up to the bathroom.
		An NA states *"Why should I be concerned about turning a patient every two hours if the RN just sits and documents and takes it easy. I am not going to worry about turning the patient either."* This patient develops stage 1 pressure ulcer by the end of the shift.
		An RN explains that she is pretty sure the vital signs the NA takes are not accurate but states, *"I don't have time to see if the NA is taking accurate vitals. I just hope they are and I take what they give me."* This patient is found to have a BP of 200/135 by the on-coming shift.
		An NA is asked to check on a patient by the RN and she ignores the request because she wants to take a break. The patient is found later gasping for breath.
2. A lack of teamness	RNs and NAs do not see themselves as a team who has the responsibility to back one another up.	The responsibilities of caring for the patients are divided into RN work and NA work. An NA asks a nurse to help her turn a patient and the RN says she will come but does not show up. The turn is not completed. (NA: *"If the RN doesn't come to help after an hour, I figure she doesn't think it is important and I just skip turning the patient."*)
		An NA requests help to ambulate a 300 lb patient from the RN, who does not respond for over two hours. The NA then tries to get the patient up by herself. The patient falls and is injured and the NA takes a medical leave for a back problem.
		NA sees a medication (Glucophage—oral insulin) left in a cup on a patient's bed stand and throws it way, never telling the RN. The patient's blood sugar is elevated on the next blood test and the RN cannot understand why. The dose of Glucophage is increased.

THEME	SUBTHEME	EXAMPLES OF RESULTANT NEGATIVE IMPACT ON QUALITY AND SAFETY
3. Inability to deal with conflict	RNs and NAs find it very difficult to confront and give/ receive feedback	RNs overlook performance problems of the NA because the NA "will refuse to help me with my patients if I do tell her anything she is not doing correctly." This NA does not inform anyone of skin reddening on a patient, who subsequently developed a pressure ulcer.
		An NA doesn't report a nurse leaving medications at the bedside because *"The manager won't believe me. I am just an aid. I couldn't talk to her about it, no way. She* [the RN] *would get mad and I can't deal with that."* This RN continues to leave medication at the bedside.
		A patient is brought up to the unit from the ED by a transporter, informs the NA. The NA fails to notify the nurse for 2 hours. In the meantime, the patient is in intense pain. The RN does not address this with the NA. A few months later, the same NA does the same thing and the patient is dead when the RN finally gets into the room.
		An NA reminds an RN multiple times not to leave medications on the counter but the RN keeps doing it and the NA lets it drop. Two weeks later this RN gives a medication meant for another patient because someone moved it.
4. Not engaging the NA in decision-making	NAs do not attend report with RNs	NA does not know that a patient is supposed to keep the head of the bed up and lowers it.
	NA not being listened to by RN	NA doesn't know the patient is going to surgery and allows patient to drink water.
	Commanding rather than asking in a respectful manner	NA doesn't know the patient's husband died last night and doesn't acknowledge it.
		An RN does not give a patient pain medication after the NA tells her that the patient is in "terrible" pain. The NA then stops telling the RN that her patient needs pain medication (*"She doesn't care what I say so I give up trying even though it really bothers me to see a patient in such pain."*)
		NA states that when she is commanded to do something by an RN "*I just don't do it and I don't tell her either.*" Another NA states: '*If she can't ask me nicely, it's not going to get done.*"

(Continued)

TABLE 12.2. **Problems in the RN–NA working relationships and resulting quality and safety problems (continued).**

THEME	SUBTHEME	EXAMPLES OF RESULTANT NEGATIVE IMPACT ON QUALITY AND SAFETY
5. Deficient delegation	Not obtaining buy-in of NA RNs not retaining accountability, not following through Not clear enough directions by RN	The RN asks an NA to measure the amount of output of a patient but does not explain how important this activity is for this patient, who has an elevated temperature of 103. The NA becomes busy and does not record fluid output for several hours.
		An RN does not follow up to be sure the NA accompanied a patient for toileting. The patient gets up on their own and falls, sustaining a hip fracture.
		An NA does not do mouth care on an elderly patient who has xerostomia and the RN does not follow up. The patient refuses to eat because of this—difficulty chewing. This patient also develops pneumonia.
		The NA doesn't say whether or not she ambulated her patients as ordered and the RN doesn't ask (she assumes she has and documents it). RN: *"What I don't know won't hurt me."*
		An RN tells an NA to "ambulate the patient" but does not specify how many times, when it should be done, or that this particular patient needs at least two people involved. The NA only ambulates the patient once by herself. The patient slips and hits her head on the door frame of the room, sustaining a cut on her forehead.
		An RN asks an NA to carefully record everything the patient drinks and any "food that turns into liquid at room temperature." The NA does not record Jell-O input because she didn't understand the directions and the RN did not ensure that the NA understood.
6. More than one "boss" for NA	NAs typically reports to two (or more) RNs and neither RN knows the full workload of the NA and whether or not it is doable.	An NA runs out of time to do all the vital signs on her patients and records the previous vital signs because she doesn't want to get in trouble with the RN. The patient's blood pressure suddenly rises and he has a stroke.
		NA: *"When one of the NAs doesn't come in, they give us all 20 patients. We can't possibly do everything for them and things are left undone, important things. The RNs don't know."*

THEME	SUBTHEME	EXAMPLES OF RESULTANT NEGATIVE IMPACT ON QUALITY AND SAFETY
7. "It's not my job syndrome"	Duties and responsibilities are strictly defined as being those of the RN or NA, thus the other does not assume responsibility.	An RN is in a patient's room and the patient needs a bedpan. Instead of getting it, she hunts for the NA to do it. In the meantime, the patient gets up, urinates on the floor, and slips and falls. An RN states vital signs are not her responsibility and she blames the NA when the patient codes.
	RNs state that ambulation, monitoring I and O, turning, bathing, mouth care, etc., are aide work and they fail to ensure that this care is completed	
	RNs report that they are not responsible for aide work	

Table reprinted with permission from Kalisch, B. (2011). The impact of RN–UAP relationships on quality and safety. Nursing Management, 42(9), 16–22.

Working in Isolation

Both RNs and NAs reported practicing almost in isolation. NAs often do not receive a report from the RN until two or more hours into the shift. As described above, the absence of briefing sessions to begin the shift and debriefing meetings during and at the end of the shifts diminishes (or makes impossible) working as a team. Both RNs and NAs expressed annoyance that when they have tasks to do that they cannot do by themselves, such as turning a heavy patient, that they have difficulty finding a team member to help. NAs reported seeking out another NA on a distant part of the unit rather than trying to engage the RN they are working with.

Inability to Deal with Conflict

Both the RNs and NAs expressed reluctance in giving feedback and engaging in conflicts with one another. They pointed to the fact that NAs and RNs do not work with the same individuals regularly, which is a deterrent to giving feedback. When the RNs were asked about how they dealt with a situation where the NA was not performing well, the vast majority stated that it is not worth the trouble of confronting them and that it is doubtful that it would help anyway (e.g., "If I say anything, the assistant will just clam up and pout. Nothing changes" [RN]). The

RNs verbalized a strong reluctance and a lack of skill in giving negative feedback to the NAs, partly because they feared retaliation from the NA, who might give less care to patients in the future (e.g., "It's a constant battle to get what you need from the NA" [RN]), but also because they detest conflict and would "avoid it at all costs." The NAs also expressed a reluctance to give feedback and deal with conflicts with each other and the RNs.

Not Engaging the NA in Decision-making

The focus group participants noted that the NA is not involved in the decisions about patient care and unit management. It starts by not having a report together at the beginning of each shift and continues with a lack of communication throughout the shift. NAs felt that they were often not listened to by the RN. Another subtheme was the nurse commanding the NA rather than asking in a respectful manner. Focus group members stated that RNs often communicate in a top-down, demanding manner. The NAs felt devalued and diminished and unwilling to be a team player because of it ("Sometimes they [RNs] look down at you like you are nothing. I am the nurse, you are an aide, and you do what I say no matter what." [NA]). When the NA was not drawn into the decisions about patient care, they did not develop an ownership of the goals of the nurse, unit, and organization. This ownership is essential for accountability ("Why should I care? No one asks me what I think" [NA]). Communication was reported to largely take place through written means.

Deficient Delegation

The RNs expressed a great deal of concern about the quality of the work of many of the NAs. They pointed to a lack of appropriate training ("I don't know how they get trained but a lot of times they just get thrown into the job" [RN]) and a poor work ethic ("I would be ecstatic if they would do their job" [RN]). The NAs were reported to not follow through on the directions of the RNs ("They kind of just develop their own routine and that is what they do" [RN]). Another issue was the extra work required of the RN when the NA did not function at a high enough level ("If she is somebody you are going to have to take by the hand, I am going to have to watch everything she does to see that she does it, or encourage her. You know, it is like on top of what I have to do, this is another load" [RN]).

RNs complained that they were the only ones capable of doing all of the tasks and responsibilities ("Secretaries cannot do our job but we can do theirs, the attendants cannot do our job but we can do theirs. No one can do our job but us" [RN]). Deficient delegation skills were consistently evident in the focus group discussions. RNs were not able to describe effective delegation when asked ("We just tell them to do it and hope they do" [RN]). The RNs repeatedly voiced practices that were the opposite of effective delegation. The NAs also did not understand their role in the delegation process ("If I don't understand what they want me to do, I don't ask them to clarify because they are too busy" [NA]).

In the first place, the RN or delegator did not complete the first step in the delegation process, which is obtaining buy-in from the delegatee (NA). Many of the focus group participants stated that the NAs do not attend shift reports with the nurses or even receive them for two or more hours into the shift, if then. Even when the NAs received reports from the RNs, there was a lack of collaborative planning as to how they would jointly care for patients during that shift, and the NA expressed reluctance to clarify responsibilities, resulting in confusion and not achieving the goals of the team. Without this type of interaction and planning for what the patient needs and who on the team will do what and at what time, the NA is unlikely to understand what needs to be done. Besides the lack of planning at the beginning of the shift, the NA focus group participants also noted that many RNs rarely checked with them during the shift to see how they were progressing and if any problems had emerged ("If I had to worry whether the NA work gets done, I wouldn't have time for my own work" [RN]).

The second issue was the RN not retaining accountability. It was very revelatory to listen to the RN focus group members refer to the fact that they believe they are accountable only for the "RN work," not the "NA work." When asked if they were accountable for all the care, they would say "Yes, but..." It appears that the majority of RNs in the focus groups functioned in a way that demonstrates non-accountability for the entire care of the patients. These RNs stated that certain tasks (measuring intake and output, turning, and ambulating, etc.) are the NA's responsibility, and if the NA does not complete these tasks, it is the NA's fault, not theirs, and they should not be expected to cover the NA in these instances ("The NAs are supposed to do the vital signs, the ambulation, turning, and I don't have time to make sure they really do these things. I have to take their word for it." [RN]).

A third problem is that some nurses would rather do the work themselves than have to deal with the issues around delegation that they feel uncomfortable with ("I can't keep my patient in a dirty bed.

I am going to make the bed myself" [RN]). A fourth delegation issue revealed was not following through to determine the outcome of the delegation. Focus groups pointed out that the RNs often do not check to see if the NA completed their work, if additional resources are needed to finish the tasks, or if there are barriers being experienced, nor do they give NAs recognition for work well done.

Other delegation problems identified by the focus group members included failing to establish rapport, not communicating positive expectations, not providing specific directions (turn the patient vs. turn the patient at 8 am, 10 am, etc.), RNs assuming the NA's knowledge and skills without verifying them, monitoring in such a way that the NAs feel they are mistrusted, and lack of RN-facilitated interaction, where the NA learns to develop solutions and solve problems.

More Than One Boss

The typical assignment involves the NA working with two or more RNs. This is necessary because there are generally fewer NAs than RNs in the staffing pattern of most units. Thus, NAs may have two or more RNs to work with, and those RNs do not talk with one another to determine the total workload of the NA. This structure contributes to the issues of holding the NA accountable and ensuring they have an appropriate workload.

- "You ask them to do something; they say they are busy with the other nurse's patients." (RN)
- "I think it all boils down to the nurses don't realize how much we have to have accomplished by 3:30." (NA)
- "All the nurses are grabbing you, 'Do this, do that, do this, do that.'" (NA)

The NAs indicate that even if one nurse explains to another one what the NA is assigned to do for her patients, they feel they do not always listen.

- "Because their mind is on just their patients, they hear the other nurse talk but they are not really listening so she is not getting the whole view of what we have to do." (NA)

On some units, the NAs stated that the RNs are so overwhelmed and "have more to do than we do," but that they "still put a lot on our shoulders that they expect us to get done." They note that this affects their communication style.

- "They are burnt out and overwhelmed. Some of them just get cold. You know, snappy. With attitude. Like they don't care." (NA)
- RNs generally stated that there are not enough NAs.
- "If we had another attendant on, we wouldn't be here two, three hours overtime. "(RN)

If one NA calls in or they were not able to staff that position for a shift, instead of reassigning the workload of the absent NA to both the remaining NAs and the RNs, the remaining NAs are assigned all of the patients. Even when the RNs acknowledged that the workload for an NA was excessive, they did not think of themselves as a team responsible for doing the work together. They conceptualized the aide work as not theirs.

It's Not My Job Syndrome
RNs report separating their work from that of the NA and focusing almost exclusively on completing their work rather than assuming leadership over the entire care of the patient ("They [the RNs] are wrapped up in their own work and their own world" [NA]). On the other hand, some of the NAs ignored the direction of the RNs or engaged in dysfunctional politics to get their intended results.

- "If you say something, they [NAs] won't do anything for your patients." (RN)
- "You ask them to do something, which is part of their job description; they will give you an attitude or just flat out say 'NO.'" (RN)

The practice of isolating aspects of work as being the sole responsibility of another person or job category is known as the "It's not my job" syndrome. RNs voiced the opinion that they should not have to, for example, take patients to the toilet, or get them water, or help ambulate them. They note that they have a great deal of work that only they can do ("If I did the NA work, I wouldn't have time for the RN work that only I can do" [RN]). As described above, it is evident that many nurses consider the work delegated to the nursing assistive personnel as the NAs work, no longer their responsibility. The NAs expressed extreme frustration about the fact that RNs did not do certain tasks even if it was logical and better for the patient for them to do so. The NAs also believe that nurses will not do what they consider dirty work.

- "I overheard two nurses talking, and one said that she had to clean up a mess and the other one said, 'Oh, no, we don't do that. That is what the NAs are for.' So I tell them that I am busy too." (NA)

- "I had one nurse call me into the room to give the guy a urinal. She was standing in the room, the urinal was on the other side of the bed but she called me in." (NA)

- "They [the RNs] don't like to get up to answer lights and that is when the NAs get really mad and frustrated." (NA)

- "The nurses have the attitude that 'That is not my job, that is your job' so that patient can sit and starve all day long if you are not able to get to them. It is not their job because they have all of this other stuff that they have to accomplish." (NA)

- "You're feeding a patient and you have another one to do, maybe even three total that have to be fed, and the nurse is telling me to go do something else, and I'm like 'Can you feed that patient?' She says, 'I have to go chart.'" (NA)

3. Development and Testing of the *Nursing Teamwork Survey (NTS)*

These studies highlighted that the Salas theory of teamwork applied to inpatient nursing teams and that there were numerous problems inhibiting teamwork on patient care units. In order to study the problem widely, we determined that we needed a quantitative tool to measure nursing teamwork and to measure whether teamwork improved or not when an intervention was tested. It would also provide a benchmark that would allow for the comparison of teams across organizations (Kalisch, Lee, & Salas, 2010).

Teamwork Measurement Tools

Many teamwork survey tools have been developed but have limitations for use with nursing teams. First of all, a number of structure problems are evident in many of the tools (e.g., unclear answer choices, no balance in positive and negative questions, etc.) Another problem is that many of these teamwork surveys are not appropriate for research but rather have been designed for consultation or education (Dimock, 1991; Glaser & Glaser, 1995; Phillips & Elledge, 1994; Wheelan, 1994). A large number of teamwork survey tools focus on specialized teams such as newly created groups (Campbell & Hallan, 1997; Dimock, 1991; Farrell, Heinemann, & Schmitt, 1992; Weisbond, 1991) or to evaluate meetings (Burns & Gragg, 1981; Harper & Harper, 1993). The most important barrier to utilizing a substantial number of existing tools is that they have not been tested for their psychometric properties (Burns & Gragg, 1981; Chartier, 1991; Francis & Young, 1992; Hall, 1988; Pfeiffer & Jones, 1974; Phillips & Elledge, 1994; Schein, 1988; Varney, 1991).

Teamwork measurement tools used in health care were reviewed by Heinemann and Zeiss (2004). They found 12 tools. Several centered on teams that care for specific patients populations such as geriatric (Farrell et al., 1992; Heinemann, Schmitt, Farrell, & Brallier, 1999; Hepburn, Tsukuda, & Fasser, 1998), psychiatric (Lichtenstein, Alexander, Jinnett, & Ullman, 1997) or rehabilitation (Heinemann & Zeiss, 2004). Although the tool *Attitudes Toward Health Care Teams* (Heinemann et al., 1999) has excellent psychometric properties, it is used to measure attitudes toward teams (for example, whether the physician should be the director of the team) as opposed to the actual behaviors of the team. Others are designed to measure collaboration between nurses and physicians (Baggs, 1994; Shortell, Rousseau, Gillies, Devers, & Simons, 1991). Using the cognitive-motivational model, Millward and Jeffries (2001) developed and tested *The Team Survey* with 10 healthcare teams and 124 professionals in the United Kingdoms' National Health Trust. Although initially promising, we found that it did not differentiate levels of teamwork with nursing teams in this country.

Development and Testing of the *NTS*
Based on this review, we determined that a new tool was needed to measure nursing teamwork and the *Nursing Teamwork Survey (NTS)* was developed and tested for its psychometric properties (Kalisch, Lee, & Salas, 2010). Items for the *NTS* were generated from the expert panels of RNs, NAs, and managers, and teamwork theory. Initially, 74 potential items were generated for the *NTS*, and this eventually was contracted down to 33 questions. Expert panels were utilized to review the questions and determine whether they were relevant and clear (Lynn, 1986).

The *NTS* utilizes a five-point Likert-type scale (1 = rarely, 2 = 25% of the time, 3 = 50% of the time, 4 = 75% of the time, and 5 = always) and is designed to be self-administered and focus on the within-team performance. The survey also contains questions about the demographic characteristics of the respondents, satisfaction, staffing adequacy, and number of patients cared for during their last shift (similar to the *MISSCARE Survey*). The *NTS* was administered to 1,758 RNs, LPNs, NAs, and USs. The ratio of sample size to number of survey items was 40:1, which exceeds the minimum 10:1 ratio recommended by Kerlinger (1978). The return rate was 56.9%.

Nursing staff survey respondents worked on a variety of units: 30% intensive care (ICUs), of which 17% were adult and 13% pediatric; 12% adult intermediate; 29% adult medical–surgical; 7% pediatric units; 7% emergency departments; 6% maternity units; and 4% other units.

Of these 1,758 participants, 68% (n = 1198) were female, 77% reported their job title as nurse, 80% worked full time, and approximately half held a baccalaureate degree. Two-thirds of the staff members were 26 to 44 years of age. The average number of years of work experience in nursing was 10.

Acceptability

The percentage of respondents completing the instrument without omitting any items was 80.4%. Another 11.5% omitted only one item, 2.9% omitted two items, and 5.2% omitted more than two items. Most respondents completed the questionnaire in 10 minutes or less.

Validity
Factor analysis and subscale development

The results from exploratory factor analysis (EFA) and confirmatory factor analysis (CFA) resulted in 33 questions in the final instrument. A five-factor solution evolved from the 33-item *NTS* scale: (a) Trust, (b) Team Orientation, (c) Backup, (d) Shared Mental Model, and (e) Team Leadership (Table 12.3). The large value calculated by the Bartlett's Test of Sphericity indicated that the correlation matrix is not an identity matrix (χ^2 = 12,860.195, df = 528, p < 0.001), and the Kaiser-Meyer-Olkin measure showed that sampling adequacy was excellent (0.961). The five factors explained 53.11% of the variance. The Trust factor was comprised of seven items with loadings greater than 0.40, the Team

TABLE 12.3. **Five-factor principal component analysis of the *Nursing Teamwork Survey* items.**

Factor	Cronbach's Alpha	Item
Team Leadership	0.744	Charge nurses or team leaders monitoring the progress of the team
		Charge nurses or team leaders balance team workload
		Extended plan to deal with changes in the workload
		Charge nurses or team leaders give clear and relevant directions

Factor	Cronbach's Alpha	Item
Team Orientation	0.831	Conflict avoidance
		Dominated by staff members with strong personalities
		Complaint by on-coming shift staff about incomplete work
		Judgmental feedback
		Defensive response
		Extra break-time
		Focusing on their own work rather than working together
		Nursing assistants and nurses not working well together
		Ignoring mistakes and annoying behavior
Backup	0.841	Noticing a member falling behind
		Pitching in together to get the work done
		Keeping an eye out for each other without falling behind
		Charge nurses or team leaders assist team members
		Knowing when assistance is needed before being asked
		Response to other team members' patients
Shared Mental Model	0.834	Understanding of own responsibilities throughout the shift
		Understanding of others' roles and responsibilities
		The shift change reports contain necessary information
		Awareness of the strengths and weaknesses of other team members
		Following through on commitment
		Working together for a quality job
		Respect
Trust	0.847	Clarifying the intended message with one another
		Constructive feedback
		Sharing ideas and information
		Engaging in changes to make improvements
		Trust
		Fair reallocation of responsibilities
		Communication of expectation

Orientation factor was comprised of nine items with loadings greater than 0.45, the Backup factor was comprised of six items with loadings greater than 0.40, the Shared Mental Model factor was comprised of seven items with loadings greater than 0.45, and the Team Leadership factor was comprised of four items with loadings greater than 0.40. The minimum possible score is 0 for each subscale, and the maximum possible scores are 35 for Trust, 35 for Team Orientation, 30 for Backup, 35 for Shared Mental Model, and 20 for Team Leadership. Higher scores indicate higher levels of trust among team members, more cohesive team orientation, more backup behaviors, more shared mental models, and better team leadership.

The Confirmatory Factor Analysis (CFA) yielded a 33-item, five-factor model that fit the data from the *NTS* very well (CFI = 0.884, RMSEA = 0.055, SRMR = 0.045). The analysis resulted in a chi-square value of 1,745.30 (df = 485, $p < 0.001$). A CFI that is close to the 0.9 criteria level indicates a close fit. Therefore, using this rule, the five-factor structure suggested by the earlier EFA was confirmed and resulted in a good model fit, thereby contributing to the stability of the tool (Kalisch et al., 2010).

Concurrent validity

To test concurrent validity, a one-way ANOVA showed that nursing staff who were very satisfied and satisfied with the level of teamwork on their unit had a significantly higher *NTS* score overall (4.10, 3.70, respectively) than the nursing staff who were dissatisfied (2.95; $p < 0.001$). As hypothesized, the overall unit teamwork score correlated significantly with the responses to this item (r = 0.633, $p < 0.001$).

Reliability

The overall test–retest coefficient with 33 items was 0.92, and each subscale had the test–retest reliability coefficients ranging from 0.77 to 0.87. For internal consistency, the alpha coefficient for the overall 33 items was 0.94, and the alpha coefficients for the subscales ranged from 0.74 to 0.85. From the analyses of intraclass correlations, significant F-statistic values inferred that the responses between nursing staff on different units were not similar at $p < 0.001$. The ICC1 and ICC2 reflect the homogeneity of the staff responses on a unit-level for each of five factors. The ICC1 values all remained in the range, indicating the reliability of an individual's assessment of the unit's teamwork. The ICC2 values were all above 0.84, indicating that the response of the unit as a whole was reliable. The computation of $r_{WG(J)}$ showed that the aggregation of the data on the unit level was feasible because the degree of congruence between individual nursing staff survey responses were shown to be correlated by unit. Every unit had a $r_{WG(J)}$ value of 0.90 and higher, with a median of 0.98 indicating that all the individuals responded to the questions in the same direction.

The analyses of acceptability, reliability, and validity demonstrated strong psychometric properties for a new tool. The results showed that the *NTS* is easy to use, as indicated by the relatively low proportion of omitted survey items. It was also verified that the *NTS* can be utilized as a unit-level variable, as indicated by the intraclass correlation result ($0.10 \leq$ ICC1 ≤ 0.16, $0.84 \leq$ ICC2). The use of the *NTS* with groups of nursing staff who work together could provide benchmark data for the performance of nursing teams.

4. Variations of Nursing Teamwork

Are there differences in hospitals and patient care units as to the level of teamwork, and do the characteristics of the staff impact teamwork? We conducted a study to determine the answers to these questions (n = 3769) (Kalisch & Lee, 2012). The study setting consisted of 95 patient care units in six hospitals (3,769 study participants). The study questions were as follows:

- What hospital, unit, and staff characteristics are associated with nursing teamwork?
- What hospital, unit, and staff characteristics are associated with the subscales of nursing teamwork (i.e., trust, team orientation, backup, shared mental model, and team leadership)?

The sample was made up of RNs (70.7%), LPNs (1.3%), NAs (17.5%), nursing leaders (3.3%), and USs (7.2%). Among participants, 90% were female, 78% were 25 to 54 years old, and 48% had a bachelor's degree or higher. The majority of the participants worked 12-hour shifts (59.2%) and were employed full time (81.7%). Almost half worked day shifts (48.4%). The nursing staff were distributed on the following types of units: medical–surgical, intermediate, and rehabilitation units (50.9%), ICUs (20.8%), pediatric and maternity (15.4%), psychiatric units (3.7%), perioperative units (3.7%), and emergency and other types of units (5.4%).

The teamwork overall score and four out of five subscales scores (trust, team orientation, backup, and shared mental model) were significantly different by hospital size. Specifically, small hospitals scored higher on teamwork overall and on trust, team orientation, backup, and shared mental model than larger hospitals. Medium-sized hospitals got higher scores on teamwork overall and on three subscales (trust, team orientation, and shared mental model) than larger hospitals. Seven variables were selected as predictors of teamwork: job title, full time equivalency, work hours, years of experience on the unit, absenteeism, perceived adequacy of staffing, and unit type. Gender, age, shift, and overtime were excluded from further analyses because there were no significant differences in teamwork scores for those variables in the univariate analysis.

Multiple regression analysis was then performed to determine the predictive ability of hospital, unit, and staff characteristics on nursing teamwork. The overall teamwork model included seven independent variables and explained 18% of the variation in teamwork overall ($p < .001$). Nurse leaders and unit secretaries had higher teamwork overall scores than RNs (both $p < .001$). Staff who rated staffing adequacy high had better teamwork overall scores ($p < .01$). The following types of units ranged from highest to lowest on teamwork: psychiatric and perioperative units as highest; ICU and pediatric and maternity units next; and medical–surgical, intermediate, and rehabilitation units and ED and other units as lowest. More specifically, those working on psychiatric units had higher overall teamwork scores than those in ICU units ($p < .001$), and those in medical–surgical, intermediate, and rehabilitation units had lower overall teamwork scores than ICU units staff ($p < .001$).

In order to determine predictors of the five subscales of teamwork, seven independent variables were included in each regression model. NAs were less likely to report team orientation than RNs. Nursing leaders and USs reported higher backup, shared mental model, and team leadership scores than RNs. For the work schedule, those who worked full time had less team orientation and shared mental model scores than those who worked part time. Staff working on night shifts had higher trust, team orientation, backup, and team leadership scores than staff working on the day shift. Those who missed two to six shifts in the past three months had lower trust, team orientation, and backup scores than those who did not miss work. The higher the staff rated the adequacy of staffing the greater the trust, team orientation, backup, shared mental models, and team leadership scores. For unit type, staff in medical–surgical, intermediate, and rehabilitation units had lower scores on trust, team orientation, backup, shared mental models and team leadership than staff working on ICU units.

In summary, the findings of this study show that teamwork varied by hospital size, perceptions of staffing levels, nursing role, and work schedules. On the other hand, there were no differences in teamwork by years of experience, amount of absenteeism, or whether the staff members were full time or part time. The studies showed that the smaller the hospital, the greater the level of teamwork. This may be accounted for by the fact that as size increases, the number of individuals that team members must communicate with increases and the complexity of relationships soars. Perceptions of staffing adequacy showed that when enough staff members were readily available, overall teamwork was higher, as well as all five teamwork subscales. When staff members are too busy to monitor and back one another up, provide leadership to team members, and develop shared mental models, teamwork is less likely to occur.

5. Staffing Levels and Teamwork

Surprisingly, we uncovered only a few studies that focused on the relationship between workload or staffing levels and teamwork, and these were in fields outside of health care, such as organizational engineering and business (Sebok, 2000; Thomas, Sexton, & Helmreich, 2003). McComb, Green, and Compton (2007) concluded that staffing quality (such as excellence in technical and professional skills and knowledge) is positively related to team members' tendency to react flexibly within a team.

In search for the answer to the question "Does the level of nurse staffing predict nursing teamwork," we conducted a cross-sectional study in four hospitals (300 to 900 beds) and 52 patient care units (Kalisch & Lee, 2011). Unit participation within hospitals ranged from 7 to 18 inpatient units (i.e., medical, surgical, intermediate care, intensive care, rehabilitation, maternal–child, and psychiatric). There were 2,545 respondents, of whom 1,741 were RNs, 41 were LPNs, 502 were NAs, and 191 were USs. The overall return rate was 55.7%. The *NTS*, unit-level Case Mix Index (CMI) as a proxy for patient acuity, and actual staffing as measured by HPPD, RN HPPD, and skill mix (definitions in Chapter 6) were collected in each of the 52 units (Kalisch, & Lee, 2013). Similar findings emerged from an earlier study (Kalisch, & Lee, 2009).

The sample characteristics were as follows: 60% were over 35 years, 46% held a bachelor's degree or higher, 89% were female, 70% were RNs, and 83% worked full time. HPPD values for participating units ranged from a low of 6.27 to a high of 21.30, with a mean of 11.02

(SD ± 4.27). The average RN HPPD value was 8.91 (SD ± 4.48), with a range of 3.75 to 20.89. The mean skill mix was 0.79 (SD ± 0.17), with a range of 0.53 to 1.00. The mean CMI was 2.28 (SD ± 1.36), with a range of 0.83 to 6.93.

Pearson correlations were calculated to determine hospital and unit characteristics significantly related to teamwork scores. A positive relationship between hospital bed size and teamwork overall scores (r = .33, p < .05) was found. Additionally, the higher the HPPD (r = .40, p < .01), RN HPPD (r = .53, p < .01), and skill mix (r = .54, p < .01), the higher the levels of nursing teamwork.

Staffing Predicts Teamwork

In order to determine if staffing predicts teamwork, a multiple regression analysis was calculated. RN HPPD was eliminated from the model due to the high correlation between HPPD and RN HPPD (r = .94, p < .01). Since the study included all levels of nurse staffing (from RN to NA), we chose HPPD rather than RN HPPD. For overall teamwork, the model included HPPD, skill mix, CMI, and bed size. The model accounted for 33.1% of the variation in overall teamwork (p = .003). After controlling for other variables, HPPD and skill mix were significantly associated with overall teamwork. The higher the HPPD, the greater the level of overall teamwork on the unit (β = .417, p = .033); the greater the skill mix, the higher the level of overall teamwork on the unit (β = .436, p = .009).

The relationship between staffing levels and the five subscales of teamwork (trust, team orientation, backup, shared mental model, and team leadership) can be found in Kalisch & Lee (2011). HPPD was significantly associated with a higher score on backup, shared mental model, and team leadership, but not trust and team orientation. Skill mix was associated with the higher scores on team orientation, backup, and team leadership, but not trust and shared mental model. Units in larger hospitals showed lower scores on team orientation, backup (β = -.40, p < .015), and team leadership (β = -.40, p < .01), but there was no difference for trust and shared mental model.

This study demonstrates that there is a relationship between the level of nurse staffing and nursing teamwork—higher levels of nurse staffing result in better nursing teamwork. This finding substantiates previous research indicating that nursing staff perceptions of staffing adequacy, as well as the number of patients they reported caring for on the previous shift, was associated with a higher level of teamwork

(Kalisch & Lee, 2009). The use of actual nurse staffing data in this study adds substantial credibility and confidence to the previous findings.

In addition to the overall scores, there were also significant relationships found with the teamwork subscales. The higher the staffing, the better the backup, shared mental model, and team leadership scores. While it is readily evident that having more staff would lead to greater availability of other team members when the need arises, it could also mean that there was less need for team members to help one another when staffing was better and they consequently had a lower workload. Perception of a shared mental model, which refers to staff having the same conception of what needs to be done and how, was also associated with better staffing. The reason for this finding might be due to having more time to communicate and conduct effective handoffs. Better staffing also resulted in a higher score on team leadership, which again might be due to the greater amount of time available to lead, but primarily because the charge nurse would be less likely to carry a patient load in addition to leadership responsibilities.

A greater proportion of RNs in the skill mix was associated with higher scores on team orientation, backup, and team leadership. These findings substantiate the results of an earlier study which compared RNs and NAs perceptions of missed care. This study showed that RNs identified significantly more missed care than NAs (both on the same unit), especially for those elements of nursing care typically completed by the NA (Kalisch, 2009). Furthermore, the RN and NA working relationships have been found to be problematic in a number of other studies (Huber et al., 1994; Kalisch, 2011; Potter & Grant, 2004; Scott-Cawiezell et al., 2004). Findings showing that teamwork is apparently more difficult to achieve in larger hospitals illustrate that perhaps the increasing complexity and the larger number of people one needs to interact with in larger institutions interferes with the creation and maintenance of effective teams even on a given patient care unit. Methods of creating hospitals within hospitals or units within units may be one solution to this problem.

The results of this study suggest that when nursing staff are stressed and overwhelmed by their workload due to insufficient staff, teamwork decreases. The need to ensure adequate staffing is obvious, but this finding also points to the importance of increasing the efficiency of care delivery in an effort to utilize staff more effectively.

6. Job Satisfaction and Teamwork

Whenever I conduct a focus group with nursing staff about working conditions and quality of care, I ask the question "Why do you work here?" The first answer for over 98% of the participants (estimated 300 groups) is "It's the people I work with." Yet we found only five research studies that specifically focused on the influence of teamwork on nurse job satisfaction (Amos, Hu, & Herrick, 2005; Chang, Ma, Chiu, Lin, & Lee, 2009; Cox, 2003; DiMeglio et al., 2005; Rafferty et al., 2001). Rafferty et al. (2001) surveyed 10,022 nurses in England and found that nurses with higher interdisciplinary teamwork scores were significantly more likely to be satisfied with their jobs, planned to stay in them, and had lower burnout scores. Chang et al. (2009) found that collaborative interdisciplinary relationships were one of the most important predictors of job satisfaction for all healthcare providers.

The relationship between group cohesion, a key process of teamwork, and nurse satisfaction before and after an intervention was studied by DiMeglio and colleagues (2005). The intervention increased both group cohesion and satisfaction among nurses. However, they did not report whether there was a relationship between group cohesion and satisfaction. Using a six-item survey instrument which measures patient care quality, nurses' work efficiency, unit morale, teamwork, willingness to help, and job satisfaction, Cox (2003) found that team performance effectiveness had a significant positive influence on staff satisfaction (n = 131). Because the measure included a variety of areas, not just teamwork, they could not evaluate if teamwork definitely predicted satisfaction. Finally, Amos et al. (2005) measured the job satisfaction of 44 nursing staff members in one patient care unit after an intervention. There was no change in satisfaction but actual teamwork was not measured. Both of these studies had small sample sizes which could have influenced their findings.

The job satisfaction of NAs has also been studied. The key problems identified were excessive workload (Crickmer 2005; Mather & Bakas, 2002; Pennington, Scott, & Magilvy, 2003), not being recognized and valued for their work (Counsell, 2002; Crickmer, 2005; Mather & Bakas, 2002; Parsons, Simmons, Penn, & Furlough, 2003; Spilsbury & Meyer, 2004), compensation (Decker, Harris-Kojetin, & Bercovitz, 2009; Parsons et al., 2003), benefits (Parsons et al., 2003) and manager support (Decker et al., 2009). The only study that examined the relationship between teamwork and NA job satisfaction showed that lower levels of coping skills in NAs was believed to contribute to higher psychological distress and decreased job satisfaction (Harrison,

Loiselle, Duquette, & Semenic, 2002). Other researchers have shown that teamwork leads to higher job satisfaction (Collette, 2004; Gifford et al., 2002; Horak, Guarino, Knight, & Kweder, 1991; Leppa, 1996). Blegen (1993) found that lower vacancy rates and turnover were associated with a higher level of teamwork

To determine the relationship between job satisfaction and teamwork, we conducted a study with a sample of 3,675 nursing staff from 5 hospitals and 80 patient care units with the aim of exploring the influence of unit characteristics, staff characteristics and teamwork on job satisfaction with current position and occupation. Participants completed the *NTS*. Hierarchical linear multiple regression analysis with the robust cluster estimation commands was conducted at the individual level to determine predictors of the satisfaction variables (Kalisch, Tschannen, & Lee, 2011b).

The satisfaction variables were significantly explained by teamwork and perceived staffing adequacy (all $p < 0.001$). For satisfaction with current position, participants' levels of satisfaction were likely to be higher when they rated their teamwork higher ($p < 0.001$), perceived their staffing as adequate more often ($p < 0.001$), were older ($p < 0.001$) and more experienced ($p < 0.01$), were RNs ($p < 0.01$), cared for fewer patients ($p < 0.05$), and worked in maternity and pediatric areas ($p < 0.05$ to $p < 0.001$). For satisfaction with occupation, in addition to their higher levels of teamwork and perceiving their staffing as adequate more often (both $p < 0.001$), being a female ($p < 0.001$), an RN (compared to NAs and USs, $p < 0.001$ and $p < 0.01$, respectively), older ($p < 0.05$), more experienced ($p < 0.05$), more educated ($p < 0.05$), caring for lower numbers of patients ($p < 0.001$), and working in psychiatric units and pediatric intensive care units ($p < 0.05$ to $p < 0.01$) were associated with a higher level of satisfaction.

Higher levels of teamwork and perceptions of staffing adequacy lead to greater job satisfaction with occupation. NAs and USs are less satisfied than nurses; men are less satisfied than women; and ICU staff members are less satisfied than medical–surgical staff members. The latter finding differs from what has been found in previous studies where intensive care nursing staff are usually found to be more satisfied, at least when the unit culture was considered supportive (Kangas, Kee, & McKee-Waddle, 1999).

The greater satisfaction of nurses as opposed to NAs and USs may be accounted for by several factors. First, nurses have a higher status and level of power, influence, and autonomy than the USs and NAs. This finding is supported by an early and well-known theory in the job design field by Hackman and Oldham, the Job Design Theory (1975). This theory indicates that performance of jobs involving higher autonomy, task significance, task identity, and skill variety result in higher levels of satisfaction. Men may be less satisfied with their occupation as an RN because of their minority status within the field. The U.S. Census Bureau (2013) reports that as of 2011, men comprise only 9.6% of the total RN population in the United States. Some researchers suggests that men may be more dissatisfied with nursing's lower pay and status than women.

7. Teamwork and Quality and Safety of Care

High-reliability organizations perform complex work that might produce errors or accidents, yet they have been successful in avoiding most accidents through a focus on error prevention (e.g., aviation and nuclear power) and teamwork. These organizations are highly complex and contain many risk factors. Health care, and within it, nursing, certainly meets the criteria for this type of organization (Sorbero, Farley, Mattke, & Lovejoy, 2008).

Teams who are functioning well make fewer errors than individuals working alone (Baker et al., 2006; Smith-Jentsch, Salas, & Baker, 1996; Volpe, Cannon-Bowers, Salas, & Spector, 1996). For example, a study was performed on two groups of pilots: one group was exhausted but had worked together as a team for some time; the other group had not worked as team but was fully rested. The study found that the tired team made fewer errors than the rested team (Carter & West, 1999). In actuality, the tired team made more errors but they were caught by their fellow team members. The Swiss cheese model (Figure 12.2) illustrates how team members help their colleagues avoid errors. Leonard, Graham, and Bonacum (2004) described an analysis of 2,455 sentinel events reported to the Joint Commission, 75% of which resulted in death (Leonard et al., 2004). Over 70% of the incidents revealed the primary root cause to be communication failure, with evidence that the team members had very different perceptions of what was supposed to happen.

Research on teamwork across industries is extensive, but within health care and nursing, it is much more limited. Even within health care, most studies of teamwork have focused on emergency (Reznek et al., 2003), perioperative, and anesthesia settings (Awad et al., 2005; Blum et al., 2004; France, Leming-Lee, Jackson, Feistritzer, & Higgins, 2008; Hansen, Uggen, Brattebo, & Winsborg, 2008; Howard, Gaba, Fish, Yang, & Sarnquist, 1992; Kurrek & Fish, 1996). There has also been a study done in the labor and delivery setting (Nielsen et al., 2007).

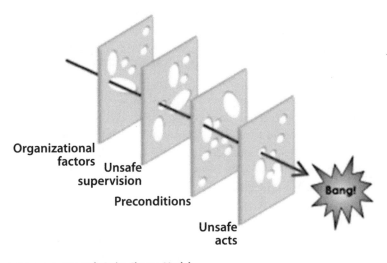

Organizational
factors Unsafe
supervision
Preconditions
Unsafe
acts
Bang!

FIGURE 12.2. **Reason's Swiss Cheese Model.**

For example, a study of intensive care staff showed that interdisciplinary teams reporting a higher level of team development had lower patient mortality rates (Wheelan, Burchill, & Tilin, 2003). Brewer (2006) found that a "group type hospital culture" resulted in fewer patient falls, and Morey and colleagues (2002) discovered that higher teamwork led to fewer errors. An intervention to improve teamwork resulted in significant improvement in micro albumin testing of diabetic patients (Taylor, Hepworth, Buerhaus, Dittus, & Speroff, 2007). Another research team found a significant positive relationship between measures of hospital teamwork culture and patient satisfaction (Meterko et al., 2004).

Schmutz and Manser (2013) completed a systematic review of 28 studies on the impact of team processes on clinical performance (e.g., fall rates, morbidity, mortality) and found that "every study reported at least one significant relationship between team processes and performance."

Leonard and colleagues (2004) emphasized the importance of effective communication and teamwork for the delivery of high-quality and safe patient care. They pointed out that communication failures are common causes of inadvertent patient harm. Salas and colleagues (2007) showed the close association of patient safety with team effectiveness and shared mindset. Shortell and Singer (2008) suggested that we need to emphasize safety over productivity and teamwork over individual autonomy to reduce errors and mistakes and to improve patient safety.

Studies specifically in nursing have shown that teamwork leads to safer care (Clark, 2009; Firth-Couzens, 2001), and raises quality of nursing care (Kalisch, Curley, & Stefanov, 2007; Leppa, 1996; Morey et al., 2002). For example, higher self-identified teamwork in the intensive care unit was found to be related to lower mortality rates (Wheelan et al., 2003), and a study by Brewer (2006) showed that a group-type hospital culture predicted fewer patient falls with injury. Kalisch and colleagues compared selected outcomes before and after an intervention to improve teamwork and found a significant decrease in patient falls, turnover, and vacancy rates after the intervention (Kalisch & Begeny, 2005; Kalisch et al., 2007).

In a systematic review by Australian researchers, 14 studies were evaluated. The results revealed that implementation of the team nursing model of care, which is popular in that part of Australia, resulted in significantly decreased incidence of medication errors and adverse intravenous outcomes, as well as lower pain scores among patients; however, there was no effect of this model of care on the incidence of falls.

In a qualitative study, presented above in the discussion of RN and NA relationships, we interviewed 20 nurses and managers to identify issues of quality and safety they have actually seen or participated in (Kalisch, 2011). The interviewees identified many examples of quality and safety problems with each of the RN–NA relationship themes, suggesting that the lack of effective working relationships between these two nursing care providers is resulting in diminished quality and increased errors. Below are some examples of situations where teamwork led to patient errors.

- A nursing assistant (NA) sees a medication (Glucophage—oral insulin) left in a cup on a patient's bed stand and throws it way, never telling the Registered Nurse (RN). The patient's blood sugar is elevated on the next blood test and the RN cannot understand why. The dose of Glucophage is increased.

- An RN requests help to ambulate a 300 lb patient from another nurse, who says she will come, but two hours later she has not shown up. The nurse then tries to get the patient up by herself. The patient falls and is injured, and the nurse has to take a medical leave for a back problem.

- An NA says she does not understand the need for the nurse to document so much of the time. She interprets this as "not putting the patient first" and decides to not answer call lights promptly because why should she do it if the RN is not doing it herself?

- A patient is brought up to the unit from the emergency department by a transporter, who informs RN #1. RN #1 fails to notify RN #2 assigned to this patient and two hours pass before RN #2 discovers that the patient has arrived on the unit. In the meantime, the patient is in intense pain. RN #2 does not address this with RN #1. A month later, RN#1 does the same thing with another patient brought to the unit, and the patient is dead when the RN assigned to the patient finally gets into the room.

8. Teamwork and Missed Nursing Care

To gain an understanding of the differences between patient care units that had the most missed nursing care and those with the least missed nursing care, we conducted a focus group study of the nursing staff on the five units with the most missed nursing care and five units with the least missed care of 110 units in our study of missed nursing care reported in Chapter 2 and 3 (Kalisch, Gosselin, & Choi, 2012). Ten themes were identified:

1. Staffing levels
2. Communication
3. Collective orientation
4. Backup
5. Monitoring
6. Leadership
7. Long tenure
8. Unit size
9. Trust
10. Accountability

Communication, collective orientation, backup, monitoring one another, leadership, and trust are all elements of teamwork in the Salas model. We concluded that this study showed that teamwork was the critical difference along with staffing levels in the amount of missed nursing care.

We then conducted a quantitative study of teamwork and missed nursing care and discovered that the level of teamwork predicts missed nursing care (Kalisch & Lee, 2010). A sample of 2,216 nursing staff members on 50 acute care patient care units in 4 hospitals completed the *Nursing Teamwork Survey* and the *MISSCARE Survey*. The response rate was 59.7%. Controlling for occupation of staff members (e.g., RN, NA) and staff characteristics (e.g., education, shift worked, experience, etc.), teamwork alone accounted for about 11% of missed nursing care.

Summary

Nursing teamwork was the focus of this chapter. We started with the results of two qualitative studies to determine what teamwork looks like (specific behaviors of teamwork) and found that the Salas framework is applicable to nursing teams. The development of a nursing teamwork survey (*Nursing Teamwork Survey*) to measure the level of teamwork was described, along with the results of studies using the NTS to determine characteristics of teamwork. Other topics included in this chapter are teamwork and staffing levels, teamwork and job and occupation satisfaction, and quality and safety, including the ability of teamwork to predict missed nursing care.

References

American Hospital Association. (2014). Fast facts on U.S. hospitals. Retrieved from http://www.aha.org/research/rc/stat-studies/fast-facts.shtml

Amos, M., Hu, J., & Herrick, C. (2005). The impact of team building on communication and job satisfaction of nursing staff. *Journal of Nursing Staff Development, 21*(1), 10–16.

Anthony, M. K., Standing, T., & Hertz, J. E. (2000). Factors influencing outcomes after delegation to unlicensed assistive personnel. *Journal of Nursing Administration, 30*(10), 474–481.

Auerbach, A. D., Sehgal, N. L., Blegen, M. A., Maselli, J., Alldredge, B. K., Vittinghoff, E., & Wachter, R. M. (2012). Effects of a multicenter teamwork and communication programme on patient outcomes: Results from the Triad for Optimal Patient Safety (TOPS) Project. *BMJ Quality & Safety, 21*(2), 118–126.

Awad, S. S., Fagan, S. P., Bellows, C., Albo, D., Green-Rashad, B., De la Garza, M., & Berger, D. H. (2005). Bridging the communication gap in the operating room with medical team training. *American Journal of Surgery, 190*(5), 770–774.

Baggs, J. G. (1994). Development of an instrument to measure collaboration and satisfaction about care decisions. *Journal of Advanced Nursing, 20*(1), 176–182.

Baker, D. P., Day, R., & Salas, E. (2006). Teamwork as an essential component of high reliability organizations. *Health Services Research, 41*(4), 1576–1598.

Barter, M., McLaughlin, F. E., & Thomas, S. A. (1997). Registered Nurse role changes and satisfaction with unlicensed assistive personnel. *Journal of Nursing Administration, 27*(1), 29–38.

Bernreuter, M. E., & Cardonna, S. (1997a). Survey and critique of studies related to unlicensed assistive personnel from 1975 to 1997, Part 1. *Journal of Nursing Administration, 27*(6), 24–29.

Bernreuter, M. E., & Cardonna, S. (1997b). Survey and critique of studies related to unlicensed assistive personnel from 1975 to 1997, Part 2. *Journal of Nursing Administration, 27*(7/8), 49–55.

Blegen, M. (1993). Nurses job satisfaction: A meta-analysis of related variables. *Nursing Research, 42*(1), 36–41.

Blegen, M. A., Sehgal, N. L., Alldredge, B. K., Gearhart, S., Auerbach, A. A., & Wachter, R. M. (2010). Improving safety culture on adult medical units through multidisciplinary teamwork and communication interventions: the TOPS Project. *Quality & Safety in Healthcare, 19*(4), 346–350.

Blum, R. H., Raemer, D. B., Carroll, J. S., Sunder, N., Felstein, D. M., & Cooper, J. B. (2004). Crisis resource management training for an anaesthesia faculty: A new approach to continuing education. *Medical Education, 38*(1), 45–55.

Brannick, M., Salas, E., & Prince, C. (1997). *Team performance assessment and measurement: Theory, methods and applications.* Mahwah, NJ: Lawrence Erlbaum Associates.

Brewer, B. B. (2006). Relationships among teams, culture, safety, and cost outcomes. *Western Journal of Nursing Research, 28*(6), 641–653.

Brown, J. P. (2004). Closing the communication loop: Using readback/hearback to support patient safety. *The Joint Commission Journal on Quality and Safety, 30*(8), 460–464.

Burns, F., & Gragg, R. (1981). Brief diagnostic instruments. In J. E. Jones & J. W. Pfeiffer (Eds.), *The annual handbook for group facilitators* (pp. 87–93). San Diego, CA: Pfeiffer & Company.

Campbell, D., & Hallan, G. L. (1997). *Team development survey.* Rosemont, IL: National Computer Systems, Inc.

Carter, A. J., & West, M. A. (1999). *Stress in health professionals.* Chichester, UK: John Wiley & Sons.

Chaboyer, W., McMurray, A., & Patterson, E. (1998) Unlicensed assistive personnel in the critical care unit: What is their role? *International Journal of Nursing Practice, 4*, 240–246.

Chang, A. M., Lam, L., & Lam, L. W. (1997). Evaluation of a health care assistant pilot programme. *Journal of Nursing Management, 5*(4), 229–236.

Chang, A. M., Lam, L., & Lam, L. W. (1998). Nursing activities following the introduction of health care assistants. *Journal of Nursing Management, 6*(3), 156–163.

Chang, W. Y., Ma, J. C., Chiu, H. T., Lin, K. C., & Lee, P. H. (2009). Job satisfaction and perceptions of quality of patient care, collaboration and teamwork in acute care hospitals. *Journal of Advanced Nursing, 65*(9), 1946–1955.

Chartier, M. R. (1991). Trust-oriented profile. In W. J. Pfeiffer (Ed.), *Annual, developing human resources* (pp. 136–148). San Diego, CA: Pfeiffer & Company.

Chase, P., & Paul, S. (1995). Integrating assistive personnel. *Nursing Management, 26*(6), 71–73.

Chassin, M. R., & Loeb, J. M. (2011). The ongoing quality improvement journey: Next stop, high reliability. *Health Affairs, 30*(4), 559–568.

Clark, P. R. (2009). Teamwork: Building healthier workplaces and providing safer patient care. *Critical Care Nursing Quarterly, 32*(3), 221–231.

Cohen, S. (2004). Delegating vs. dumping: Teach the difference. *Nursing Management, 35*(10), 14–18.

Collette, J. (2004). Retention of staff: Team-based approach. *Australian Health Review, 28*(3), 349–356.

Counsell, C. M. (2002). Consider this...Inspiring support staff employees. *Journal of Nursing Administration, 32*(3), 120–121.

Cox, K. B. (2003). The effects of intrapersonal, intragroup, and intergroup conflict on team performance effectiveness and work satisfaction. *Nursing Administration Quarterly, 27*(2), 153–163.

Crickmer, A. (2005). Who wants to be a CNA? *Journal of Nursing Administration, 35*(9), 380–381.

Davis, J. M., & Farrell, M. (1995). Factors affecting the delegation of tasks by the registered nurse to patient care assistants in acute care settings. *Journal of Nursing Staff Development, 11*(6), 301–306.

Decker, F. H., Harris-Kojetin, L. D., & Bercovitz, A. (2009). Intrinsic job satisfaction, overall satisfaction, and intention to leave the job among nursing assistants in nursing homes. *The Gerontologist, 49*(5), 596–610.

DiMeglio, K., Padula, C., Piatek, C., Korber, S., Barrett, A., Ducharme, M., ... Corry, K. (2005). Group cohesion and nurse satisfaction: Examination of a team-building approach. *The Journal of Nursing Administration, 35*(3), 110–120.

Dimock, H. G. (1991). Survey of team development. In J. W. Pfieffer (Ed.), *Encyclopedia of team-development activities* (pp. 243–246). San Diego, CA: Pfeiffer & Company.

Eppich, W. J., Brannen, M., & Hunt, E. A. (2008). Team training: Implications for emergency and critical care pediatrics. *Current Opinion in Pediatrics, 20*(3), 255–260.

Farrell, M. P., Heinemann, G. D., & Schmitt, M. H. (1992). A measure of anomie in health care teams. In J. R. Snyder (Ed.), *Interdisciplinary health care teams: Proceedings of the Fourteenth Annual Conference in Chicago* (pp. 186–197). Indianapolis, IN: School of Allied Health Sciences, Indiana University School of Medicine, Indiana University Medical Center.

Firth-Couzens, J. (2001). Cultures for improving patient safety through learning: The role of teamwork. *Quality Health Care, 10*(2), 26–31.

Fisher, M. (1999). Do your nurses delegate effectively? *Nursing Management, 30*(5), 23–26.

France, D. J., Leming-Lee, S., Jackson, T., Feistritzer, N. R., & Higgins, M. S. (2008). An observational analysis of surgical team compliance with perioperative safety practices after crew resource management training. *American Journal of Surgery, 195*(4), 546–553.

Francis, D., & Young, D. (1992). *The team review survey.* San Diego, CA: Pfeiffer & Company.

Gifford, B. D., Zammuto, R. F., & Goodman, E. A. (2002). The relationship between hospital unit culture and nurses' quality of work life. *Journal of Healthcare Management, 47*(1), 13–26.

Glaser, B. G., & Strauss, A. L. (1967). *Discovery of grounded theory: Strategies for qualitative research.* Chicago, IL: Aldine.

Glaser, R., & Glaser, C. (1995). *Team effectiveness profile.* King of Prussia, PA: Organization Design and Development, Inc.

Hackman, J. R., & Oldham, G. R. (1976). Motivation through the design of work: Test of a theory. *Organizational Behavior and Human Performance, 16*(2), 250–279.

Hall, J. (1988). *Team index: An assessment of your team's readiness for effective team work.* The Woodlands, TX: Teleometrics International.

Hansen, K. S., Uggen, P. E., Brattebo, G., & Winsborg, T. (2008). Team-oriented training for damage control surgery in rural trauma: A new paradigm. *Journal of Trauma, 64*(4), 949–953.

Harper, A., & Harper, B. (1993). *Skill-building for self-directed team members.* Yorktown, NY: MW Co.

Harrison, M., Loiselle, C. G., Duquette, A., & Semenic, S. E. (2002). Hardiness, work support and psychological distress among nursing assistants and registered nurses in Quebec. *Journal of Advanced Nursing, 38*(6), 584–591.

Heinemann, G. D., & Zeiss, A. M. (Eds.). (2004). *Team performance in health care: Assessment and development.* New York, NY: Kluwer Academic/Plenum.

Heinemann, G. D., Schmitt, M. H., Farrell, M. P., & Brallier, S. A. (1999). Development of an attitudes toward health care teams scale. *Evaluation & the Health Professions, 22*(1), 123–142.

Hepburn, K., Tsukuda, R. A., & Fasser, C. (1998). Teams skills scale. In E. L. Siegler, K. Myer, T. Fulmer, & M. Mazey (Eds.), *Geriatric interdisciplinary team training* (pp. 264–265). New York, NY: Springer.

Horak, B. J., Guarino, J. H., Knight, C. C., & Kweder, S. L. (1991). Building a team on a medical floor. *Health Care Management Review, 16*(2), 65–71.

Howard, S. K., Gaba, D. M., Fish, K. J., Yang, G., & Sarnquist, F. H. (1992). Anesthesia crisis resource management training: Teaching anesthesiologist to handle critical incidents. *Aviation, Space, and Environmental Medicine, 63*(9), 763–770.

Huber, D. G., Belgen, M. A., & McCloskey, J. C. (1994). Use of nursing assistants: Staff nurse opinions. *Nursing Management, 25*(5), 64–68.

Institute of Medicine. (2000). *To err is human: Building a safer health system.* Washington, DC: National Academies Press.

Kalisch, B. J. (2011). The impact of RN–UAP relationships on quality and safety. *Nursing Management, 42*(9), 16–22.

Kalisch, B. J., Gosselin, A., & Choi, S. H. (2012). A comparison of patient care units with high versus low levels of missed nursing care. *Health Care Management Review, 37*(4), 320–328.

Kalisch, B., & Lee, H. (2009). Nursing teamwork, staff characteristics, work schedules and staffing. *Health Care Management Review, 34*(4), 323–333.

Kalisch, B., & Lee, K. (2010). The impact of teamwork on missed nursing care. *Nursing Outlook, 58*(5), 233–241.

Kalisch, B., & Lee, K. (2011). Nurse staffing levels and teamwork: A cross sectional study of patient care units in acute care hospitals. *Journal of Nursing Scholarship, 43*(1), 82–88.

Kalisch, B., & Lee, K. (2013). Variations of nursing teamwork by hospital, patient unit, and staff characteristics. *Applied Nursing Research, 26*(1), 2–9.

Kalisch, B., Lee, H., & Rochman, M. (2010). Nursing staff teamwork and job satisfaction. *Journal of Nursing Management, 18*, 938–947.

Kalisch, B., Lee, H., & Salas, E. (2010). The development and testing of the nursing teamwork survey. *Nursing Research, 59*(1), 42–50.

Kalisch, B., & Schoville, R. (2012). It takes a team. *The American Journal of Nursing, 112*(10), 50–54.

Kalisch, B., Weaver, S., & Salas, E. (2009). What does nursing teamwork look like? A qualitative study. *Journal of Nursing Care Quality, 24*(4), 298–307.

Kangas, S., Kee, C. C., & McKee-Waddle, R. (1999). Organizational factors, nurses' job satisfaction, and patient satisfaction with nursing care. *Journal of Nursing Administration, 29*(1), 32–42.

Keeney, S., Hasson, F., McKenna, H., & Gillen, P. (2005). Nurses', midwives' and patients' perceptions of trained health care assistants. *Journal of Advanced Nursing, 50*(4), 345–355.

Kupperschmidt, B. R. (2002). Unlicensed assistive personnel retention and realistic job previews. *Nursing Economics, 20*(6), 279–283.

Kurrek, M. M., & Fish, K. J. (1996). Anaesthesia crisis resource management training: An intimidating concept, a rewarding experience. *Canadian Journal of Anaesthesia, 43*(5 Pt 1), 430–434.

Leonard, W., Graham, S., & Bonacum, E. (2004). The human factor: The critical importance of effective teamwork and communication in providing safe care. *Quality and Safety in Health Care, 13*(Suppl 1), i85–i90.

Leppa, C. J. (1996). Nurse relationships and work group disruption. *The Journal of Nursing Administration, 26*(10), 23–27.

Lichtenstein, R., Alexander, J. A., Jinnett, K., & Ullman, E. (1997). Embedded intergroup relations in interdisciplinary teams: Effects on perceptions of level of team integration. *Journal of Applied Behavioral Science, 33*(4), 413–434.

Liedtka, J., & Whitten, E. L. (1997). Building better patient care services: A collaborative approach. *Health Care Management Review, 22*(3), 16–24.

Lynn, M. R. (1986). Determination and quantification of content validity. *Nursing Research, 35*(6), 382–385.

Mather, K. F., & Bakas, T. (2002). Nursing assistants' perceptions of their ability to provide continence care. *Geriatric Nursing, 23*(2), 76–81.

Mather, K. F., & Bakas, T. (2002). Nursing assistants' perceptions of their ability to provide continence care. *Geriatric Nursing, 23*(2), 76-81.

Mathieu, J. E., Heffner, T. S., Goodwin, G. F., Salas, E., & Cannon-Bowers, J. A. (2008). The influence of shared mental models on team process and performance. *Journal of Applied Psychology, 85*(2), 273-283.

McComb, S. A., Green, S. G., & Compton, W. D. (2007). Team flexibility's relationship to staffing and performance in complex projects: An empirical analysis. *Journal of Engineering and Technology Management, 24*, 293-313.

McKenna, H., Hasson, F., & Keeney, S. (2004). Patient safety and quality of care: the role of the health care assistant. *Journal of Nursing Management, 12*(6), 452-459.

Meek, I. (1998). Evaluation of the role of the health care assistant within a community mental health intensive care team. *Journal of Nursing Management, 6*(1), 11-19.

Meterko, M., Mohr, D. C., & Young, G. J. (2004). Teamwork culture and patient satisfaction in hospitals. *Medical Care, 42*(5), 492-498.

Millward, L. J., & Jeffries, N. (2001). The Team Survey: A tool for health care team development. *Journal of Advanced Nursing, 35*(2), 276-287.

Morey, J. C., Simon, R., Jay, G. D., Wears, R. L., Salisbury, M., Dukes, K. A., & Berns, S. D. (2002). Error reduction and performance improvement in the emergency department through formal teamwork training: Evaluation results of the MedTeams Project. *Health Services Research, 37*(6), 1553-1581.

Nielsen, P. E., Goldman, M. B., Mann, S., Shapiro, D. E., Marcus, R. G., Pratt, S. D., ... Sachs, B. P. (2007). Effects of teamwork training on adverse outcomes and process of care in labor and delivery: A randomized controlled trial. *Obstetrics and Gynecology, 109*(1), 48-55.

Nielsen, P., & Mann, S. (2008). Team function in obstetrics to reduce errors and improve outcomes. *Obstetrics and Gynecology Clinics of North America, 35*(1), 81-95.

Parsons, L. C. (1999). Building RN confidence for delegation decision-making skills in practice. *Journal for Nurses in Staff Development, 15*(6), 263-269.

Parsons, S. K., Simmons, W. P., Penn, K., & Furlough, M. (2003). Determinants of satisfaction and turnover among nursing assistants. The results of a statewide survey. *Journal of Gerontological Nursing, 29*(3), 51-58.

Pennington, K., Scott, J., & Magilvy, K. (2003). The role of certified nursing assistants in nursing homes. *Journal of Nursing Administration, 33*(11), 578-584.

Pfeiffer, J. W., & Jones, J. E. (1974). Post meeting reaction form. In J. W. Pfeiffer (Ed.), *A handbook of structured experiences for human relations training* (Vol. 3; pp. 30). San Diego, CA: Pfeiffer & Company.

Phillips, S. L., & Elledge R. L. (1994). *Team building for the future: Beyond the basics.* San Diego, CA: Pfeiffer & Company.

Potter, P., & Grant, E. (2004). Understanding RN and unlicensed assistive personnel working relationships in designing care delivery strategies. *Journal of Nursing Administration, 34*(1), 19-25.

Rafferty, A. M., Ball, J., & Aiken, L. H. (2001). Are teamwork and professional autonomy compatible, and do they result in improved hospital care? *Quality and Safety in Health Care, 10*(Suppl 2), ii32–ii37.

Reznek, M., Smith-Coggins, R., Howard, S., Kiran, K., Harter, P., Sowb, Y., ... Krummel, T. (2003). Emergency medicine crisis resource management (EMCRM): Pilot study of simulation-based crisis management course for emergency medicine. *Academic Emergency Medicine, 10*(4), 386–389.

Rondeau, K. V., & Wagar, T. H. (1998). Hospital chief executive officer perceptions of organizational culture and performance. *Hospital Topics, 76*(2), 14–21.

Salas, E., Sims, D. E., & Burke, C. S. (2005). Is there a "big five" in teamwork? *Small Group Resarch, 36*(5), 555–599.

Salas, E., Stagl, K., & Burke, C. S. (2004). 25 years of team effectiveness in organizations: Research themes and emerging needs. In C. L. Cooper & I. T. Robertson (Eds.), *International review of industrial and organizational psychology* (Vol. 19; pp. 47–91). New York, NY: John Wiley & Sons.

Salmond, S. W. (1995a). Models of care using unlicensed assistive personnel, Part 1: Job scope, preparation and utilization patterns. *Orthopaedic Nursing, 14*(5), 20–30.

Salmond, S. W. (1995b). Models of care using unlicensed assistive personnel Part II. Perceived effectiveness. *Orthopaedic Nursing, 14*(6), 47–58.

Schein, E. H. (1988). *Process consultation: Its role in organization development* (2nd ed., Vol. 1, pp 76–83). Reading, MA: Addison Wesley Publishing Company.

Schmutz, J., & Manser, T. (2013). Do team processes really have an effect on clinical performance? A systematic literature review. *British Journal of Anesthesia, 100*(4), 529–544.

Schulman-Green, D., Harris, D., Xue, Y., Loseth, D. B., Czaplinski, C., Donovan, C., & McCorkle, R. (2005). Unlicensed staff members' experiences with patients' pain on the inpatient oncology unit. *Cancer Nursing, 28*(5), 340–347.

Scott-Cawiezell, J., Schenkman, M., Moore, L., Vojir, C., Connolly, R. P., Pratt, M., & Palmer L. (2004). Exploring nursing home staff's perceptions of communication and leadership to facilitate quality improvement. *Journal of Nursing Care Quality, 19*(3), 242–252.

Sebok, A. (2000). Team performance in process control: influences of interface design and staffing levels. *Ergonomics, 8*(43), 1210–1236.

Shortell, S. M., O'Brien, J. L., & Carman, J. M. (1995). Assessing the impact of continuous quality improvement/total quality management: Concept versus implementation. *Health Services Research, 30*(2), 377–401.

Shortell, S. M., Rousseau, D. M., Gillies, R. R., Devers, K. J., & Simons, T. L. (1991). Organizational assessment in intensive care units (ICUs): Construct development, reliability, and validity of ICU nurse–physician questionnaire. *Medical Care, 29*(8), 709–726.

Shortell, S. M., & Singer, S. J. (2008). Improving patient safety by taking systems seriously. *Journal of the American Medical Association, 299*(4), 445–447.

Shortell, S. M., Zimmerman, J. E., Rousseau, D. M., Gilles, R. R., Wagner, D. P., Draper, E. A., ... Duffy, J. (1994). The performance of intensive care units: Does good management make a difference? *Medical Care, 32*(5), 508-525.

Sil´en-Lipponen, M., Tossavainen, K., Turunen, H., & Smith, A. (2005). Potential errors and their prevention in operating room teamwork as experienced by Finnish, British and American nurses. *International Journal of Nursing Practice, 11*(1), 21-32.

Smith-Jentsch, K. A., Salas, E., & Baker, D. P. (1996). Training team performance-related assertiveness. *Personnel Psychology. 49*(4), 909-936.

Sorbero, M. E., Farley, D. O., Mattke, S., & Lovejoy, S. (2008). *Outcome measures for effective teamwork in inpatient care: Final report.* Arlington, VA: RAND Corporation.

Spilsbury, K., & Meyer, J. (2004). Use, misuse and non-use of health care assistants: Understanding the work of health care assistants in a hospital setting. *Journal of Nursing Management, 12*(6), 411-418.

Standing, T., Anthony, M. K., & Hertz, J. E. (2001). Nurses' narratives of outcomes after delegation to unlicensed assistive personnel. *Outcomes Management for Nursing Practice 5*(1), 18-24.

Taylor, C. R., Hepworth, J. T., Buerhaus, P. I., Dittus, R., & Speroff, T. (2007). Effect of crew resource management on diabetes care and patient outcomes in an inner-city primary care clinic. *Quality and Safety in Health Care, 16*(4), 244-247.

Tourangeau, A. E., White, P., Scott, J., McAllister, M., & Giles, L. (1999). Evaluation of a partnership model of care delivery. *Canadian Journal of Nursing Leadership, 12*(2), 4-20.

Thomas, E. J., Sexton, J. B., & Helmreich, R. L. (2003). Discrepant attitudes about teamwork among critical care nurses and physicians. *Critical Care Medicine,* 31(3), 956-9.

U. S. Census Bureau. (2013). *Men in nursing occupations: American community survey highlight report.* Retrieved from http://www.census.gov/people/io/files/Men_in_Nursing_Occupations.pdf

Varney, G. H. (1991). In G. H. Varney (Ed.), *Building productive teams* (pp. 29-30). San Francisco: Jossey-Bass.

Volpe, C. E., Cannon-Bowers, J. A., Salas, E., & Spector, P. E. (1996). The impact of cross-training on team functioning: An empirical investigation. *Human Factors: The Journal of the Human Factors and Ergonomics Society, 38*(1), 87-100.

Weaver, S. J., Lyons, R., Diaz Granados, D., Rosen, M. A., Salas, E., Oglesby, J., ... King, H. B. (2010). The anatomy of health care team training and the state of practice: A critical review. *Academic Medicine, 85*(11), 1746-1760.

Weisbond, M. R. (1991). Team development rating form. In J. W. Pfieffer (Ed.), *Encyclopedia of team-development activities* (pp. 249-250). San Diego, CA: Pfeiffer & Company.

Wheelan, S. A. (1994). *The group development questionnaire: A manual for professionals.* Provincetown, MA: GDQ Associates.

Wheelan, S. A., Burchill, C. N., & Tilin, F. (2003). The link between teamwork and patients' outcomes in intensive care units. *American Journal of Critical Care, 12*(6), 527–534.

Young, G. J., Charns, M. P., Desai, K., Khuri, S. F., Forbes, M. G., Henderson, W., & Daley, J. (1998). Patterns of coordination and clinical outcomes: A study of surgical services. *Health Services Research, 33*(5), 1211–1236.

PART 2

STRATEGIES TO DECREASE MISSED NURSING CARE

— 13 —

Culture and Leadership Strategies

In this chapter, culture and leadership and their relationship to the quality and safety of patient care are reviewed along with the presentation of approaches that are likely to reduce missed nursing care.

Organizational Culture

Before any organizational change can be made, the culture needs to be aligned to the desired vision. Like every individual, each organization has its own personality and way of behaving. Organizational culture, although not easy to define, has been described in several ways (Braithwaite, Hyde, & Pope, 2010; Martin, 2002). Sociological approaches define it as the values, attitudes, beliefs, customs, and practices shared by a group (Alvesson, 2002; Ashkanasy, Wilderom, & Peterson, 2000). Others talk about rituals, ceremonies, and rites of an organizational culture (Islam & Zyphur, 2009). It has also been defined as the overall behavior pattern of a group (Islam & Zyphur, 2009). Organizational culture is defined by Drennan (1992, p. 3) as "the way things are done around here," and encompasses a shared understanding of beliefs and actions that are obtained through group learning and socialization (Cooke, Rousseau, & Lafferty, 1988).

Schein (1985) describes culture exercising a coordinating function. Lou Gerstner, the CEO who saved IBM from near ruin in the 1990s, said "culture is everything" (Arizona State University, 2011). It is the thinking, behaving, and believing that members have in common. The overall organizational culture creates parameters as to how subgroups function, but each subgroup within an organization has its own culture as well.

Take the example of a new nurse on a patient care unit. She asks another staff member to help her walk a patient and that staff member says, "We don't do that. We don't have time to ambulate." This is the beginning of the new nurse's socialization to the group. As another example, she observes a call light going off and no one getting up to answer it. It is as if she is the only person who hears it. This is another lesson about this unit's culture and what is valued by the staff. An RN doesn't wash her hands before caring for a patient and the NA who sees it says nothing. This is yet another indication that there is a hierarchy in which lower-ranked staff members are not supposed to, or are not expected to, identify and address problems. The new nurse also watches another nurse prepare her medications in a designated area that she is told is a safe area in which the nurse is not to be disturbed. However, she sees that the nurse is repeatedly interrupted by other staff. Yet another lesson is learned: safety in medication administration is not a priority. This is an example of how the culture is transmitted to new people on the team:

- "If the culture of your floor allows [being distracted] to be ok. If I'm a new nurse on a floor, I may be hesitant to get my phone out. But then I see every other nurse that's around me doing it, then I'm going to say, this is the culture of the floor. It's fine. Everybody does it. Of course I'm going to do it." (RN)

- "There is a space designated around where we give medications and no one is to enter it and no one is supposed to talk with the person. But we do it all the time." (RN)

Consequently, by the end of the first day on the unit, the new nurse has learned a great deal about the culture and in a couple of weeks, she will be well grounded in the values of unit.

Safety Culture

Developing a patient safety culture was one of the recommendations made by the Institute of Medicine to assist hospitals in improving patient safety. In recent years, a great deal of evidence has been published on patient safety culture. What do we know about the impact of organizational culture on patient, staff, and organizational outcomes? Studies of organizational cultures and their impact on the performance of healthcare organizations have focused primarily on the role of leadership (Davies, Mannion, Jacobs, Powell, & Marshall, 2007; Hartmann et al., 2009). Clarke (2006), in a review of the subject in the Annual Review of Nursing Research, summarized by noting that although positive organizational climate and culture have been associated with safer health care by many, the state of the science is not as strong as one might hope. In another review of studies about the influence of organizational culture on healthcare performance, the researchers uncovered some evidence to suggest that organizational culture may be a relevant factor in the performance of healthcare organizations (El-Jardali, Dimassi, Jamal, Jaafar, & Hemadeh, 2011; Gregory, Harris, Armenakis, & Shook, 2009; Williams, Manwell, Konrad, & Linzer, 2007). For example, in a study of more than 3,000 coronary artery bypass patients from 16 hospitals, a supportive group culture characterized by trust was associated with higher physical and mental functional health-status scores six months after discharge (Shortell, Bennett, & Byck, 1998).

Fair and Just Culture

Just culture refers to a model of shared accountability between an organization and the employees within it. It's a culture that holds organizations accountable for the systems they design and implement and for how they respond to staff behaviors. In turn, staff members are accountable for the quality of their choices and for reporting both their errors and system vulnerabilities (Griffith, 2009). A just culture recognizes that individual providers should not be held accountable for errors that are caused by system failings over which they have no control (e.g., nurse fails to give a medication because pharmacy has not delivered it). Brunt (2010) points out that a just culture also recognizes that many individual errors represent "predictable interactions between human operators and the system in which they work." However, in contrast to a no-blame culture, Brunt discusses that a just culture "does not tolerate conscious disregard of clear risks to patients or gross misconduct, such as falsifying a record, performing professional duties while intoxicated, etc."

Human error that causes harm to patients has traditionally led to discipline and even termination. However, for us to develop an understanding of what leads to errors and learn from those mistakes, we have to promote a culture where mistakes are reported in a non-punitive environment. In order for staff to have the greatest positive impact on patient care and achieve the highest level of excellence possible, they must feel compelled and supported to speak about problems, errors, conflicts, and misunderstandings in an environment where to do so with curiosity, honesty, and respect is both a shared goal and a shared responsibility. Makin individuals pay for their mistakes when they had little control over them does nothing to solve the problem. It only makes it more likely that employees will not report their mistakes, making it impossible to learn what went wrong. In other words, the focus is not on blame, but transparency. Yet errors caused by staff members who are careless, intoxicated, or malicious constitute an obvious and valid exception to a blame-free culture.

Leape (2009) indicated that in the organizational environment in most hospitals, at least six major changes are required to begin the journey to a culture of safety:

1. Acknowledge that errors are primarily caused by system failures
2. Eliminate punitive environments
3. Move from secrecy to transparency
4. Move from provider-centered to patient-centered
5. Change our models of care to team-based collaborative work
6. Ensure that accountability is universal and reciprocal, not top-down

These principals apply to errors of omission as much as errors of commission. Nursing staff members need to be encouraged to report care that is missed. At the end of each shift, for example, if nursing staff were to routinely discuss what nursing care they missed or were unable to provide during the shift, this would be an important first step toward dealing with the overarching problem. When there is an accumulation of data highlighting specific areas of nursing care that are being missed, an analysis of the root causes of these omissions can be made. In an organization with a strong safety culture, these errors of omission are considered valuable insights into vulnerabilities that exist and are therefore key learning opportunities.

Culture Change

The question becomes, how can we change the culture to ensure that safe practices are adopted by the organization? Changing a culture is very difficult and takes time, but it can and must be done. When it comes to quality and safety problems, what choice do we have but to start on the road toward change? Changing a workplace culture is best started with the development of a strategic plan, a process by which an organization envisions its ideal future and develops the necessary procedures and operations to achieve that future. It starts with a clarification of core values (i.e., what the organization stands for, its culture, philosophies, and enduring beliefs that determine behavior and significantly relate to decision-making) held by staff members, managers, senior leadership, and the Board. This involves a process of self-examination, the confrontation of difficult choices, and the setting of priorities.

The next step in the process of change is to develop a vision statement—a compelling picture of the organization at some point in the future that breaks with current thinking and assumptions and is achievable, inspirational, understandable, and preferably 100 words or less. Kotter (2007, p. 101) notes that if you cannot "communicate the vision in five minutes or less and get a reaction that signifies both understanding and interest," it will not be effective. In many healthcare organizations, the values and vision are determined by a small group of the top leadership. In other cases, some or all managers throughout the organization are engaged in the process of vision development. However, it is rare that the determination of values and the development of a vision statement have included members of the front ine staff. Typically, staff members are given the values and vision, but given little help as to how to implement them in their area of the organization.

If they are written well, as Kotter says, they should be understood in five minutes. Even when this is the case, if the values and vision are to penetrate the organization, most, if not all, of the staff need to be actively engaged in the development process by being asked for their input. One way this can be achieved is to seek out reviews of and input into the drafts of these documents. By doing this, the organization avoids the phenomenon of a "vision in a vacuum" wherein a small group tasked with the development these statements communicates that they know what is best for everyone and do not ask for input from others in the organization. Once the values and vision are determined, each unit within the organization needs to clarify and adopt them for their particular service or unit. This means that the overall department or division of nursing, as well as each patient care unit within the division of nursing, needs to engage in the planning process in some way.

Case Study: The Transformation Process

To illustrate the process, a case study of a hospital nursing organization that underwent a transformation is presented (Kalisch & Curley, 2008).[1]

The process started with an assessment of the current status, including a study of available organizational data (e.g., market share, financial status, staffing, turnover, etc.), followed by focus groups with the staff and making observations on the units. A number of weaknesses and threats were identified. Previous administrators treated nursing "as a necessary [and expensive] evil" and had little appreciation as to how nursing could contribute to the bottom line as well as to the quality of the organization. The nursing staff tended to be task-oriented with varying levels of critical-thinking skills. Evidence-based nursing practice was rare. The staff was also not particularly service-oriented. Many nurses had spent their entire career in this organizational structure and, consequently, had difficulty thinking about doing things differently. Staff–manager relationships were parental in nature, and accountability was low for both staff and managers. The nurse managers had not been adequately prepared for their leadership roles. Effective communication was lacking both among nurses and between nursing staff and other departments and physicians. Staff nurses felt that they lacked a voice in decision-making, and many had adopted the "Why bother?" attitude. Trust was low. There was a high frequency of missed nursing care and a lack of teamwork. There was also a sizable number of nurses with negative attitudes who tended to propagate their viewpoints widely to other staff, including new nurses. "It is not my job" syndrome was rampant. Staff felt that they were not recognized for their contributions and that no one would care if they left. New nurses were not appropriately mentored and often left prematurely because of this. Many of the physician–nurse relationships were disrespectful and lacked collegiality, and inappropriate behavior occurred regularly. Physicians were dissatisfied with the knowledge level of many nurses. The patient assignments worked against continuity of care (staff rarely had the same patients for more than one shift) and teamwork (staff did not work consistently with the same people).

Based on this assessment, a transformation of the nursing organization was undertaken. It took place in five phases:

1. Setting the stage for change
2. Management training
3. Strategic planning
4. Developing and implementing changes at the nursing organization level
5. Developing and implementing changes at the nursing unit level

Phase 1: Setting the stage for change

Once the assessment was completed, the vice president of nursing felt that it was important to set the stage for change. An all-day session was held with what would become the "leadership group"—50 staff nurses and managers drawn from all patient care units in the hospital. The major focus of this session was on change and innovation, but the group also engaged in their own SWOT (strengths, weaknesses, opportunities, and threats) analysis, building on the data collected in the assessment referred to above.

Phase 2: Management training

The next phase was management training for the directors, nurse managers, and assistant nurse managers since it was evident that there were problems in this area. It was decided that management training was an essential preliminary step because of the critical role that the managers would assume in the transformation project. Sessions focused on high-involvement management, working effectively on teams, building trust, dealing with conflict, recruiting and selecting, delegating, process improvement, and developing accountability. These particular areas were selected on the basis of needs identified in the initial organizational assessment.

Phase 3: Strategic planning

The third phase in the transformation process focused on strategic planning. A steering committee, made up of nurse managers/directors and clinical specialists, was appointed to provide oversight, plan the group meetings, resolve issues, and make key decisions as needed. The leadership group (referred to above) convened for a series of sessions over several months to develop a strategic plan for nursing. Four workshops focused on a step-by-step development of a plan:

1. Values and vision
2. Goals
3. Objectives
4. Implementation planning

In the first workshop, a series of exercises and planning tools were used to conduct a stakeholder analysis and to analyze what currently drives decision-making in the nursing organization. They also identified the distinctive competencies or the qualities and attributes that would set them apart from their competitors (superior service and being an employer of choice). Based on these analyses and overall values and vision for the organization, the values and vision statements for nursing were developed.

After this workshop, the leadership team members shared the values and vision with all of the nursing staff in the organization for review and input. Staff (RNs, NAs, USs) were encouraged to add to the vision and values and "make them better." The idea was to get as many staff members on the playing field and engaged in the process as possible.

Workshop 2 was devoted to the development of goals. Although there are many different terms used in strategic planning, in this project, goals refer to what the nursing organization wanted to accomplish. Objectives, developed in the next session, were defined as the specific strategies with timelines and measures required to reach each goal. The first step in goal identification was to conduct a gap analysis (the gap between where they were at the current time and where they hoped to be in the future). A list of potential goal areas were then prioritized according to need, potential impact, and resources required, and then the selection of six goals was finalized (Figure 13.1). The third workshop was devoted to the development of specific objectives for each goal (Figure 13.1) along with measures for each objective, which were to be used to evaluate the progress and outcomes of the teams.

The aim of the fourth workshop was to create the implementation plan. The first task was to create the teams that would implement the goals and objectives. The leadership group was divided into eight action teams for each goal or objective:

1. Teamwork
2. Empowerment
3. Missed nursing care
4. Critical thinking
5. Mentoring
6. Up-down and down-up communication
7. Shift report communication
8. Interdepartmental communication

The physician–nurse relationship team was not formed due to an overall hospital project addressing all physician relationship issues.

After an orientation to the process, the teams developed their team name, motto, and structure (meeting times and places, ground rules, measures, etc.) for their upcoming bimonthly meetings. They also

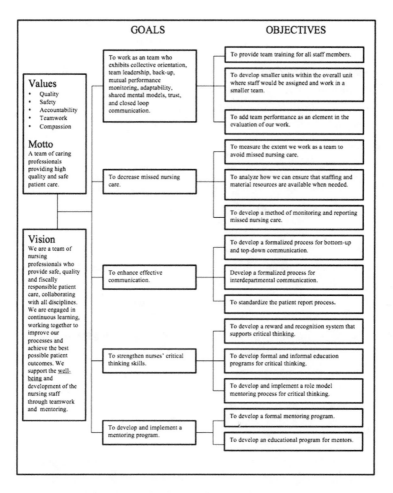

FIGURE 13.1. **Example strategic plan for a nursing organization.**

determined what additional people should be added to the teams. For example, the interdepartmental communication team determined that they would need to add staff members from the other departments, as did the teamwork and up-down, down-up communication teams.

Phase 4: Developing and implementing changes at the organization level

After the fourth workshop, the action teams met twice monthly. Just-in-time training methods in meeting management, generating creativity, process improvement techniques, and action plan development were provided when the teams were ready to engage in these activities. About once every other month, half-day meetings were held with the entire strategic planning leadership group. At these sessions, each action team presented the results of their work to date and received feedback. These meetings served as a motivating force for the action teams to stay on target and demonstrate progress. They were also opportunities to celebrate their achievements.

Selected accomplishments of the action teams included:

- Formation of a nurse practice council
- Establishment of a yearly exemplar conference that has evolved into reports on sophisticated evidence-based studies
- Development of a mentoring program
- Establishment of a rapid response team, critical-thinking education for every nurse
- Action plans for enhancing critical-thinking developed jointly by each nurse and his or her manager
- Integration of critical-thinking education into the orientation program, evidence based practice education
- Real-time nurse staff assignments directory on the intranet available to all departments (Kalisch et al., 2006)
- An online Kardex and oral shift report process and form (Kalisch et al., 2007)
- Refinement of the nurse of the year award to include critical thinking and evidence-based practice criteria

Phase 5: Developing and implementing changes at the unit level

Once the organization-wide changes were well underway, the efforts turned to the patient unit or grassroots level. This turned out to be the most challenging and far-reaching aspect of the transformation project. It also was the phase that led to deep and sustained change. Starting with one unit (medical–oncology), a process to achieve staff engagement and teamwork was implemented. This process was then repeated sequentially with the other units in the hospital (surgical–orthopedic, cardiac, intensive care, emergency department, and finally, perioperative services).

The first step in the unit-based efforts was to conduct focus groups with all staff members and former patients and interviews with key physicians who practiced on the unit. The focus groups and interviews were transcribed and analyzed for key themes. The second step was to present these results first to the unit managers and then to the unit staff. Integrated into these presentations were the results of an analysis of existing data on unit staffing, clinical outcomes (patient fall rate, skin integrity, infection rates, etc.), and staff satisfaction (turnover, vacancy, agency usage, call-ins, etc.). A network analysis of staff inter-actions and data about the number of different staff members they work with was also presented (Kalisch & Begeny, 2005a, 2005b). At this point, the unit staff and managers were asked if they were willing to commit to change and participate in a project designed to improve unit functioning, with particular emphasis on teamwork and engage-ment. All of the unit staff members agreed to participate, although an occasional person expressed doubt about the possibility of success.

The third step was to engage the entire unit staff in developing their core values, vision, and goals and building on the nursing organization and the overall hospital values and visions. This was accomplished by meeting with one-half of the staff at a time. Each half participated in two sessions, one to discuss the values and vision and one to discuss goals. Splitting up the staff was necessary because it was not feasible to pull all of the staff from the unit at one time. A coordinating committee made up of three staff members from each of the two sessions inte-grated the results from both groups and drafted a list of values, a vision statement, and goals. It turned out that there was an amazing amount of overlap between the two groups on every unit. The integrated list of values, vision, and goals were posted in the unit lounge, and everyone was encouraged to offer suggestions for changes. Through an iterative process, a final version was agreed upon.

The fourth step was to appoint a guiding team of staff and managers on each unit. To capture the range of strengths of the staff, they each completed the I-Opt survey, which measures information processing styles. These were used along with other information about staff (i.e., role, years of experience, shift worked, and so on) to select members for the Guiding Team. The use of processing styles data assisted us in gaining a range of action-oriented and innovative thinking on the teams. The membership varied somewhat from unit to unit but included seven to ten individuals (nurses, nursing assistants, managers, and unit secretaries).

The fifth step was to initiate the work of the guiding teams in a day and a half long session we labeled a "deep dive" (Robert Wood Johnson Foundation, 2011). The agenda for these meetings included time to reflect on and share an ideal workday on the unit and what made it so positive. It also included content and experiences on generating creative ideas, including time to visit parts of the hospital they did not work on and observe "with new eyes." The next step was to review all of the available data about the current status of the unit focus group and interview results, unit staffing, clinical outcomes, and staff satisfaction data and to generate a list of problem areas (e.g., staff relationships, retention, pain management, and others). The next step was an extensive brainstorming session where staff envisioned working on a unit where patients received outstanding care and every staff member was flourishing and then listed what specific elements were present in that scenario. They were also encouraged to include "wild ideas" and engage in humor. The next step was to clarify the meaning of each item on the list and then to categorize these items under the unit goals. What resulted was a solution list for each goal. These were then placed into a four-by-four table ranging from easy to hard on the vertical axis and high cost to low cost on the horizontal axis.

By testing and implementing the items listed in the low-cost, easy quadrant first, the guiding team was able to achieve "quick wins," which was important to the rest of the staff. The next steps involved detailed planning and rapid-cycle implementation for each solution. The teams were encouraged to pilot test ideas on a limited basis (e.g., on one wing of the unit or on one shift) in order to refine a particular idea as well as facilitate the change process (because the limited basis would not be as threatening to the staff). Some of the changes initiated by the guiding teams have taken a considerable amount of time to work out the details, but this stems primarily from having to deal with the staff's fear of and resistance to change.

Through this process, the nursing organization achieved significant improvements. Nurses are now engaged in evidence-based practice projects, they have gained a major voice in decisions both at the unit level and overall organization, teamwork on the units has greatly improved, physician relationships are more respectful and collegial, most of the "negative" staff members have left the organization, and those that remain do not have the influence they once did. A large number of individual staff members have flourished in leadership roles, and the status and image of nursing has been transformed from a "necessary evil" to a vital and respected contributor to the success of the hospital.

Critical Success Factors of Culture Change Projects

Transforming a nursing organization is a major undertaking. Essential ingredients found to be necessary for the success of the project are support from top administration, provision of necessary resources, willingness to face the brutal facts, early and ongoing attention to sustainability, infusion into the grassroots, unrelenting communication, emphasis on building and maintaining trust, not declaring success too soon, and recognizing that you cannot fully know how.

First, *support from the top* is absolutely critical. The literature on organizational change emphasizes the importance of strong support from the CEO and the leadership team, and this was a major factor in the success of this project (Quinn, 2004). The second ingredient for success is *adequate resources*. A major transformation is costly, although if successful, may be cost-reducing in the long run (less staff turnover, decreased use of agency and travel staff, fewer litigations, shorter length of stays, fewer adverse events, fewer readmissions, better reimbursement from Medicare and other payers, etc.).

The third necessary ingredient was a *willingness to face "the brutal facts,"* a phrase used by Collins (2001) in his best seller, *Good to Great*. The need for change requires that the "brutal facts" be recognized (e.g., missed nursing care, high staff turnover, poor patient satisfaction scores, etc.). The importance of conducting an assessment as was carried out in this case study is essential. It is the natural inclination for people to de-emphasize their problems once confronted with the challenge of change. Even people who think change is great often change their minds when confronted with actually implementing said change. To deal with this, the results of the focus groups (staff members' own words) about problems they were experiencing were reviewed. These served to remind staff of the problems that existed which led to a need for change. Using the data collected in the assessment phase can be very useful in refocusing the staff on the need to change.

The fourth element was *early attention and ongoing to sustainability*. It is common to address sustainability at the end of a project implementation (Doppelt, 2003). Sustainable change, explains Collins, follows "a predictable pattern of buildup and breakthrough . . . it takes a lot of effort to get the thing moving at all, but with persistent pushing in a consistent direction over a long period of time," momentum builds and breakthroughs occur (p. 186).

Infusion into the grassroots is the fifth essential ingredient. There are two levels of change in any project: strategic and grassroots. As Galpin (1996) notes, "grassroots change is the effort that drives change deep into the organization." Leadership did not tell managers and staff what to do to achieve excellence but asked the questions that would assist nursing staff and managers to develop answers and provide the data that would help them see alternate ways of functioning, information they could not ignore. They did not just give staff members the opportunity to give their opinions, but worked hard to really hear them. They actively worked against asking staff to say what they thought simply for the purpose of getting them to buy into changes they thought would work.

Extensive involvement of staff and managers at all levels of the nursing organization is critical to any project's success. Unleashing the power of individuals and teams of staff members leads them to believe that their voice matters, and consequently, they are more likely to be committed and supportive of changes. The project needs to tap into the hearts, as well as the minds, of the staff members, generating excitement and exhilaration about the possibilities (O'Malley, 2000). Specifically, the leadership provided by members of the guiding team on each unit was absolutely critical. As pointed out by Holman, Devane, and Cady (2007), "what is needed for effective, sustainable change are sessions in which people collectively explore each other's assumptions, seek and expand common ground, shape a desired future, and jointly take ownership of the solutions to the issues at hand."

Unrelenting communication is the sixth critical ingredient for a successful transformation. As Kotter (2007, p. 100) points out, "without credible communication, the hearts and minds of the troops are never captured." In the strategic planning phase, each member of the planning group were assigned a group of constituents (typically their own unit staff) for which they were responsible for sharing the activities and discussion occurring in the planning meetings and also gaining input about the issues being discussed and considered. Preparation of talking points and questions to take back to their constituents will help the planning group members synthesize the discussion and decisions, and it also will ensure that everyone is communicating the same message. In the case study above, the talking points were communicated within 24 to 48 hours after each meeting. In addition, newsletters were published each month and attached to the paychecks of all staff, emails were sent out, project bulletin boards were placed in each unit staff lounge, and time was devoted to the project in each unit meeting.

The seventh essential ingredient is *emphasis on building and maintaining trust* (Covey & Merrill, 2006; Reina & Reina, 2006). This means telling the truth, even when it is something the staff or managers do not want to hear, and by creating an environment where the truth can be heard. It is important to avoid promises that might not materialize, and consistent follow-through on promises needs to be meticulously attended to. Every effort to be predictable and to make decisions that

are fair needs to be made. Openness needs to be promoted by extensive communication.

Ensuring early wins is the eighth essential ingredient in any transformation project. It is important to have early wins or achievements.
As Kotter explains, transformation takes time, and "a renewal effort
risks losing momentum if there are no short-term goals to meet and
celebrate. Most people won't go on the long march unless they see
compelling evidence in 12 to 24 months that the journey is producing
expected results" (2007, p. 102).

The ninth element is *not declaring success too soon.* There are no
shortcuts to this type of transformation. Declaring success too soon is
a mistake made in many transformation projects. Kotter (2007, p. 102)
notes "after a few years of hard work, managers may be tempted to
declare victory with the first clear performance improvement. While
celebrating a win is fine, declaring the war won can be catastrophic."
Any undertaking like this one requires a very long time for results to
become a part of the culture. It is essential for changes to be reempha-
sized and time taken to work through the issues that have led to going
back to the old ways.

In addition, a study of nurses' information processing styles uncovered the fact that nursing staff as a group tend to be resistant to change
and risk averse (Kalisch & Begeny, 2006). Compared to teachers, information specialists, scientists, and others, nurses were significantly
more likely to be in the conservator quadrant, which is characterized
by avoidance of change. To convince people with this pattern of information processing to change, a great deal of time, along with detailed
scenarios and data, is required. This can be discouraging to leadership
and could potentially derail a project.

Recognizing that you cannot fully know how is the tenth and final
essential element in transformation projects. It is impossible in the
beginning of a transformation process to fully know how to get there.
This means that nurse leaders undertaking major changes will inevi-
tably feel a combination of fear, hope, and dread. If the transformation
project is to succeed, however, he or she has to keep doing what he or
she thinks is right despite criticism, conflict, and organizational politics. Quinn (2004, p. 9) refers to this process as "building the bridge
as you walk on it" or "learning how to walk through hell effectively."
Transformation is very difficult, yet the future belongs to the adap-
tive. Transformation is a journey that has no end because nursing like
other organizations win by constantly adapting and changing.

Leadership

Former U.S. President Harry S. Truman said, "In periods where there is no leadership, society stands still." The same can be applied to organizations. Leadership is essential for progress and improvement. Leaders and managers provide guidance and support, they motivate and create confidence, they build morale and an improved work environment, and they coordinate the work. One of the most consistent findings in research about what it takes to build a safety culture is that managerial and leader commitment constitutes a very strong factor. Specifically, leadership is considered an essential element in guaranteeing a safety-driven organization. Safe patients, safe workers, and safe systems are interrelated and interconnected.

There is a difference between leadership and management. Said simply, leadership is setting a new direction or vision for a group or spearheading a new direction. On the other hand, management directs people/resources according to values and standards that have been established. Often the same people play both leader and manager roles at different points in time. Although not essential, it certainly helps a manager if he/she is also a good leader. Conversely, leaders do well if they have some degree of management skills because it helps them envision the implementation of their strategic vision.

There have been hundreds of theories of leadership developed, but the transactional and transformational one is most frequently referred to. Transactional leadership, also known as managerial leadership, focuses on the role of supervision, organization, and group performance. The individuals who function in this manner are interested in increasing the efficiency of established routines and procedures. In active transactional leadership, the leader promotes compliance through both rewards and punishments that are contingent upon the performance of the followers. The leader views the relationship between managers and subordinates as an exchange (the employee is paid to provide the nursing care). Unlike transformational leadership, leaders using the transactional approach are not looking to change the future, they are interested in maintaining the current status according to the rules. Transactional leaders pay attention to followers' work in order to find deviations and they provide constructive feedback to keep everybody on task.

Burns (1978) introduced the concept of transformational leadership in his book, *Leadership*. He defined transformational leadership as a process where "leaders and their followers raise one another to higher levels of morality and motivation." Bass developed the concept further in *Leadership and Performance Beyond Expectations* (1985), pointing out that transformational leaders have high levels of integrity and fairness, have expectations, provide encouragement, support, inspiration, and recognition to those they lead, and motivate people to buy into the future vision for the organization. These leaders have a way of motivating the people around them, instilling a feeling that everyone is accountable, and that everyone is in it together. These leaders are proactive, challenge long-held assumptions, and do not accept answers like "because this is the way we've always done it." By asking questions, transformational leaders challenge the status quo and are not afraid of failure. They foster an environment where it is safe to have conversations, be creative, and voice ideas, and where all team members feel valued. They challenge cultural norms and work to inspire passion with their teams. Transformational leaders assume the best of their employees. They believe them to be trusting, respectful, and self-motivated. The leaders help to supply the followers with tool they need to excel.

Using a sample of managers across different industries, a study was conducted of the underlying processes through which transformational and active transactional leadership affects followers' organizational identification. They found that transformational leadership resulted in higher organizational identification and psychological empowerment above and beyond active transactional leadership. Transformational leadership demonstrates a motivational mechanism through which followers identify with their organizations (Zhu, Sosik, Riggio, & Yang, 2012). Other studies have also found that transformational leadership is more effective and results in greater staff empowerment than transactional leadership (Breevaart et al., 2014; Ivey & Kline, 2010).

In a study of leadership in health care and its relationship to outcomes, it was found that participative leadership (i.e., a style of leadership that involves all members of a team in identifying goals and strategies and relies on the leader functioning as a facilitator rather than issuing orders or making assignments), a form of transformational leadership, was positively related to staff perceptions of better patient safety climate (Zaheer, Ginsburg, Chuang, & Grace, 2013). Although it did not identify a particular style of leadership, a study of hand hygiene and leadership compared two infectious disease units. In the first unit, a multimodal intervention including educational training, leadership engagement, distribution of individualized hand sanitizer bottles, and an advertising campaign promoting hand hygiene was implemented and data was collected for four years after the intervention. Researchers found adherence declined slightly from year 1 (84.2%) to year 4 (71.0%) but remained much higher than before the intervention. On the second unit, which did not participate in the previous intervention, adherence dropped (from 50.7% to 5.7%) after a hand hygiene leader stepped down from his leadership position (Lieber et al., 2014).

Although there is a paucity of research evidence to answer the question "What is the best leadership style to achieve an environment that promotes safety and quality?" empirical work has suggested a significant association between leadership style and perceived safety climate. For example, a safety-specific transformational leadership style has been shown to be related to a more positive safety climate (Barling, Loughlin, & Kelloway, 2002), and passive leadership has demonstrated a relationship with poorer safety climate (Kelloway, Mullen, & Francis, 2006). Clarke (2012) completed a meta-analysis of research on transformational and transactional leadership styles as predictors of safety climates. Active transactional leadership had a positive correlation with perceived safety climate, safety participation, and safety compliance. The findings suggest that active transactional leadership is important in ensuring compliance with rules and regulations, whereas transformational leadership is primarily associated with encouraging employee participation in safety (Clarke, 2012). Therefore, in line with the augmentation hypothesis of leadership, a combination of both transformational and transactional styles appears to be most beneficial for quality of care and patient safety.

This finding was underlined by Bohan (2014), who conducted a qualitative study of leadership, quality, and safety in health care. He found that executives see themselves as transformational but identified that this style requires adapting to the needs of the situation or outcome required. Thus, at times autocratic and transactional leadership were required in order to achieve of targets (time it takes to answer call lights) and patient outcomes (numbers of hospital acquired infections, pressure ulcers, falls, etc.).

Within health care, a few studies have been completed. Kunzle, Kolbe, and Grote (2010) conducted a systematic review of the findings of effective leadership strategies in critical care teams. Since team and leadership skills are increasingly recognized as important for patient safety, a body of literature on leadership in critical care has emerged. An input–process–output model of leadership was used to systemize the findings. The results of this review clearly show that effective leaders play a pivotal role in promoting team performance and safety. Effective leadership is characterized by clear and unambiguous behavior that is adaptable to situational demands and shared between team members.

Visibility of Leadership
Leadership is vital for culture change and maintenance. For a safety culture to be ingrained in the DNA of the organization, leaders need to model safety and facilitate an environment where safety can be implemented (Vogelsmeier, Scott-Cawiezell, Miller, & Griffith, 2010). They need to be visible and knowledgeable about what is actually happening on the front line. Vogelsmeier and colleagues (2010) found that there are differences in perceptions of safety culture between healthcare leaders and staff. Nurses and other team members who are closest to the patient were found to more accurate in their assessment of patient safety. Closing this gap is important for the appropriate allocation of resources and support to create and maintain a safety culture. We found a similar situation in the discrepancies of reports of managers versus nursing staff as to the amount and type of missed nursing care (see Chapter 5).

Leadership at all levels of the organization needs to be visible so that employees will believe that they and their circumstances are understood. Leadership must also care about the work their employees do and what motivates them to it well, and understand what employees need to make their work more satisfying. This cannot happen if managers and leaders are stuck in their office and rarely see firsthand how people function or what obstacles they confront in their workspaces.

There have been several studies of "WalkRounds," a practice where executives make weekly visits to areas in the hospital. This had been promoted for decades but typically did not have an organized structure. Frankel and colleagues (2003) describe weekly visits by senior executives where they are joined by one of two nurses and other available staff. They ask specific questions about adverse events and systems that led to these occurrences. They are entered into a database along with the contributing factors, which are collated with priority scores attached. These are used to determine quality projects. Sexton and colleagues (2014) studied WalkRounds in neonatal intensive care units and found that they led to better patient safety culture and less caregiver burnout.

One researcher screened over 2,000 articles on strategies to improve safety culture. Only 21 studies met the inclusion criteria. There was some evidence to support that leadership Walk Rounds ($p = 0.02$) and multifaceted unit-based programs ($p < 0.05$) may have a positive impact on patient safety climate. Pronovost and colleagues (2005) studied the effectiveness of a structured multifaceted unit-based safety program (structured framework for assessing, identifying, reporting, and improving patient safety concerns). This intervention had a positive effect on safety climate scores ($p < 0.05$). Six other studies supported these positive findings of the effectiveness for multi-faceted unit-based programs (Blegen et al., 2010; Paine et al., 2010; Pronovost et al., 2008; Sexton et al., 2011; Timmel et al., 2010; Wolf, Way, & Stewart, 2010). All studies reported varying levels of improvements in at least one dimension of patient safety climate over time. Other patient safety culture studies reported positive impact with other patient safety culture strategies, surgical safety checklists, and improvement approach strategies (Haynes et al., 2011).

Summary

This chapter contains a discussion of organizational culture and leadership styles that promote safety and are needed to reduce missed nursing care. The change process and strategic planning are explained as methods to systematically change a culture to the desired safe, quality-oriented one. Transactional and transformational leadership styles are contrasted, and their relationship to the development of a safety culture explained.

References

Alvesson, M. (2002). *Understanding organizational culture.* London: Sage Publications, Ltd.

Arizona State University: W. P. Carey School of Business. (2011). Culture clash: When corporate culture fights strategy, it can cost you. Retrieved from http://research.wpcarey.asu.edu/management-entrepreneurship/culture-clash-when-corporate-culture-fights-strategy-it-can-cost-you/

Ashkanasy, N., Wilderom, C., & Peterson, M. (Eds.). (2000). *Handbook of organizational culture and climate.* Thousands Oak, CA: Sage Publications, Inc.

Barling, J., Loughlin, C., & Kelloway, E. K. (2002). Development and test of a model linking safety-specific transformational leadership and occupational safety. *Journal of Applied Psychology, 87*(3), 488–496.

Bass, B. M. (1985). *Leadership and performance beyond expectations.* New York, NY: Free Press.

Blegen, M. A., Sehgal, N. L., Alldredge, B. K., Gearhart, S., Auerbach, A. A., & Wachter, R. M. (2010). Improving safety culture on adult medical units through multidisciplinary teamwork and communication interventions: the TOPSProject. *Quality & Safety in Health Care, 19*(4), 346–50.

Bohan, P. (2014). Can leadership behavior affect quality and safety (Q & S) in complex healthcare environments? *American Journal of Public Health Research, 2*(2), 56–61.

Braithwaite, J., Hyde, P., & Pope, C. (Eds.). (2010). *Culture and climate in healthcare organizations.* New York, NY: Palgrave Macmillan.

Breevaart, K., Bakker, A., Hetland, J., Demerouti, E., Olsen, O. K., & Espevik, R. (2014). Daily transactional and transformational leadership and daily employee engagement. *Journal of Occupational and Organizational Psychology, 87*(1), 138–157.

Brunt, B. A. (2010). Developing a just culture. *HealthLeaders Media.* Retrieved from http://www.healthleadersmedia.com/page-2/NRS-251182/ Developing-a-Just-Culture

Burns, J. M. (1978). *Leadership.* New York, NY: Harper & Row, Publishers.

Clarke, S. (2012). Safety leadership: A meta-analytic review of transformational and transactional leadership styles as antecedents of safety behaviors. *Journal of Occupational and Organizational Psychology, 86*(1), 22–49.

Clarke, S. P. (2006). Organizational climate and cultural factors. *Annual Review of Nursing Research, 24*, 255–272.

Collins, J. (2001). *Good to great: Why some companies make the leap... and others don't.* New York, NY: Harper.

Cooke, R. A., Rousseau, D. M., & Lafferty, J. C. (1988). Personal orientations and their relation to psychological and physiological symptoms of strain. *Psychological Reports, 62*, 223–238.

Covey, S. M. R., & Merrill, R. R. (2006). *The speed of trust: The one thing that changes everything.* New York, NY: Free Press.

Davies, H. T., Mannion, R., Jacobs, R., Powell, A. E., & Marshall, M. N. (2007). Exploring the relationship between senior management team culture and hospital performance. *Medical Care Research and Review, 64*(1), 46–65.

Doppelt, B. (2003). *Leading change toward sustainability.* Sheffield, UK: Greenleaf Publishing Limited.

Drennan, D. (1992). *Transforming company culture.* London: McGraw-Hill.

El-Jardali, F., Dimassi, H., Jamal, D., Jaafar, M., & Hemadeh, N. (2011). Predictors and outcomes of patient safety in hospitals. *BMC Health Services Research, 11*, 45.

Frankel, A., Graydon-Baker, E., Neppl, C., Simmonds, T., Gustafson, M., & Gandhi, T. K. (2003). Patient safety Leadership WalkRounds. *The Joint Commission Journal on Quality and Safety, 29*(1), 16–26.

Frankel, A., Grillo, S. P., Baker, E. G., Huber, C. N., Abookire, S., Grenham, M., ... Gandhi, T. K. (2005). Patient safety Leadership WalkRounds at Partners Healthcare: Learning from implementation. *The Joint Commission Journal on Quality and Safety, 31*(8), 423–437.

Galpin, T. J. (1996). *The human side of change.* San Francisco, CA: Jossey-Bass.

Gregory, B. T., Harris, S. G., Armenakis, A. A., & Shook, C. L. (2009). Organizational culture and effectiveness: A study of values, attitudes, and organizational outcomes. *Journal of Business Research, 62*(7), 673–679.

Griffith, K. S. (2009). Column: The growth of a just culture. *The Joint Commission Perspectives on Patient Safety, 9*(12), 8–9.

Hartmann, C. W., Meterko, M., Rosen, A. K., Shibei, Z., Shokeen, P., Singer, S., & Gaba, D. M. (2009). Relationship of hospital organizational culture to patient safety climate in the Veterans Health Administration. *Medical Care Research and Review, 66*(3), 320–338.

Haynes, A. B., Weiser, T. G., Berry, W. R., Lipsitz, S. R., Breizat, A. H., Dellinger, E. P., ... Gawande, A. A. (2011). Changes in safety attitude and relationship to decreased postoperative morbidity and mortality following implementation of a checklist-based surgical safety intervention. *BMJ Quality & Safety, 20*(1), 102–107.

Holman, P., Devane, T., & Cady, S. (2007). *The change handbook: The definitive resource on today's best methods for engaging whole systems* (2nd ed.). San Francisco, CA: Berrett-Koehler Publishers, Inc.

Islam, G., & Zyphur, M. J. (2009). Rituals in organizations: A review and expansion of current theory. *Group & Organization Management, 34*(1), 114–139.

Ivey, G. W., & Kline, T. J. B. (2010). Transformational and active transactional leadership in the Canadian military. *Leadership & Organization Development Journal, 31*(3), 246–262.

Kalisch, B. J., & Begeny, S. (2005a). Improving nursing unit teamwork. *The Journal of Nursing Administration, 35*(12), 550–556.

Kalisch, B. J., & Begeny, S. (2005b). Improving patient care in hospitals, creating team behavior. *Organizational Engineering Institute, 6*(1), 1–11.

Kalisch, B. J., & Begeny, S. (2006). The information processing styles of nurse and nurse managers: Impact on change and innovation. *Nursing Administration Quarterly, 30*(4), 330–339.

Kalisch, B. J., & Curley, M. (2008). Transforming a nursing organization: A case study. *The Journal of Nursing Administration, 38*(2), 76–83.

Kalisch, B. J., Hurley, P., Hodges, M., Landers, D., Richter, G., Stefanov, S., & Curley, M. (2007). PI tool patches broken communication. *Nursing Management, 38*(4), 16–18.

Kalisch, B. J., Myer, K. A., Mackey, D. M., Aiken, S. A., McNerney, M. J., Beauchesne, P. A., ... Wallace, B. D. (2006). Online patient assignments enhance horizontal communication. *Nursing Management, 37*(6), 51.

Kelloway, E. K., Mullen, J., & Francis, L. (2006). Divergent effects of transformational and passive leadership on employee safety. *Journal of Occupational Health Psychology, 11*(1), 76–86.

Kotter, J. P. (2007, January). Leading change: Why transformation efforts fail. *Harvard Business Review, 85*(1), 96–103.

Kunzle, B., Kolbe, M., & Grote, G. (2010). Ensuring patient safety through effective leadership behavior: A literature review. *Safety Science, 48*(1), 1–17.

Leape, L. L. (2009). Errors in medicine. *Clinica Chimica Acta, 404*(1), 2–5.

Lieber, S. R., Mantengoli, E., Saint, S., Fowler, K. E., Fumagalli, C., Bartolozzi, D., ... Bartoloni, A. (2014). The effect of leadership on hand hygiene: Assessing hand hygiene adherence prior to patient contact in 2 infectious disease units in Tuscany. *Infection Control and Hospital Epidemiology, 35*(3), 313–316.

Martin, J. (2002). *Organizational culture: Mapping the terrain.* Thousand Oaks, CA: Sage Publications, Inc.

O'Malley, M. N. (2000). *Creating commitment.* New York, NY: John Wiley.

Paine, L. A., Rosenstein, B. J., Sexton, J. B., Kent, P., Holzmueller, C. G., & Pronovost, P. J. (2010). Assessing and improving safety culture throughout an academic medical centre: a prospective cohort study. *Quality & Safety in Health Care, 19*(6), 547–554.

Pronovost, P. J., Berenholtz, S. M., Goeschel, C., Thom, I., Watson, S. R., Holzmueller, C. G., ... Sexton, J. B. (2008). Improving patient safety in intensive care units in Michigan. *Journal of Critical Care, 23*(2), 207–221.

Pronovost, P., Weast, B., Rosenstein, B., Sexton, J. B., Holzmueller, C. G., Paine, L., ... Rubin, H. R. (2005). Implementing and validating a comprehensive unit-based safety program. *Journal of Patient Safety, 1*(1), 33–40.

Quinn, R. E. (2004). *Building a bridge as you walk on it: A guide for leading change.* San Francisco, CA: Jossey-Bass.

Reina, D. S., & Reina, M. L. (2006). *Trust and betrayal in the workplace: Building effective relationships in your organization* (2nd ed.). San Francisco, CA: Berrett-Koehler Publishers, Inc.

Robert Wood Johnson Foundation. (2011). *Transforming care at the bedside. An RWJF national program.* Retrieved from http://www.rwjf.org/content/dam/farm/reports/program_results_reports/2011/rwjf70624

Schein, E. H. (1985). *Organizational culture and leadership.* San Francisco, CA: Jossey-Bass.

Sexton, J. B., Berenholtz, S. M., Goeschel, C. A., Watson, S. R., Holzmueller, C. G., Thompson, D. A., ... Pronovost, P. J. (2011). Assessing and improving safety, climate in a large cohort of intensive care units. *Critical Care Medicine, 39*(5), 934–939.

Sexton, J. B., Sharek, P. J., Thomas, E. J., Gould, J. B., Nisbet, C. C., Amspoker, A. B., ... Profit, J. (2014). Exposure to Leadership WalkRounds in neonatal intensive care units is associated with a better patient safety culture and less caregiver burnout. *BMJ Quality & Safety.* Advance online publication. doi: 10.1136/bmjqs-2013-002042

Shortell, S. M., Bennett, C. L., & Byck, G. R. (1998). Assessing the impact of continuous quality improvement on clinical practice: What it will take to accelerate progress. *The Milbank Quarterly, 76*(4), 593–624.

Timmel, J., Kent, P. S., Holzmueller, C. G., Paine, L., Schulick, R. D., & Pronovost, P. J. (2010). Impact of the comprehensive unit-based safety program (CUSP) on safety culture in a surgical inpatient unit. *Journal on Quality and Patient Safety, 36*(6), 252–260.

Vogelsmeier, A., Scott-Cawiezell, J., Miller, B., & Griffith, S. (2010). Influencing leadership perceptions of patient safety through just culture training. *Journal of Nursing Care Quality, 25*(4), 288–294.

Williams, E. S., Manwell, L. B., Konrad, T. R., & Linzer, M. (2007). The relationship of organizational culture, stress, satisfaction, and burnout with physician-reported error and suboptimal patient care: Results from the MEMO study. *Health Care Management Review, 32*(3), 203–212.

Wolf, F. A., Way, L. W., & Stewart, L. (2010). The efficacy of medical team training: Improved team performance and decreased operating room delays: a detailed analysis of 4863 cases. *Annals of Surgery, 252*(3), 477–483.

Zaheer, S., Ginsburg, L., Chuang, Y. T., & Grace, S. L. (2013). Patient safety climate (PSC) perceptions of frontline staff in acute care hospitals: Examining the role of east of reporting, unit norms of openness, and participative leadership. *Health Care Management Review.* Advance online publication. doi:10.1097/HMR/0000000000000005

Zhu, W., Sosik, J. J., Riggio, R. E., & Yang, B. (2012). Relationships between transformational and active transactional leadership and followers' organizational identification: The role of psychological empowerment. *Journal of Behavior and Applied Management 13*(3), 186–212.

Endnote

1   This analysis has been previously published in part and permission to reprint it has been obtained from the following. Kalisch, B., & Curley, M. (2008). Transforming a nursing organization: A case study. *Journal of Nursing Administration, 38*(2), 76–83.

— 14 —

Teamwork Strategies

There have been many studies testing strategies to improve teamwork outside of the healthcare industry, and to a lesser degree, within health care. Very few studies, however, have focused on teamwork within nursing. After a thorough review of the research on interventions to enhance teamwork, Buljac-Samardzic, Dekker-van Doorn, van Wijngarrden, and van Wijk concluded that one of the key gaps in research on healthcare teamwork is due to the lack of studies of mono-disciplinary (single discipline) teamwork. This does not take away from the fact that interdisciplinary teamwork in health care is a critical area that needs major attention. Both are important. In this chapter, we will address strategies to enhance teamwork under the topics of culture, leadership, size of team, physical space, training, tools, structured protocols, systems redesign, handovers, and staff engagement.

Culture

In addition to the just culture and the safety culture described in Chapter 13, there is a need for a team culture. Having teamwork as a strong value and having it embedded in the mission and vision of the organization is essential for achieving teamwork in an organization. As discussed earlier, team culture refers to the social and cognitive environment, the shared view of reality, and the collective beliefs and values reflected in a consistent pattern of behaviors among team members. In this purview, culture is associated with the attitudes that team members develop toward the team, teamwork, and social loafing (Chatman & Flynn, 2001; Chen, Chen, & Meindl, 1998; Hui, Yee, & Eastman, 1995; Klein, Bigley, & Roberts, 1995; McDaniel & Stumpf, 1995; Rousseau, 1995). The process of culture change is not easy but it can and is being done. An approach for such a change was described in Chapter 13.

Leadership

As presented in Chapter 13, meta-analyses that have been completed support the idea that transformational leaders, by inspiring staff members to transcend self-interest and focus on group goals, promote their commitment to work, effort, and performance (Bass, Avolio, Jung, & Berson, 2003; DeGroot, Kiker, & Cross, 2000; Judge & Piccolo, 2004; Lowe & Galen, 1996). As teamwork involves performing tasks through joint work and interaction between individual members (Sundstrom, DeMeuse, & Futrell, 1990), transformational leadership has been found to have especially powerful effects on team performance (DeGroot et al., 2000; Dionne, Yammarion, Atwater, & Spangler, 2004).

Studying how conflict is handled in a team has been identified as a valuable factor to consider in understanding how transformational leadership fosters teamwork, as well as other positive outcomes (De Dreu & Gelfand, 2008; Jehn & Bendersky, 2003; Jehn & Mannix, 2001; Tipsvold, 2008). A study of conflict management approaches adopted in teams showed that transformational leadership promotes team coordination and thereby team performance by encouraging them to adopt a cooperative, as opposed to competitive, approach to conflict management. This is an important mechanism through which transformational leadership enhances team coordination, and in turn, achieves higher levels of team performance.

Training and post-training support is needed for leaders and managers in an organization in order to make the necessary changes to adopt a team culture and transformational leadership. The charge nurse, who has largely been neglected in terms of leadership training in most healthcare organizations, is a key nursing team leader on inpatient units. The nurse manager is drawn into many other activities and provides the overall leadership for the unit. However, the charge nurse is at the point of care delivery and leads teams on an hour-to-hour basis. In many hospitals, the charge nurse role is rotated among all or many of the staff members on a unit. This critical role should be a permanent position and an investment should be made in their leadership development. They require training in leadership, teamwork, team facilitation, conflict management, performance management, and other areas, just like all managers.

Team Size

As introduced in Chapter 12, team size is one of the more obvious environmental factors that impacts the level of teamwork. The average number of individuals in a team across industries and countries is five to twelve people (Kalisch, Begeny, & Anderson, 2008). One organization has collected data on over 2,000 teams doing everything from oil drilling to developing new medical devices over the past decade and has found that the most frequent size of teams is nine people (Kalisch et al., 2008). The average federal group size is eight people (Friel, 2001); the U.S. Army National Guard manual reports an average group size of about nine (U.S. Army Field Artillery Center, 2003). Yet nursing teams in acute care hospitals range from 20 to over 150 nursing staff members, with most having teams of 80 or more.

Of the previous studies on teamwork and team size, the majority support smaller teams. For example, an investigation of the relationship between team size and quality of group experience, as well as the mediating role of counterproductive behaviors (i.e., parasitism, interpersonal aggression, boastfulness, and misuse of resources), was conducted with a sample of 97 work teams in a public safety organization (Aube, Rousseau, & Tremblay, 2011). The results support the idea that the smaller the team, the better the teamwork. In addition, each of the four categories of counterproductive behaviors played a mediating role in this relationship. Reports of interdisciplinary teamwork at Veterans hospitals demonstrated that components of team cooperation and team functioning were negatively impacted when size increased (Guzzo, Salas, & Associates, 1995; Stahelski & Tsukuda, 1990).

Research supports the conclusion that smaller teams lead to better teamwork. This is due to the fact that larger teams have more linkages among members and therefore have greater difficulty developing and maintaining role structures. They also encounter greater coordination and communication challenges and are susceptible to decreased motivation (Hoegl, 2005; LePine, Piccolo, Jackson, Mathieu, & Saul,

2008; Sundstrom, DeMeuse, & Futrell, 1990). Members of larger teams are also found to be less attached to the group and there are more instances of social loafing (team members not carrying their workload) (Alexander, Lichtenstein, Jinnet, D'Aunno, & Ulman, 1996; Guzzo et al., 1995; Hakenes & Katolnik, 2013; Hoegl, 2005; Keyton & Beck, 2008; Cox, 2003).

Within the nursing field, we conducted a study of 2,265 direct care nursing providers (RNs, NAs, LPNs, and USs) working on 53 units in 4 hospitals that examined the relationship between teamwork and unit size (Kalisch, Russell, & Lee, 2013a). Four measures of unit size were utilized: average daily census, number of RNs, number of NAs, and number of total staff. Pearson correlation coefficients (measures of the linear correlation [dependence] between two variables) were calculated to determine which of the four variables measuring unit size correlated with teamwork overall and/or with the five teamwork subscales (trust, team orientation, backup, shared mental model, and leadership). A significant negative correlation was found between nursing teamwork overall and the number of NAs (more NAs, less teamwork) and between teamwork overall and the average daily census (the larger the census, the lower the teamwork) (Kalisch et al., 2013a). On the other hand, no significant relationship was found between teamwork and the number of RNs or the number of staff overall.

From these findings, it appears that more patients on a unit lead to less teamwork. Conversely, fewer patients on a unit generate higher teamwork. This finding may be due to the fact that larger units have bigger spaces and layouts, making it difficult for staff to monitor and assist one another. The fact that a larger number of NAs (but not a larger number of RNs) leads to lower teamwork points to a presence of problems in the RN–NA relationship, previously discussed in Chapter 12. It appears that the key problem in nursing teamwork is caused by the difficulties that occur within these dyads. When RNs work with other RNs, they usually have their own patients, but when RNs work with NAs, they share responsibilities for patients.

The significant measures of unit size were also negatively correlated with each of the five nursing unit teamwork subscales. We calculated the strengths of r for the significant unit size variables using Cohen's (1988) guidelines (small = .10–.29, medium = .30–.49, large = .50–1.0). The largest shared variance and the strongest negative correlation between the significant independent variables was found with the Backup subscale. The number of NAs explained 37% of the variance in the Backup subscale. The more NAs as a proportion of the staff, the less backup reported. The implications of these findings regarding team size and teamwork are that consideration needs to be given to not only decreasing team size but also to developing strategies that enhance the teamwork between RNs and NAs.

Redesigning Care Teams

Overly large teams appear to be unable to develop a high level of teamwork, partly because of the greater likelihood of counterproductive behaviors, inability to communicate, lack role clarity, and the lack of knowledge about one another's strengths and weaknesses. Redesign is needed.

One method to reduce the size of an inpatient unit nursing staff that I have found to be successful is to divide the typical 30 or 40 bed unit into four 10-bed subunits, assigning the staff to one of these subunits on a permanent basis (6 months or more) rather than to the entire unit. This creates teams of 12 to 14 staff members for each of the subunits (around the clock). In another hospital, three wings became subunits, reducing the number of staff (around the clock) to 16 individuals for each subunit. These smaller teams led to better teamwork, more satisfied patients, and a higher continuity of care. To handle vacations and absences, a separate team was created to fill this role for all of the smaller teams on the unit.

If the team is smaller, it is harder for team members to engage in loafing and easier to monitor and communicate with one another (Cusumano, 1997). If the same people work together consistently, they will be more motivated to give feedback about performance to one another. In the traditionally large team, we found that nursing staff work together about every other week (Kalisch, Begeny, & Anderson, 2008). This leads to sweeping problems under the rug rather than addressing and resolving them with coworkers because they don't work with any given staff member very often. If they do work together and report off to the same staff members day after day, week after week, they are more motivated to give feedback because they will be experiencing the problems repeatedly if they do not.

Many nursing staff members believe that the way to impact the performance of another team member is to tell the manager and let him or her take care of it. The manager cannot possibly monitor the day-to-day work of staff members. Firstly, no one person can watch 80 or more staff members. Secondly, they are not there 24 hours a day, 7 days a week. Also, they have many other responsibilities. Performance relies on coworker feedback (positive and negative). Think about how you would feel if someone reported a problem about you to a supervisor and had not discussed it with you beforehand. This leads to greater problems with teamwork. The only way to affect the behavior of coworkers is to address problems directly with them (using effective feedback techniques). If a staff member fails to alter their behavior after two or three reminders, then say: "I notice you have not ____ even though I have mentioned it several times. I need to go to the manager with this problem. Do you want to come with me?"

Besides creating smaller teams, the RN–NA relationship needs special attention and intervention. The method of assigning an NA to report to two or more RNs is fundamentally positioned to create problems. I have found that there is more teamwork if it is possible to create teams of two (maybe three) RNs and one NA caring for a group of patients, working together regularly. The RNs need to receive training in delegation and leadership and both the RNs and NAs need to be taught the best methods for giving feedback. If there is one dominant skill that gets in the way of teamwork, it is the inability to give effective feedback.

Physical Layout

The layout of the work space is also a contributor to the quality of teamwork. Li and Robertson (2011) conducted field studies with cancer teams at three hospitals. Their results highlight how factors such as room size, team size, seating arrangements, display configuration, and variations in preparing and presenting medical information clearly influence the dynamics of the conversation and information sharing in multidisciplinary cancer teams.

One of the major emphases in recent years as to the design of hospitals is a shift toward what is called "patient-centered design." There is a growing emphasis on creating supportive, aesthetically pleasing, and comfortable healing environments developed with the patients' and families' needs in mind. The Planetree model of patient-centered care is one example. Planetree's philosophy is based on the premise that care should be organized first and foremost around the needs of patients (Planetree, 2014). Another example is the Pebble Project, which is a collaboration of providers who aim to create better healthcare facilities that "improve patient and worker safety and clinical outcomes, while maximizing environmental performance and operating efficiency" (Pebble Project, 2014). The experiences of Planetree, Pebble, and others indicate that there are a number of design factors that affect the patient and staff experiences as well as the quality of care (Ulrich et al., 2008).

However, some of these design elements are actually causing problems with nursing teamwork. New construction often produces very large rooms and hallway spaces. While this is very helpful to patients and families, it makes teamwork very difficult, and in some cases, impossible for nursing staff. Nursing staff note that they cannot see one another because they "are so spread out." One nurse asked, "How do you monitor one another, how do you back one another up, how do we communicate with these large spaces? How can we share our competencies when we never see each other?"

Becker notes that the relationship between communication and space layout has been studied very little (2007, 2010). He points out that a lot of communication occurs around the nurses' station, medication rooms, and lounges. Circumstantial and often chance communication creates occasions for on-the-job mentoring, learning, and behavioral modeling as well as the sharing of knowledge and expertise. Most patient care units have neither the space available for teams to meet formally and share information nor the technologies and resources to support collaboration in shared spaces.

If teamwork is to be achieved, new construction and renovation of hospitals and other healthcare facilities needs to take these factors into consideration. Patient comfort and satisfaction is of critical importance but so is the facilitation of teamwork that is needed to provide safe, quality care. It is critical that nurses and other providers be involved in the design of units. Redden and Evans point out that to achieve success, a partnership between the architect and the nurse is needed along with the critical operational processes and knowledge of evidence-based design (Redden & Evans, 2014).

Teamwork Training

A 2008 meta-analysis of 45 published and unpublished studies concluded that team training is "useful for improving cognitive outcomes, affective outcomes, teamwork processes, and performance outcomes" (Salas et al., 2008). This and other meta-analyses have resulted in the conclusion that team training is an effective and essential strategy.

Salas and his colleagues evaluate training on Kirkpatrick's four types of evaluation, as follows (Kirkpatrick, 1994; Salas & Cannon-Bowers, 2001; Van Buren & Erskine, 2002):

1. Reaction of trainees (affective and attitudinal responses; how well did the learners like the training process?)
2. Learning (the extent to which knowledge and skills are acquired)
3. Behavior (changes in performance of the newly learned knowledge and skills while on the job)
4. Results (tangible results of the learning process in terms of reduced cost, improved quality, increased production, efficiency, etc.)

The reaction level is operationalized by using self-report measures. However, there is very little reason to believe that how trainees feel about a training program says much about what they actually learned and if their behavior or job performance changed (greater teamwork) as a result or if the organization benefited (e.g., decreased infection rates, decreased falls, decreased pressure ulcers, lower costs, fewer readmissions, etc.). To assess the learning that occurred as the result of training, knowledge tests can be utilized. Observations of the behavior of the team members at work are the most effective ways to determine if teamwork behaviors are being implemented. The results can be measured by patient outcome data (e.g., number of patient falls, time it takes to answer call lights, etc.) along with measures of organizational effectiveness (e.g., how many medications are available to the nurse when she is ready to administer them.)

Crew Resource Management Training
In health care, several training programs have been developed using simulation- or classroom-based approaches. Crew Resource Management (CRM) training, which evolved from commercial and military aviation is an often used approach that has been adapted to health care. CRM training has been used in aviation for almost three decades. It has been defined as a set of "instructional strategies designed to improve teamwork in the cockpit by applying well-tested training tools (e.g., performance measures, exercises, feedback mechanisms) and appropriate training methods (e.g., simulators, lectures, role playing, videos) targeted at specific content (i.e., teamwork knowledge, skills, and attitudes)" (Salas, Fowlkes, Stout, Milanovich, & Prince, 1999, p. 163). The emphasis on this training is not on technical skills but on teamwork, communication, leadership, situation awareness, and decision-making. There are major differences between pilots and nursing staff however.

Along with the recognition of the importance of enhanced teamwork in health care to improve safety, there has also been the realization that health care should be a high-reliability organization (HRO). An HRO is an organization that has succeeded in avoiding catastrophes in an environment where normal accidents can be expected due to risk factors and complexity (e.g., aviation, nuclear power plants, etc.). Health care is certainly a complex, risky, high-consequence industry where accidents can be expected. However, the safety record in health care does not lend itself to being called highly reliable at this point in time.

In 2006, Salas, Wilson, Burke, and Wightman published an updated review of studies of CRM training and concluded that current evidence shows that it produces "positive reactions, enhanced learning, and desired behavioral change in a simulated or real environment" (Salas et al., 2006). However, "what cannot be answered with certainty is whether CRM training has an effect on the bottom line: safety" (p. 408).

Medical Team Training

Another approach to team training in health care is TeamSTEPPS, an interdisciplinary program developed by the Department of Defense and the Agency for Healthcare Research and Quality. Although variations occur with its implementation, it generally involves a train-the-trainer portion of two to three days of didactic and inter-active workshops designed to create a cadre of teamwork instructors with the skills to train other staff members in 4 to 16 hours (Agency for Healthcare Research and Quality, 2014). It also includes a 1 to 2 hour condensed version of the course, specifically designed for non-clinical support staff. The training program is accompanied by a manual, training videos, and advice on how to successfully imple-ment the program in an organization. Research testing the efficacy of TeamSTEPPS has shown some positive outcomes. A customized 2.5 hour TeamSTEPPS program was given to PICU, SICU, and respiratory therapy staff. Reports of improved teamwork and observations of team performance were higher after training. From pre- to post-training, the average time for placing patients on extracorporeal membrane oxygenation (ECMO) decreased significantly. The rate of nosocomial infections at post-implementation was below the upper control limit for seven out of eight months in both the PICU and the SICU (Mayer et al., 2011).

A study of TeamSTEPPS training showed significant improve-ments in team structure, leadership, situation monitoring, mutual support, and communication ($p < .001$) (Sheppard, Williams, & Klein, 2013; Weaver et al., 2010). In addition, challenges by nurses to scripted medication order errors doubled from 38% to 77% after the training. Detection and correction of inadequate chest compressions increased from 62% to 85% after the training (Sawyer, Laubach, Hudak, Yamamura, & Pocrnich, 2013). Weaver and colleagues (2010) conducted a study in the operating room using TeamSTEPPS. They found that the trained group demonstrated significant increases in the quantity and quality of pre-surgical procedure briefings and the use of quality teamwork behaviors during cases.

A host of other teamwork training approaches have been developed, including Team Oriented Medical Simulation (TOMS), Multidisciplinary Obstetric Simulated Emergency Scenarios (MOSES), Geriatric Interdisciplinary Team Training (GITT), and Dynamic Outcomes Management (DOM).

Hughes and colleagues (2014) did a meta-analysis on all types of training programs in health care, calling them Medical Teamwork Training (MTT). The sample was 87 studies containing 100 independent samples. Each study analyzed the four levels of evaluation (reaction, learning, behavior, and results) described above. Using the Kirkpatrick criteria, they found that trainees believed that it was effective and useful. The training was also found to achieve an increase in knowledge. In regard to the third level, behaviors, they found that training had a significant effect on the behavioral transfer of competencies to the job. They also found that teamwork training had a positive and significant impact on patient outcomes such as mortality rates, complications rates, and patient satisfaction.

Teamwork Training in Nursing

Although interdisciplinary teamwork is vital, teamwork within nursing is also critical to the reduction of errors and the improvement of the quality of care. As noted above, one of the key gaps in research in healthcare teamwork is the lack of studies of mono-disciplinary teamwork. They found only three such studies (two in nursing and one in anesthesiology). DiMeglio and colleagues (2005) tested a team building intervention with staff nurses and found an improvement in group cohesion and nurse-to-nurse interaction. Gibson (2001) discovered that a goal-setting intervention was not related to group effectiveness.

A study evaluating an intervention (a combination of training, an engaged guiding team, and coaching) to increase teamwork and engagement resulted in a significant decrease in patient falls, staff vacancy, and turnover rates, and a significant rise in staff ratings of the level of teamwork (Kalisch, Curley, & Stefanov, 2007). The drawback to this intervention was the considerable length of time and the amount of resources required (i.e., staff time, facilitator time, etc.). Finally, comparing a group of nurses who participated in a TeamSTEPPS workshop with those who had not, leadership was found to have improved significantly but communication, mutual support, situation monitoring, and team structure did not improve (Castner, Foltz-Ramos, Schwartz, & Ceravolo, 2012). These data suggest that TeamSTEPPS as it is currently configured is insufficient to address nursing care delivery problems in inpatient settings.

Another study on one medical–surgical patient care unit tested an intervention for team training using virtual simulation (using Second Life). Nursing staff (RNs and NAs) in groups of three or four individuals underwent one hour of training using scenarios that occur regularly on patient care units. The *Nursing Teamwork Survey* and the *MISSCARE Survey* were administered pre- and post-intervention to determine the efficacy of the training program (Kalisch, Abersold, McLaughlin, Tschannen, & Lane, 2014). Although 44 staff members participated in the training, only 16 completed both the pre- and the posttest. Despite the small sample size, paired t-tests revealed that the intervention significantly improved overall teamwork as well as three out of five subscales of the *Nursing Teamwork Survey*. The effect size was large ($d = .93$). In addition, overall missed nursing care was slightly improved ($d = .24$), although it did not reach statistical significance ($p = .476$). The major obstacles to the use of virtual simulation are technical difficulties.

Teamwork Tactics

In another study, a quasi-experimental design with repeated measures taken at pretest, posttest, and two months after completion of an intervention (TEAM TACTICS) resulted in positive results (Kalisch, Xie, & Ronis, 2013b). The framework for the study is contained in Figure 14.1. The intervention was a train-the-trainer type and is a customization of the approach used with TeamSTEPPS. The sample for the study was the nursing staff on three medical–surgical units in three separate acute care hospitals (one unit in each hospital). Three nurses (two from day and evening shifts and one from the night shift) from each unit underwent a training program for two days to prepare them to train all the staff on their own units in three one-hour-long sessions. There were four to five staff members per training group, and it was repeated as many times (typically 18 to 20) as needed to accommodate

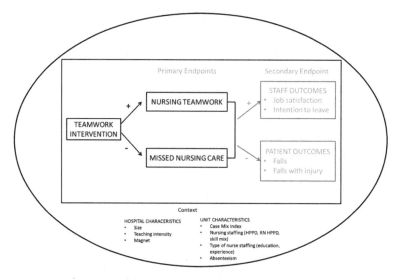

FIGURE 14.1. **The teamwork intervention model.**
(Kalisch et al., 2013b)

the size of the nursing staff on a given unit. The training actually took place on the patient units with coverage for the hour from managers, educators, and clinicians to allow nursing staff to participate in the training during work hours. If the patient load was heavy, the session would be cancelled. Because staff nurses were conducting the actual training, this did not result in a loss of funds for the trainer since they could participate in needed patient care.

The training was scenario-based and focused on staff role-playing scenarios based on teamwork and missed care problems that occur regularly on inpatient units in acute care hospitals. Examples of teamwork training scenarios can be found in Tables 14.1 and 14.2. The training was followed by debriefing that applied teamwork behaviors (e.g., leadership, team orientation, backup, performance monitoring, etc.) and missed nursing care (Figures 14.2 and 14.3).

Three measures were used to test the efficacy of this intervention: The *Nursing Teamwork Survey,* the *MISSCARE Survey,* and a knowledge test on teamwork. Return rates for the surveys ranged from 73% to 84%. Follow-up tests that individually compared pretest, posttest, and delayed posttest were conducted within the mixed model and used the Bonferroni correction for multiple comparisons. The intervention resulted in a significant increase in teamwork (F = 6.911, *p* = 0.001) and a significant decrease in missed nursing care (F = 3.592, *p* = 0.029) (Figure 14.4). Satisfaction with teamwork also increased significantly (F = 6.62, df = 283.08, *p* = .002).

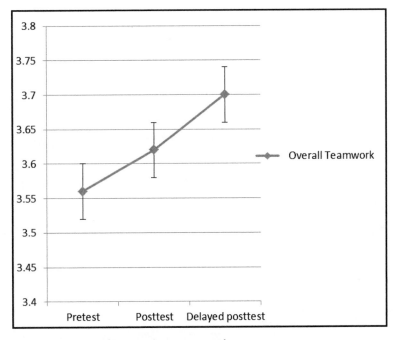

FIGURE 14.2. **Impact of intervention on teamwork.**
(Kalisch et al., 2013b)

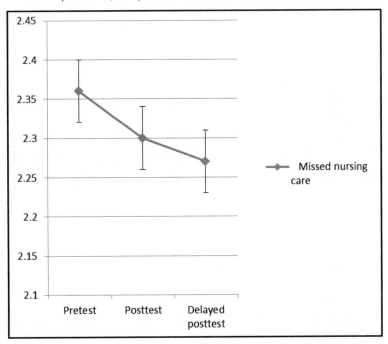

FIGURE 14.3. **Impact of intervention on missed nursing care.**
(Kalisch et al., 2013b)

TABLE 14.1. **Example teamwork training scenario 1.**

Roles

1. RN A
2. Unit Secretary (US)
3. Radiology Technician (RT)
4. RN B

Background

At 12:00 P.M., Mr. Jones, a 75-year-old male, is admitted to a medical–surgical unit with a diagnosis of pneumonia. He has a history of cardiovascular disease, hypertension, and dementia and is a smoker. Mr. Jones is assigned to RN B, but she is at lunch. RN A is covering for RN B.

The following roles will be given on slips of paper to the four players but are not be known by the other player.

RN A: You are admitting Mr. Jones because the RN B is at lunch. There is no armband sent up with the paperwork and you ask the US to obtain it. Then, you are called to respond to an emergent patient situation off the unit. You assume that the US will place the armband on the patient.

Unit Secretary: When RN A told you there is no armband for Mr. Jones, you print out the armband and place it on top of the counter where the patient charts are located. You assume the nurse will pick it up and place it on the patient. You are slammed with orders that need to be addressed (act them out and talk to yourself if necessary).

Radiology Technician: You receive Mr. Jones for an x-ray. He does not have an armband. He is alert and oriented to name only. You call the unit and tell RN B that you are sending him back to the unit because you have no way to identify him for the x-ray.

RN B: RN A is doing the admission since you are gone. When you get back to the unit, Mr. Jones has been taken to radiology. You get a call from the radiology technician who tells you that Mr. Jones does not have an armband and they are going to send him back. You go to ask the US about what happened.

Debriefing

1. In what way were the elements of teamwork (present or absent) evident in this scenario?

Teamwork Elements	Example of Presence	Example of Absence
Team leadership		The US and RN A assume that the other person would take care of the armband placement. The opportunity for them to take a leadership role was missed.

(*Continued*)

Teamwork Elements	Example of Presence	Example of Absence
Team orientation		The US and RN A assume that the other person would take care of the armband placement. Each team member viewed themselves as an isolated individual only accountable for their specific role (as opposed to everyone believing that the work of the team is everyone's).
Mutual performance monitoring		The US and RN A did not keep track of one another's work while completing their own work.
Backup	Once RN B was confronted with the problem of no arm-band, she went and discussed it with the US and RN A (as opposed to ignoring it and not saying anything).	US did not back up the RN A after she has asked her to print the armband.
Shared mental model		The US and RN A had different ideas as to what should be done in this type of situation. RN A assumed that the US would put the armband on the patient and the US assumed RN A would do it, even though it sat on the counter where the US could probably see it.
Closed-loop communication		RN A did not use closed-loop communication in asking the US to print out the name band. She should have specified to print it and place it on patient. The US did not clarify what RN A wanted her to do.
Mutual trust	RN B trusted RN A to cover her patients and RN A trusted the US to put the armband on the patient.	After this instance, trust among those involved would be diminished and would have to be rebuilt.

2. How did the lack of nursing teamwork lead to missed nursing care?

   ◆ No armband placed on patient (potential safety problem)
   ◆ X-ray could not be completed
   ◆ Could have resulted in the patient getting the wrong test

(Continued)

Scenario 1: Examples of feedback

1. Feedback from RN B to US

    When you leave the armband for the patient on the counter for a long period of time,

    I feel frustrated

    Because the patient is at risk when he doesn't have his armband on and I was busy with other things.

    I would like you to put the patient's armband on when it sits on the counter more than a few minutes

    Because then the patient will be safe.

    What do you think?

2. Feedback from US to RN B

    When you ask me to print the armband for the patient and don't tell me you want me to put it on him,

    I feel upset

    Because I assume you will put the armband on the patient and that it is not my job.

    I would like you to be clear about everything you want me to do

    Because then I can do my job.

    What do you think?

3. Feedback from RN A to RN B

    When you do not complete the entire admission process,

    I feel worried

    Because this could result in the patient receiving the wrong care.

    I would like you to figure out a way to make sure the armband is placed on the patient when you are admitting him

    Because we would avoid any safety issues.

    What do you think?

TABLE 14.2. **Example teamwork training scenario 2.**

Roles

1. RN

2. Nursing assistant A (NA A)

3. Nursing assistant B (NA B)

Background

The setting is a medical–surgical unit where a 66-year-old male, Mr. Sullivan, needs to be ambulated. He is 6 feet tall and weighs 250 pounds. The chart indicates he has not been out of bed for 2 days. The RN asks NA A to help her ambulate Mr. Sullivan. The food trays just arrived in the unit.

The following roles will be given on slips of paper to the three players but are not be known by the other players.

RN: You ask NA A to help you ambulate Mr. Sullivan. NA A does not come to help you right away, so you continue to take care of your other patients. At the end of the shift, you realize that Mr. Sullivan has not been ambulated.

Nursing Assistant A: You are busy administering food trays with NA B and you tell NA B that the RN wants you to help her with ambulating a patient.

Nursing Assistant B: NA A is administering food trays with you. She tells you that the RN wants her to help with ambulating a patient. You tell NA A that this RN never helps the NAs when the NAs request her help because "she is always busy charting." You feel the RN does not have to spend all that time documenting. You tell NA A, "Don't bother. She can wait or do it by herself."

Debriefing

1. In what way were the elements of teamwork (present or absent) evident in this scenario?

Teamwork Elements	Example of Presence	Example of Absence
Team leadership		Although an appropriate task to request help, the RN does not find out what other work the NAs have and how they could work together to make it happen.
		NA A did not report back to the RN.
Team orientation		The RN does not consider the work of the NAs.
		NA A does not tell the RN that she cannot help her ambulate the patient.
		NA B acts out her anger toward the RN in a passive-aggressive manner rather than letting the RN know how she feels.
Mutual performance monitoring		The RN is not aware of the current responsibilities of the NAs. The NAs do not consider the work of the RN or the goals the RN has for the patient.

(Continued)

Teamwork Elements	Example of Presence	Example of Absence
Backup		Neither the RN nor the NAs support one another. The NAs do not back up the RN. The RN does not inquire about the workload of the NAs.
Adaptability		The NAs do not inform the RN that they are not available. NA B stubbornly refuses to offer help because she is angry.
Shared mental model		The RN and NAs have different ideas about what their role should be in this situation. The NAs feel they should pass the trays while the RN is solely focused on ambulating a patient rather than the whole picture.
Closed-loop Communication		The RN did not find out if and when the NA was going to come help her. NA A did not tell the RN that she could not help her.
Mutual trust		The RN will probably not be able to trust the NAs to complete delegated tasks in the future. The NAs do not trust the RN and feel that the RN does not help them carry out their responsibilities or is unaware of their work demands.

2. How did the lack of nursing teamwork lead to missed nursing care?

   ◆ Ambulation
   ◆ Passing food trays and feeding patients when food is still warm

Scenario 2: Examples of feedback

1. Feedback from RN to NA A
   When you did not come back to help me ambulate the patient and did not tell me you were not coming,
   I felt frustrated
   Because I thought you were going to help me.
   I would like you to let me know if you are not going to help me,
   Because then I can find someone else to help.
   What do you think?

2. Feedback from NA A to RN
   When you ask me to leave all the trays and feeding to NA B,
   I felt angry
   Because she cannot possibly pass 20 trays and feed two patients by herself.
   I would like you to find out what I am involved in before you ask me to help you,
   Because this would give us the opportunity as a team to figure out how we could get all the work done.
   What do you think?

Model of Care

Over the past 100 years, nursing has utilized a number of different models of nursing care (Fernandez, Johnson, Tran, & Miranda, 2012). In the 1920s, private duty nursing was practiced. Students provided all the labor for hospitals. The Great Depression of the 1930s led to a decrease in private duty job opportunities, which led to more nurses being employed by hospitals (as opposed to self-employed in private duty). During World War II, the country experienced its first major shortage of nurses when supply could not meet demand. As a result, a new way of delivering nursing care was required, one that leaned much more heavily on the use of NAs and LPNs to compensate for the fewer RNs available to work in hospitals.

At that time, functional nursing was the standard model of care, in which each staff member was assigned one or more tasks, such as medication delivery, dressing changes, procedures, or hygiene care. Tiedeman and Lookinland (2004) described this delivery system as an assembly line approach in which the head nurse acted much like today's charge nurse, making assignments, receiving and giving report on all patients, coordinating care, and participating in rounds with physicians. Functional nursing was said to result in fragmentation of care, a lack of accountability, and an inability to develop in-depth relationships with patients and families. At the same time, nursing school curricula began to emphasize a holistic—as opposed to task-oriented—approach to patient care. Graduating nurses were unfulfilled by not being able to provide comprehensive nursing care, taking into account the physical, social, and psychological issues facing patients.

Team nursing was introduced in the 1950s. This approach called for an RN team leader to oversee the care of a group of patients with the assistance of LPNs and NAs. Each patient was assigned to a team member, who was supposed to perform total patient care except for responsibilities requiring an RN license, such as giving medications (Daeffler, 1975; Glandon, Colbert, & Thomasma, 1989). The RN team leader obtained the patient report from the head (or charge) nurse at the beginning of the shift and then gave the report to team members (Manthey, 2002; Tiedeman & Lookinland, 2004).

The hallmark of this nursing care delivery system, a daily team conference about the patients, was meant to ensure that everyone on the team knew the status of all patients cared for by the team. The RN team leader might be responsible for a team that provided care to as many as 25 patients (Manthey, 2002; Shukla & Turner, 1984; van

Servellen & Mowry, 1985). This large number of patients alone inhibited the delivery of quality patient care, and nursing teams almost always reverted back to the functional nursing approach in which each team member took on specific tasks.

So-called team nursing was then replaced by primary nursing to provide the nurse with his or her own patients and a more satisfying nursing experience. Manthey (2002), in her book on primary nursing, said that team nursing was characterized by fragmentation, major communication issues, and a lack of accountability. The real problem with this team nursing model was that it was implemented with a functional approach (one giving all medications, another the treatments, another the baths and vital signs, etc.). Consequently, teamwork acquired a negative reputation, and even today, the mention of team nursing is responded to negatively ("Don't tell me we are going back to team nursing" [RN].

The premise behind primary nursing is that one nurse would be the key nurse for the patient throughout the hospital stay (Ciske, 1979; Hegyvary, 1977; Zander, 1985). While appealing, it was not possible because nurses work three or five shifts a week if they are full-time, leaving the patients in the hands of other nurses for the rest of the time. Nursing staff also take breaks (or should). Hence, no one nurse can provide all or even a large proportion of the care of a hospitalized patient. Just as important, no nurse has all the knowledge and skills necessary to provide the full scope of care needed by any given patient (Kalisch & Schoville, 2012). Also, nursing staff members need to monitor one another and back each other up in order to provide safe, quality nursing care. For example, if a nursing staff member does not change his or her patient's IV tubing (anyone can forget), if they are practicing as a team, another staff member will remind them to do so (not in a non-judgmental way) and the error will be avoided.

Yet we found in a qualitative study consisting of interviews with RNs with varying years of experience that the belief still persists among nurses that each patient "should" be cared for by just one nurse. The term primary nursing is still widely used by nurses, often describing themselves as being a patient's primary nurse or primary. Interestingly, when we conducted an informal Web search for the models of care utilized in hospitals across the country, we found that many facilities list primary nursing as their model of care delivery but actually appear to be using a mixture of several nursing models. This philosophical belief system (which may not be evident to the nurse herself) causes the nursing staff of most acute care hospital units to not follow a model of care that emphasizes teamwork (Kalisch, Begeny, & Anderson, 2008). It stresses individual responsibility, with RNs being assigned several patients (although the assigned patients may change from day to day). What became evident to us, as we spoke to nurses about the various care models, was that it wasn't team nursing per se that failed but the implementation of this model of care. Team nursing was rarely, if ever, practiced as it was envisioned. Yet, the negative view of working as a team persists.

Handoffs

Handovers and handoffs are critical communication events that impact teamwork and occur regularly in hospitals and other health-care organizations. The Joint Commission defines this as "a process in which information about patient/client/resident care is communicated in a consistent manner" from one healthcare provider to another (Riesenberg, Leitzsch, & Cunningham, 2010). Patients are routinely transferred from one service to another, from one level of care to another, or from one provider to another (Arora et al., 2009). As patient care responsibility is transferred or shared among various services (e.g., ED, OR, intensive care, medical–surgical units, etc.) and among different healthcare professionals (e.g., technicians, nurses, physicians, etc.) during various work shifts, the communication of pertinent patient care information is of critical importance.

Patient care units utilize a variety of methods for conducting inter-shift handoffs, ranging from face-to-face verbal reports in a conference room or at the patient's bedside to taped and written reports. Some shift reports have a formal structure while others do not. There have been a few studies that compare methods of shift report. Two studies found incomplete information in verbal handoffs compared to formal documentation (Sexton et al., 2004) or a taped report (O'Connell & Penney, 2001).

In one experimental study, researchers varied handoff style (task-centered versus patient-centered) and content (consistent versus inconsistent) to test recall. They reported low recall rates ranging from 20% to 34% (Dowding, 2001). Richard listened to taped and face-to-face shift reports, checked the actual condition of patients, and then analyzed the data for omissions leading to incongruence (Richard, 1988). (An omission was defined as information that, if left out of the shift report, could lead to increased inefficiency; incongruence was defined as occurring when information given during the report was not the same as the actual condition, and the difference could result in negative medical or legal outcomes.) The taped reports were significantly more likely to lead to omissions than face-to-face reports, but were less likely to produce incongruence. In another study, Barbera and colleagues eliminated taped reports and instituted a system whereby all relevant information for each patient was recorded in a binder located directly outside her or his room (Barbera, Conley, & Postell, 1998). Comparing the old system with the new one, the investigators demonstrated that the recording of medical histories improved from 55% to 100%, compliance with flow-sheet documentation increased from 45% to 100%, and the recording of IV catheter insertion dates improved from 75% to 95%.

Communication breakdown at these moments can endanger patients and lead to fragmented care (Cohen, Hilligoss, & Kajdacsy-Balla Amaral, 2012). Shift reports that are incomplete, inaccurate, biased, or misinterpreted have the potential to create problems in patient safety and quality, including missed nursing care (Anthony & Preuss, 2002; Ebright, Patterson, Chalko, & Render, 2003; Institute of Medicine, 2004).

Nursing inter-shift handoffs involve communicating essential patient information between the outgoing and the oncoming nursing staff during shift changes. Nursing staff depend on the content and the accuracy of these reports to base their clinical decisions on and to plan their patients' care. There are other handoffs experienced by nursing staff as well, such as during breaks and times that a nurse must be away from the unit (e.g., securing supplies, attending a class, or when a patient is transferred to or from areas such as the ED, the perioperative area, or a diagnostic setting) (Ong & Coiera, 2011). Each of these types of handoffs has similar as well as different challenges. For example, handoffs in intra-hospital transports present challenges that are not experienced in inter-shift handoffs (Ong & Coiera, 2011).

Errors
Handoffs can and often do create significant information gaps, errors, and omissions in patient care and are considered a weak link in patient care (Chang, Arora, Lev-Ari, D'Arcy, & Keysar, 2010; Patterson & Wears, 2010; Riesenberg, Leitzsch, & Little, 2009). An examination of 10 years of sentinel events found that communication breakdowns, including handoffs, were involved two-thirds of the time (Croteau, 2005). Pezzolesi and colleagues (2010) found that 45% of all handoff incidents were incomplete, and 29% of the time, there was no handoff report at all. Ebright, Urden, Patterson, and Chalko studied novice

nurses' near misses and adverse events and found that, in seven of eight cases, inadequate handoffs—characterized by either a lack of information or confusion—were involved (Ebright et al., 2004).

Strople and Ottani (2006) concluded that current methodologies used to collect and convey patient information are ineffective and may contribute to adverse events. A total of 425 inpatient handoffs were observed in a study by Goff and colleagues: 48% by residents, 33% by nurses, 13% by attending obstetricians, and 6% by midwives. Only 40% of all handoffs met criteria for high quality (Goff, Knee, Morello, Grow, & Bsat, 2014). In a study of information lost during shift reports in 68 hospitals in Lebanon, 57% of the 6,807 responding hospital employees agreed that pertinent patient information—such as abnormal vital signs, laboratory values or radiology test findings, pain management, allergy, fall risk, and functional status—are often not reported during shift change (El-Jardali, Jaafar, Dimassi, Jamal, & Hamdan, 2010). A subsequent review of reported patient safety incidents showed that medication errors, delays in treatment, wrong treatment, duplication of laboratory tests, and near-miss events were caused by patient information omissions during inter-shift handoffs (Younan & Fralic, 2013). Nagpal, Vats, Ahmed, Vincent, and Moorthy (2010) found that only 44% of key information was retained by the time patients were transferred from the operating room to the gastroenterology inpatient unit and 75% of patients experienced incidences of error. Staggers and Jennings (2009) found several themes during handoffs with facts and professional judgments being only second and third in frequency. Handoffs were unstructured, replete with interruptions and high noise levels, and nurses did not use available electronic health records.

Several systematic reviews of studies on handoffs have been completed (Arora et al., 2009; Cohen & Hilligoss, 2010; Halm, 2013; Hays, 2003; Matic, Davidson, & Salamonson, 2011; Messam & Pettifer, 2009; Patterson & Wears, 2010; Riesenberg et al., 2010; Strople & Ottani, 2006). A list of barriers to effective handoffs was developed by Riesenberg and colleagues (2010). These barriers include communication problems such as incomplete, wrong, or disorganized information, being interrupted, personal chatting, failure to report the current status of the patient (in addition to what is documented), routinized presentation, and not being able to contact the handoff nurse for questions that arise after the report. Other problems include interpersonal problems, hierarchy, role confusion, language and cultural differences, equipment failures, time constraints, and fatigue.

The findings of these studies and others concerning accurate and complete information transfer has led to such policy changes as the Joint Commission requiring U.S. hospitals to standardize the way handoffs are conducted (TJC, 2006). Approaches that have been used to improve handoffs include the use of mnemonics, reframing the purpose of the handoff, creating a protected environment for handoffs, and using a combination of written and verbal reports. These will be described below.

Mnemonics

One strategy for improving handoffs is the use of mnemonics (memory assistants). Riesenberg and colleagues (2009) conducted a systematic review of published articles on the use of mnemonics. They uncovered 46 studies describing 24 mnemonics. SBAR (Situation, Background, Assessment, and Recommendation) was the most frequently cited mnemonic (70%). Another mnemonic is "I PASS the BATON":

- Introduction
- Patient
- Assessment
- Situation
- Safety concerns
- Background
- Actions
- Timing
- Ownership
- Next

HANDOFFS is another example:

- Hospital location, room number
- Allergies, adverse reactions, medications
- Name, age, gender
- DNAR, diet
- Ongoing medical/ surgical problems
- Facts about this hospitalization
- Follow-up
- Scenarios (Brownstein & Schleyer, ND)

Still another mnemonic is SIGNOUT from Johns Hopkins University (2011):

- **S**ick or DNR?
- **I**dentifying data (name, age, gender, diagnosis)
- **G**eneral hospital course
- **N**ew events of the day
- **O**verall health status/clinical condition
- **U**pcoming possibilities with plan, rationale
- **T**asks to complete overnight with plan, rationale

Reframing Purpose

Another strategy offered by Cohen and colleagues involves changing the underlying belief that the essential function of a handoff is only a one-way information transmission. This fails to recognize that handoffs are an opportunity to create what they call co-constructions of the patient's condition and needs. They make the case that the more important purpose of these handoffs is to create a greater comprehension of the most important and uncertain aspects of the patient's status in the mind of the oncoming party. Focusing only on transmitting information (many times this is simply repeating what is available in the written records) does not create a full understanding of the patient for the oncoming provider. They note that "what matters most is the effect of handoff interaction on the mind of the receiver, on the subsequent ability to make sense of the patient's unfolding episode of illness and treatment and to take the appropriate actions" (Cohen, Hilligoss, & Kajdacsy-Balla Amaral, 2012, p. 2). They recommend that the outgoing staff member take the perspective of the one beginning their shift (Epley & Caruso, 2009). In situations where the nurse handing off information has control of the knowledge about the patient, a handoff may be a simple narrative of what was done and why. However, this report may not be what the oncoming nurse really needs. A description of potential problems and the unresolved issues may be more important for the nurse taking over the responsibility of caring for the patient.

Protected Environment

Since it has been shown that handoffs are often interrupted, causing miscommunication and loss of valuable information, creating an environment which eliminates interruptions and other distractions would be helpful.

Combination of Written and Verbal Reports

In one study, researchers compared three handoff styles (written, verbal, and a combination of these). Although the combination style yielded good recall rates (96% or higher), the styles that were solely verbal or written did not, with rates varying from 0% to 58% (Pothier, Monteiro, Mooktiar, & Shaw, 2005).

Summary

Strategies for enhancing teamwork are examined in this chapter, including the redesign of patient units, team training, and making changes in the model of nursing care delivery. Because the most critical forms of communication in hospitals are handoffs, methods for improving these processes are presented.

References

Agency for Healthcare Research and Quality. (2014). Implementation at a glance: TeamSTEPPS instructor manual. Retrieved from http://www.ahrq.gov/professionals/education/curriculum-tools/teamstepps/instructor/reference/implglance.html

Alexander, J. A., Lichtenstein, R., Jinnet, K., D'Aunno, T. A., & Ullman, E. (1996). The effects of treatment team diversity and size on assessments of team functioning. *Hospital & Health Services Administration, 41*(1), 37–50.

Anthony, M. K., & Preuss, G. (2002). Models of care: The influence of nurse communication on patient safety. *Nursing Economics, 20*(5), 209–215.

Armour Forse, R., Bramble, J. D., & McQuilan, R. (2011). Team training can improve operating room performance. *Surgery, 150*(4), 771–778.

Arora, V., Manjarrez, E., Dressler, D., Basaviah, P., Halasyamani, L., & Kripalani, S. (2009). Hospitalist handoffs: A systematic review and task force recommendations. *Journal of Hospital Medicine, 4*(7), 433–440.

Aube, C., Rousseau, V., & Tremblay, S. (2011). Team size and quality of group experience: The more the merrier? *Group Dynamics: Theory, Research, and Practice, 15*(4), 357–375.

Barbera, M. L., Conley, R., & Postell, M. (1998). A silent report. *Nursing Management, 29*(6), 66–67.

Bass, B., Avolio, B., Jung, D., & Berson, Y. (2003). Predicting unit performance by assessing transformational and transactional leadership. *Journal of Applied Psychology, 88*(2), 207–288.

Becker, F. (2007). Nursing unit design and communication patterns: What is "real" work? *Health Environments Research & Design Journal, 1*(1), 58–62.

Becker, F. (2010). Nursing unit design, communication, and teamwork: An ecological approach to integrated healthscape strategies. Proceedings from *The 3rd Annual Conference of The Health and Care Infrastructure Research And Innovation Center*. Edinburgh, Scotland.

Brownstein, A., & Schleyer, A. (N.d.). The art of HANDOFFS: A mnemonic for teaching the safe transfer of critical patient information. Retrieved from http://healthcare-professionals.sw.org/resources/docs/authorized/ome/TheArtOfHandoffs.pdf

Buljac-Samardzic, M., Dekker-van Doorn, C. M., van Wijngarrden, J. D., & van Wijk, K. P. (2010). Interventions to improve team effectiveness: A systematic review. *Health Policy, 94*(3), 183–195.

Castner, J., Foltz-Ramos, K., Schwartz, D. G., & Ceravolo, D. J. (2012). A leadership challenge: Staff nurse perceptions after an organizational TeamSTEPPS initiative. *The Journal of Nursing Administration, 42*(10), 467–472.

Chang, V. Y., Arora, V. M., Lev-Ari, S., D'Arcy, M., & Keysar, B. (2010). Interns overestimate the effectiveness of their hand-off communication. *Pediatrics, 125*(3), 491–496.

Chatman, J. A., & Flynn, F. J. (2001). The influence of demographics heterogeneity on the emergence and consequences of cooperative norms in work teams. *Academy of Management Journal, 44*(5), 956–974.

Chen, C. C., Chen, X., & Meindl, J. R. (1998). How can cooperation be fostered? The cultural effects of individualism-collectivism. *Academy of Management Review, 23*(2), 285–304.

Ciske, K. L. (1979). Accountability—the essence of primary nursing. *The American Journal of Nursing, 79*(5), 890–894.

Cohen, J. (1988). *Statistical power analysis for the behavioral sciences* (2nd ed.). Hillsdale, NJ: Lawrence Erlbaum.

Cohen, M. D., & Hilligoss, P. B. (2010). The published literature on handoffs in hospitals: Deficiencies identified in an extensive review. *Quality and Safety in Health Care, 19*(6), 493–497.

Cohen, M. D., Hilligoss, P. B., & Kajdacsy-Balla Amaral, A. C. (2012). A handoff is not a telegram: An understanding of the patient is co-constructed. *Critical Care, 16*(1), 303.

Cox, K. (2003). The effects of intrapersonal, intragroup, and intergroup conflict on team performance effectiveness and work satisfaction. *Nursing Administrative Quarterly, 27*(2), 52–163.

Croteau, R. (2005). JCAHO comments on handoff requirement. *OR Manager, 21*(8), 8.

Cusumano, M. A. (1997). How Microsoft makes large teams work like small teams. *Sloan Management Review, 39*, 9–20.

Daeffler, R. J. (1975). Patients' perception of care under team and primary nursing. *The Journal of Nursing Administration, 5*(3), 20–26.

De Dreu, C. K. W., & Gelfand, M. J. (Eds). (2008). *The psychology of conflict and conflict management in organizations*. New York, NY: Lawrence Erlbaum.

DeGroot, T., Kiker, D. S., & Cross, T. C. (2000). A meta-analysis to review organizational outcomes related to charismatic leadership. *Canadian Journal of Administrative Science, 17*(4), 356–372.

DiMeglio, K., Padula, C., Piatek, C., Korber, S., Barrett, A., Ducharme, M., ... Corry, K. (2005). Group cohesion and nurse satisfaction: Examination of a team-building approach. *Journal of Nursing Administration, 35*(3), 110–120.

Dionne, S. D., Yammarion, F. J., Atwater, L. E., & Spangler, W. D. (2004). Transformational leadership and team performance. *Journal of Organizational Change Management, 17*(2), 177–193.

Dowding, D. (2001). Examining the effects that manipulating information given in the change of shift report has on nurses' care planning ability. *Journal of Advanced Nursing, 33*(6), 836–846.

Ebright, P. R., Patterson, E. S., Chalko, B. A., & Render, M. L. (2003). Understanding the complexity of registered nurse work in acute care settings. *Journal of Nursing Administration, 33*(12), 630–638.

Ebright, P. R., Urden, L., Patterson, E., & Chalko, B. (2004). Themes surrounding novice nurse near-miss and adverse-event situations. *The Journal of Nursing Administration, 34*(11), 531–538.

El-Jardali, F., Jaafar, M., Dimassi, H., Jamal, D., & Hamdan, R. (2010). The current state of patient safety culture in Lebanese hospitals: A study at baseline. *International Journal for Quality in Health Care, 22*(5), 386–395.

Epley, N., & Caruso, E. M. (2009). Perspective taking: Misstepping into others' shoes. In K. D. Markman, W. M. P. Klein, & J. A. Suhr (Eds.), *Handbook of imagination and mental simulation* (pp. 295–309). New York, NY: Psychology Press.

Evans, A. (1993). Accountability: A core concept for primary nursing. *Journal of Clinical Nursing, 2*(4), 231–234.

Fernandez, R., Johnson, M., Tran, D. T., & Miranda, C. (2012). Models of care in nursing: A systematic review. *International Journal of Evidence-Based Healthcare, 10*(4), 324–337.

Friel, B. (2001). Drop in projected retirements puts Bush management cuts at risk. Retrieved from http://www.govexec.com/dailyfed/0501/052201b1.htm

Gibson, C. (2001). Me and us: Differential relationships among goal-setting training, efficacy and effectiveness at the individual and team level. *Journal of Organizational Behavior, 22*(7), 789–808.

Glandon, G., Colbert, K. W., & Thomasma, M. (1989). Nursing delivery models and RN mix: Cost implications. *Nursing Management, 20*(5), 30–33.

Goff, S. L., Knee, A., Morello, M., Grow, D., & Bsat, F. (2014). Handoff quality for obstetrical inpatients varies depending on time of day and provider type. *Journal of Reproductive Medicine, 59*(3-4), 95–102.

Guzzo, R. A., Salas, E., & Associates. (1995). *Team effectiveness and decision making in organizations.* San Francisco, CA: Jossey-Bass.

Hakenes, H., & Katolnik, S. (2013). Optimal team size and overconfidence. Retrieved from http://dx.doi.org/10.2139/ssrn.2355731

Halm, M. A. (2013). Nursing handoffs: Ensuring safe passage for patients. *American Journal of Critical Care, 22*(2), 158–162.

Hays, M. M. (2003). The phenomenal shift report: A paradox. *Journal for Nurses in Staff Development, 19*(1), 25–33.

Hegyvary, S. T. (1977) Foundations of primary nursing. *Nursing Clinics of North America, 12*(2), 187–196.

Hoegl, M. (2005). Smaller teams—better teamwork: How to keep project teams small. *Business Horizons, 48*(3), 209–214.

Hughes, A. M., Gregory, M. E., Sonesh, S. C., Benishek, L. E., Joseph, D. L., Marlow, S., … Salas, E. (2014). Transforming healthcare one team at a time: A meta-analysis of medical team training. Under Review.

Hui, C. H., Yee, C., & Eastman, K. L. (1995). The relationship between individualism-collectivism and job satisfaction. *Applied Psychology: An International Review, 44*(3), 276–282.

Institute of Medicine. (2004). *Keeping patients safe: Transforming the work environment of nurses.* Washington, DC: National Academies Press.

Jehn, K., & Bendersky, C. (2003). Intragroup conflict in organizations: A contingency perspective on the conflict-outcome relationship. *Research in Organizational Behavior, 25,* 187–242.

Jehn, K., & Mannix, E. (2001). The dynamic nature of conflict: A longitudinal study of intragroup conflict and age performance. *Academy of Management Journal, 44*(2), 238–251.

Johns Hopkins University Graduate Medical Education. (2011). *Guidelines for patient handoffs.* Retrieved from http://www.hopkinsmedicine.org/medpeds_urban_health/policies/xfer_handoff.pdf

Judge, T. A., & Piccolo, R. F. (2004). Transformational and transactional leadership: A meta-analytic test of their relative validity. *Journal of Applied Psychology, 89*(5), 755–768.

Kalisch, B. J., Abersold, M., McLaughlin, M., Tschannen, D., & Lane, S. (2014). An intervention to increase nursing teamwork using virtual media. *Western Journal of Nursing Research.* Advance online publication. doi:10.1177/0193945914531458

Kalisch, B. J., & Begeny, S. M. (2005a). Improving nursing unit teamwork. *Journal of Nursing Administration, 35*(12), 550–556.

Kalisch, B. J., & Begeny, S. M. (2005b). Improving patient care in hospitalsKalisch, B. J., Begeny, S. M., & Anderson, C. (2008). The effect of consistent nursing shifts on teamwork and continuity of care. *Journal of Nursing Administration, 38*(3), 132–137.

Kalisch, B. J., Curley, B., & Stefanov, S. (2007). An intervention to enhance nursing teamwork and engagement. *Journal of Nursing Administration, 37*(2), 77–84.

Kalisch, B. J., Russell, K., & Lee, K. H. (2013a). Nursing teamwork and unit size. *Western Journal of Nursing Research, 35*(2), 214–225.

Kalisch, B. J., & Schoville, R. (2012). It takes a team. *The American Journal of Nursing, 112*(10), 50–54.

Kalisch, B. J., Xie, B., & Ronis, D. (2013b). A train the trainer intervention to increase teamwork and decrease missed nursing care in acute care patient units. *Nursing Research, 62(6),* 405-413.

Keyton, J., & Beck, S. J. (2008). Team attributes, processes, and values: A pedagogical framework. *Business Communication Quarterly, 71*(4), 488-504.

Kirkpatrick, D. L. (1994). *Evaluating training programs.* San Francisco, CA: Berrett-Koehler.

Klein, R. L., Bigley, G. A., & Roberts, K. H. (1995). Organizational culture in high reliability organizations: An extension. *Human Relations, 48*(7), 771-793.

LaCrosse, S. (2008). Exploring nursing practice using RROHC as a model. *Nurse Leader, 6*(6), 42-45.

LePine, J., Piccolo, R., Jackson, C., Mathieu, J., & Saul, J. (2008). A meta-analysis of teamwork processes: Tests of a multidimensional model and relationship with team effectiveness criteria. *Personnel Psychology, 61*(2), 273-308.

Li, J., & Robertson, T. (2011). Physical space and information space: Studies of collaboration in distributed multi-disciplinary medical team meetings. *Behavior and Information Technology, 30*(4), 443-454.

Lowe, K. B., & Galen, K. K. (1996). Effectiveness correlates of transformational and transactional leadership: A meta-analytic review of the MLQ literature. *Leadership Quarterly, 7*(3), 385-425.

Manthey, M. (2002). *The practice of primary nursing* (2nd ed.). Minneapolis, MN: Creative Health Care Management.

Matic, J., Davidson, P. M., & Salamonson, Y. (2011). Review: Bringing patient safety to the forefront through structured computerisation during clinical handover. *Journal of Clinical Nursing, 20*(1-2), 184-189.

Mayer, C. M., Cluff, L., Lin, W. T., Willis, T. S., Stafford, R. E., Williams, C., ... Amoozegar, J. B. (2011). Evaluating efforts to optimize TeamSTEPPS implementation in surgical and pediatric intensive care units. *The Joint Commission Journal on Quality and Patient Safety, 37*(8), 365-374.

McDaniel, C., & Stumpf, L. (1995). The organizational culture: Implications for nursing service. *The Journal of Nursing Administartion, 23*(4), 54-60.

Messam, K., & Pettifer, A. (2009). Understanding best practice within nurse intershift handover: What suits palliative care? *International Journal of Palliative Nursing 15*(4), 190-196.

Nagpal, K., Vats, A., Ahmed, K., Vincent, C., & Moorthy, K. (2010). An evaluation of information transfer through the continuum of surgical care: A feasibility study. *Annals of Surgery, 252*(2), 402-407.

O'Connell, B., & Penney, W. (2001). Challenging the handover ritual. Recommendations for research and practice. *Collegian, 8*(3), 14-18.

Ong, M. S., & Coiera, E. (2011). A systematic review of failures in handoff communication during intrahospital transfers. *The Joint Commission Journal on Quality and Patient Safety, 37*(6), 274-284.

Patterson, E. S., & Wears, R. L. (2010). Patient handoffs: Standardized and reliable measurement tools remain elusive. *The Joint Commission Journal on Quality and Patient Safety, 36*(2), 52–61.

Pebble Project. (2014). About. Retrieved from http://www.healthdesign.org/pebble/about

Pezzolesi, C., Schifano, F., Pickles, J., Randell, W., Hussain, Z., Muir, H., & Dhillon, S. (2010). Clinical handover incident reporting in one UK general hospital. *International Journal of Quality in Health Care, 22*(5), 396–401.

Planetree. (2014). Homepage. Retrieved from http://planetree.org/

Pothier, D., Monteiro, P., Mooktiar, M., & Shaw, A. (2005). Pilot study to show the loss of important data in nursing handover. *British Journal of Nursing, 14*(20), 1090–1093.

Redden, P., & Evans, J. (2014). It takes teamwork ... the role of nurses in ICU design. *Critical Care Nursing Quarterly, 37*(1), 41–52.

Richard, J. A. (1988). Congruence between intershift reports and patients' actual conditions. *The Journal of Nursing Scholarship, 20*(1), 4–6.

Riesenberg, L. A., Leitzsch, J., & Cunningham, J. M. (2010). Nursing handoffs: A systematic review of the literature. *American Journal of Nursing, 110*(4), 24–34.

Riesenberg, L. A., Leitzsch, J., & Little, B. W. (2009). Systematic review of handoff mnemonics literature. *The American Journal of Medical Quality, 24*(3), 196–204.

Rousseau, D. M. (1995). *Psychological contracts in organizations: Understanding written and unwritten agreements.* Thousand Oaks, CA: Sage.

Salas, E., & Cannon-Bowers, J. A. (2001). The science of training: A decade of progress. *Annual Review of Psychology, 52,* 471–499.

Salas, E., DiazGranados, D., Klein, C., Burke, C. S., Stagl, K. C., Goodwin, G. F., & Halpin, S. M. (2008). Does team training improve team performance? A meta-analysis. *Human Factors, 50*(6), 903–933.

Salas, E., Fowlkes, J. E., Stout, R. J., Milanovich, D. M., & Prince, C. (1999). Does CRM training improve teamwork skills in the cockpit? Two evaluation studies. *Human Factors, 41, 326–343.*

Salas, E., Wilson, K. A., Burke, C. S., & Wightman, D. C. (2006). Does crew resource management training work? An update, an extension, and some critical needs. *Human Factors, 48*(2), 392–412.

Sawyer, T., Laubach, V. A., Hudak, J., Yamamura, K., & Pocrnich, A. (2013). Improvements in teamwork during neonatal resuscitation after interprofessional TeamSTEPPS training. *Neonatal Network: The Journal of Neonatal Nursing, 32*(1), 26–33.

Sexton, A., Chan, C., Elliott, M., Stuart, J., Jayasuriya, R., & Crookes, P. (2004). Nursing handovers: do we really need them? *Journal of Nursing Management, 12*(1), 37–42.

Shukla, R. K., & Turner, W. E. (1984). Patients' perception of care under primary and team nursing. *Research in Nursing and Healthy, 7*(2), 93–99.

Sheppard, F., Williams M., & Klein, V. (2013). TeamSTEPPS and patient safety in healthcare. *Journal of Healthcare Risk Management, 32*(3), published ahead of print. doi: 10.1002/jhrm

Staggers, N., & Jennings, B. M. (2009). The content and context of change of shift report on medical and surgical units. *The Journal of Nursing Administration, 39*(9), 393–398.

Stahelski, A., & Tsukuda, R. (1990). Predictors of cooperation in health care teams. *Small Group Research, 21*(2), 220–233.

Strople, B., & Ottani, P. (2006). Can technology improve intershift report? What the research reveals. *Journal of Professional Nursing, 22*(3), 197–204.

Sundstrom, E., DeMeuse, K. P., & Futrell, D. (1990). Work teams: Applications and effectiveness. *American Psychologist, 45*(2), 120–133.

The Joint Commission. (2006). *National patient safety goals: 2006 critical access hospital and hospital national patient safety goals.* Oakbrook Terrace, IL: The Joint Commission.

Tiedeman, M. E., & Lookinland, S. (2004). Traditional models of care delivery: What have we learned? *The Journal of Nursing Administration, 34*(6), 291–297.

Tipsvold, D. (2008). The conflict-positive organization: It depends upon us. *Journal of Organizational Behavior, 29*(1), 19–28.

U.S. Army Field Artillery Center. (2003). Field Artillery Proponency Briefing 13; Career Management Field. Retrieved from http://sill-www.army.mil

Ulrich, R. S., Zimring, C., Zhu, X., DuBose, J., Seo, H. B., Choi, Y. S., ... & Joseph, A. (2008). A review of the research literature on evidence-based healthcare design. *Health Environments Research and Design Journal, 1*(3), 61–125.

Van Buren, M. E., & Erskine, W. (2002). The 2002 ASTD state of the industry report. Alexandria, VA: American Society of Training and Development.

van Servellen, G. M., & Mowry, M. M. (1985). DRGs and primary nursing: Are they compatible? *The Journal of Nursing Administration, 15*(4), 32–36.

Weaver, S. J., Rosen, M. A., DiazGranados, D., Lazzara, E. H. Lyons, R., Salas, E., ... King, H. B. (2010). Does teamwork improve performance in the operating room? A multilevel evaluation. *The Joint Commission Journal on Quality and Patient Safety,* 36(3), 133–142.

Younan, L. A., & Fralic, M. F. (2013). Using "best-fit" interventions to improve the nursing intershift handoff process at a medical center in Lebanon. *The Joint Commission Journal on Quality and Patient Safety, 39*(10), 460–467.

Young, G. J., Charns, M. P., Desai, K., Khuri, S. F., Forbes, M. G., Henderson, W., & Daley, J. (1998). Patterns of coordination and clinical outcomes: A study of surgical services. *Health Services Research, 33*(5), 1211–1236.

Zander, K. (1985). Second generation primary nursing. A new agenda. *Journal of Nursing Administration, 15*(3), 18–24.

— 15 —

Patient and Family Engagement

The patient's perspective in regards to their safety in health care has been largely ignored in the past. However, it is increasingly being advocated as an essential means to improve the quality of care as well as a method to decrease patient errors. It has been referred to in a variety of ways: as a necessary aspect of a continuously learning health system; as the holy grail of health care; as a vital ingredient for reforming the healthcare system; and as the next "blockbuster drug of the century" (Al-Shorbaji & Geissbuhler, 2012; Chase, 2012; Institute of Medicine, 2011; Wilkin, 2012). It is also being recognized as essential to the redesign of the healthcare system.

The American Hospital Association recently reported that patient engagement is the key to achieving the "triple aim" of health reform (improved health outcomes, better patient care, and lower costs) (Rodak, 2013). The London Declaration, endorsed by the World Health Organization World Alliance for Patient Safety, calls for a greater role for patients to improve the safety of health care worldwide (Longtin, et al., 2010; World Health Organization, 2005). Involvement of patients in safety management and the reporting of incidents has also been recommended by the Council of Europe and the World Alliance for

Patient Safety, and several organizations now provide educational materials to patients that are designed to motivate them to engage in ensuring their safety (Perneger, 2008; World Health Organization, 2008). For example, the "Speak Up" initiative of The Joint Commission, started a number of years ago, offers brochures for patients that include instructions on how to participate in the prevention of medication errors, nosocomial infections, and other issues (TJC, 2008).

Why Patient Engagement?

Schwappach (2008) noted that there are a number of reasons why patient engagement is a valid approach to increasing patient safety and quality of care. Patient engagement can lead to better health outcomes, save costs, and increase quality and safety (Charmel & Frampton, 2008; Epstein & Street, 2008). For example, patient and family engagement facilitates the transition from acute care hospitals to home or other settings. Currently, patients and their families leave the acute care hospital ill-prepared to carry out the required care, and as a result, the patient is often readmitted.

Another key reason for patient involvement, as Unruh and Pratt (2006) point out, is that patients are the only ones who are physically present during all aspects of treatment and care; thus, they are an essential resource because they have significant contextualized information about their specific care (Unruh & Pratt, 2006). It has been noted that many patients prefer to be involved in their own care (Davis, Jacklin, Sevdalis, & Vincent, 2007). Lyons points out that patients are highly motivated to decrease the risk of harm and ensure good outcomes (2007).

A review of the existing literature on patient involvement and safety in health care reveals correlating themes to this new field, highlighting key challenges. (Sutton, Eborall, & Martin, 2014). Insights from the wider literature illuminate key issues for involvement in patient safety and suggest promising ways to circumvent these challenges and achieve involvement in patient safety in a way that maximizes impact while avoiding unintended consequences.

Many safety problems occur at the point of delivery or at the frontline (e.g., hand washing, medication administration, ambulation, etc.). Due to this fact, they are observable by the patient and their families. Patients are potentially capable of recognizing that wrong medications or wrong doses are being given, or that devices such as infusion pumps are malfunctioning (Muller, 2003; Schulmeister, 1999). Patients experience the same procedures repeatedly and observe the treatments and actions of the providers. For example, patients detect drugs and doses that do not match their experience at home or that deviate from one medication administration to the next. They also can determine when infusion pumps are not working appropriately (Muller, 2003; Schulmeister, 1999). They notice deviations from routines, and at times, they act to avoid harm (Hurst, 2001; Unruh & Pratt, 2006).

Levels of Engagement

According to an American Institutes for Research framework, there are three patient engagement levels. In the first level, patients engage in their own care, while in the second level, patients actively give providers their input. The third level refers to instances when patients work to improve the care delivery at the institutional and regulatory levels (Carman et al., 2013).

Patient and Family as Team Members

Making the patient a part of the healthcare team is a critical ingredient to patient engagement. As Martin and Finn (2011) note, "increasingly policy encourages partnerships between users and professionals" (p. 1050). Salas, Wilson, Murphy, King, and Baker (2007) emphasized that team training in health care will not work if the patient is not a part of the team. Patient and family engagement requires motivating and empowering patients to work with providers and be active participants in their care. One of the greatest challenges associated with this change is transitioning from viewing patients and families as passive recipients of care to active and engaged partners at all levels of care and decision-making. Patients (and families) can help make their healthcare experience safer by becoming active, involved, and informed members of the team.

What Does Patient Engagement Achieve?

Although there has been limited research to date to answer the question "Can patients improve their own safety and quality of care?" a number of researchers have studied the subject and have reported promising results. Weingart and colleagues discovered that patient engagement in their own care reduced the risk of errors (2007a). Others have found that patients can help reduce medical errors by informing providers about their medical histories, drug allergies, and side effects as well as lapses in care that may have led to an adverse event (Basch et al., 2005; Beckjord et al., 2007; Friedman, Provan, Moore, & Hanneman, 2008; Wald et al., 2004; Wasson, MacKenzie, & Hall, 2007; Weingart et al.,

2005a, 2008; Weingart, Rind, Tofias, & Sands, 2006). It has also been demonstrated that patient engagement can foster collaboration and empowerment, and in turn, enhance patients' ratings of the quality of their care (Greenfield, Kaplan, & Ware, 1985; Hibbord, Mahoney, Stock, & Tusler, 2007; Taylor et al. 2008).

Providing patients with complete information and involving them in their care can serve not only as an important safeguard against errors, but also as an expression of providers' commitment to ensuring patients' safety and a demonstration of their respect for patients (Entwistle & Quick, 2006). Failing to meet such expectations, then, would have the potential to erode patients' trust in their providers. A review of studies showed that self-efficacy, preventability of incidents, and effectiveness of actions seem to be central to patients' intention to engage in error prevention. Patient engagement is necessary for successful transitions home and to avoid readmissions. If patients and families are not prepared to care for themselves after discharge, the likelihood of readmission is much higher. Currently, 20% of patients are readmitted, costing Medicare $26 billion annually with more than $17 billion paying for unnecessary readmissions. Since CMS penalizes hospitals for high readmission rates, this also impacts the financial status of the hospitals. Of course, not all readmissions are due to a lack of patient and family engagement, but case studies and other reports suggest that it is a substantial causative factor.

Transparency and Patient Voice

Two essential ingredients for successful patient/family engagement are transparency and the patient's voice. Transparency functions in such a way that it is easy for others to see what actions are performed. It has been defined simply as "the perceived quality of intentionally shared information from a sender" (Schnackenberg & Tomlinson, 2014). There are numerous examples in our current healthcare industry that point to a lack of transparency, including the cost of health care, the patient record, patient outcomes, the level of staffing, and others.

Once transparency is achieved, patients have to speak up regarding their healthcare treatment. In the book *The Empowered Patient*, the author urges patients to realize that there are times they have to advocate for themselves and their loved ones (Cohen, 2010). One of the key obstacles to patient involvement is that speaking up may be difficult for patients who are overwhelmed or confused by the healthcare milieu. Also, it can be hard to speak up if the caregiver is perceived as hurried, distracted, or ready to move to the next patient, or if their phone or pager is sounding frequently.

While patients are apprehensive or concerned about the safety of their care and are able to report adverse events (Agoritsas, Bovier, & Perneger, 2005; Schwappach, 2008; Weingart et al., 2005b; Weingart et al., 2007b), it does not mean that they are willing to engage in safety measures. Some patients already observe and intercept errors during their hospital stay without being explicitly told or educated to do so (Frey et al., in press; Kuo, Phillips, Graham, & Hickner, 2008; Parnes et al., 2007). Patients or family members who experience procedures repeatedly often monitor them, detecting deviations from routines and occasionally intervening to avoid harm (Hurst, 2001; Unruh & Pratt, 2006). Schwappach (2010) completed a systematic review of engaging patients as "vigilant partners" in safety. He concluded that patients have a positive attitude about "engaging in their safety at a general level, but their intentions and actual behaviors vary considerably" (2010, p. 11).

Example: Patients' Role in Improving Hand Hygiene

New CMS payment rules penalize hospitals for preventable HAIs, which cost the industry nearly $30 billion per year and cause 100,000 patient deaths. However, studies have found that, without being prompted, hospital workers wash their hands as little as 20% of the time they spend with patients (Erasmus et al., 2010).

There are several examples of how, in an effort to decrease HIAs, hospitals are empowering patients to ask providers if they washed their hands. The Center for Disease Control (CDC) provided 16,000 copies of the video, "Hand Hygiene Saves Lives," a five-minute patient education tool emphasizing the importance of hand washing, to facilities nationwide for patients to view during their admission to the hospital. Showing patients a video on hand hygiene at the time of their admission dramatically increased instances of patients asking hospital employees to wash their hands and hospital employees complying with their requests (Allegranzi, Conway, Larson, & Pittet, 2014; Allegranzi et al., 2013). Other hospitals have seen success by displaying posters or having staff wear buttons that say, "Ask me if I've washed my hands" in the hopes of getting patients to feel comfortable. Interestingly, studies have shown that patients are more likely to ask nurses than physicians to wash their hands (Allegranzi et al., 2013; Sax, Uckay, Richet, Allegranzi, & Pittet, 2007; Davis, Koutantji,

& Vincent, 2008; Duncan, 2007; Duncanson & Pearson, 2005; Swift, Koepke, Ferrer, & Miranda, 2001).

Potential Negative Effect of Patient Engagement

Involving patients in their own care has the potential to erode trust and confuse relationships between healthcare staff and patients in a number of ways. Patients may feel that responsibility for their safety is being pushed toward them inappropriately (Entwistle & Quick, 2006). Patients may fear negative consequences if they fail to fulfill the recommended actions. Trust may be diminished if patients observe suboptimal care practices and have the skills and knowledge to evaluate them. There may also be circumstances in which patients' engagement may lead to risks (e.g., in emergency situations). The involvement of patients could also lure professionals into a false sense of safety, and other safety barriers may be relaxed (Lyons, 2007). Interventions to educate patients may also increase inequalities among patients (e.g., education, age, language, communication skills, etc.) (Johnstone & Kanitsaki, 2006). Finally, patient involvement may be costly and there may be more cost-effective alternatives to increase safety.

Strategies to Facilitate Patient Engagement

Methods of enhancing patient engagement include: liberal visitation; interdisciplinary rounds at the patient's bedside; including family members in rounds; permitting patients to access and write on their own healthcare records; change of shift report at the patients' bedside; putting a patient advocate on the care team; developing training programs and tools; creating patient councils; and involving patients and families in committee memberships.

Liberal Visitation

Controversy over hospital visitation has been seriously debated for a long time. Traditionally, visiting hours in hospitals have been restricted for several reasons: physiological stress, interference with the delivery of care by nurses and physicians, noise level, patients' rest is disturbed, a higher workload for nurses, and a greater risk of infection (Tang, Chung, Lin, & Wan, 2009). Tang and associates found that the measured values for all indoor air characteristics, except bacterial concentrations, were higher after patient visitation than before patient visitation. Berwick and Kotagal (2004), however, provide evidence that the impact on physiological stress and the interference to the delivery of care are not sustained by research. They conclude that restricting visiting in ICUs is "neither caring, compassionate, nor necessary" (Berwick & Kotagal, 2004). Roland, Russell, Richards, and Sullivan (2001) reviewed the literature and found that open visitation policies enhance patient and family satisfaction, and patients and families desire more open visitation policy (Kleinpell, 2008).

A national survey of nurses caring for acute myocardial infarction patients revealed that more hospitals have adopted open visitation policies (Carlson, Riegel, & Thomason, 1998). Studies have shown that nurses, however, rarely enforce restrictive visiting hours. A study of nurses' perceptions about open versus restricted visiting hours and the effects on the patient, the family, and the nurse, found that 70% of official visitation policies were restrictive; yet in practice, 78% of nurses were nonrestrictive in their visitation practices (Simon, Phillips, Badalamenti, Ohlert, & Krumberger, 1997). Restricted hours were perceived to decrease noise (83%) and promote patients' rest (85%). Open visitation practices were perceived to beneficially affect the patient (67%) and the patient's family (88%), and to decrease anxiety (64%). Perceptions of ideal visiting hours included restrictions on the number of visitors (75%), hours (57%), visits by children (55%), and duration of visits (54%), but no restrictions on visitation by immediate family members (60%). As evidenced by the data, the decisions made by nurses about visitation rights require complex judgment.

Interdisciplinary Rounds at the Patient's Bedside
In Chapter 9 (patient outcomes), we reviewed research studies that show how interdisciplinary rounds are beneficial for patient safety and quality of care. For example, one research team conducted a qualitative study that used team rounds to identify safety issues and identified 88 problems in 1,000 minutes of observations (Lamba, Linn, & Fletcher, 2014). Yet this is one of the most missed elements of patient care by nursing staff. Conducting these rounds at the bedside allows patients to learn about the plans for them and participate in the discussion (Rosen, Stenger, Bochkoris, Hannon, & Kwoh, 2009). This practice offers the potential to enhance transparency and patient engagement. Patients prefer to interact with the care team at the bedside (Lehmann, Brancati, Chen, Roter, & Dobs, 1997).

Another example is a study by Simon and colleagues (1997) on the effects of bedside case presentations on 20 patients. Blood pressure and pulse rate were monitored, and plasma norepinephrine concentrations were assessed. These measures indicated that the bedside presentation was not physiologically stressful. Scores on the

State-Trait Anxiety Inventory and interview results after rounds also suggested that patients did not find them psychologically stressful. Many patients felt the bedside rounds were supportive experiences that increased their knowledge of their illnesses, enabled them to see providers' concern for their well-being, and allowed them to ask questions (Simons, Baily, Zelis, & Zwillich, 1989).

Including Family Members in Rounds

Studies about family presence in patient rounds is one of the least studied issues in the patient-centered movement (Davidson et al., 2007). Most studies have been in intensive care, especially pediatric ICUs. Cypress conducted a review of studies and found only two were conducted in the adult ICU settings (Cypress, 2012). A study of hospitalized pediatric patients revealed that, when given the option to attend bedside rounds, 85% of parents did so (Muething, Kotagal, Schoteetker, Gonzalez del Ray, & DeWitt, 2007). Lewis and colleagues (1988) noted that participation in bedside rounds gives family members the opportunity to obtain valuable information and that these types of communication practices can positively impact patient outcomes. A quality improvement initiative permitting parents to be present at bedside rounds in a pediatric ICU found that this practice was perceived to be beneficial by physicians, nurses, and parents (Kleiberg, Davenport, & Freyenberger, 2006; Wanzer, Booth-Butterfield, & Gruber, 2004). A study surveying intensive care staff—physicians, nurses, allied health personnel, and managers—about their attitudes toward having family present during bedside rounds revealed that physicians and managers agreed with the practice but nurses disagreed. Over half of the respondents felt the presence of family members would prolong rounds, reduce the team's education, and restrict delivery of negative healthcare information (Santiago, Lazar, Jiang, & Burns, 2014).

Permitting Patients' Access and Ability to Write on Their Own Healthcare Records

Giving patients access to their records during hospitalization and in other care settings is another strategy to increase patient participation (Gladwin, 2007). The patient chart has traditionally been one of the most guarded (by providers) documents in health care. Most healthcare providers have objected even to sharing the written results of routine matters such as blood cholesterol testing. The traditional belief was that patients were not supposed to see their records, much less contribute to them. In some cases, this was viewed as helpful to patients. Keeping the truth from dying patients, for example, was seen as a kindness—as it sometimes still is. Even when the prognosis isn't so serious, physicians and nurses determine what to say and when to say it; many are uneasy about letting patients see what they consider to be sensitive narratives. While some healthcare organizations have created electronic portals through which patients can schedule appointments, email their healthcare providers, and see lab and other test results, the narrative notes made by physicians and nurses have remained secret.

Keeping the patient record from the patient's view can be seen as a power and control issue. Paternalism is the policy or practice in which people in positions of authority restrict the freedom and responsibilities of those subordinate to them; this is generally thought to be in the subordinates' best interest. Information is power. Transparency changes the power dynamics and can be very disturbing in the hierarchical healthcare culture.

There are several reasons why patients benefit from having access to their healthcare records. Often patients cannot remember what their physician and nurse told them but have no access to the written record to refresh their memory, such as what medications they are to take. Having access to their medical records would enable patients (and their families) to monitor accuracy and fill in clinically relevant gaps in information.

A national project called OpenNotes experimented with including patients in clinical communications about their own diagnoses and treatments, with the goal of engaging them as partners in achieving and sustaining health (Wielawski, 2014). The idea was to give all team members, including the patient, access to the same information. As mentioned previously, information is power, and giving patients their own information empowers them. It serves to engage them in their own health care.

One key problem that came up with the OpenNotes project was in regard to the quality and communicative value of physicians', nurses', and other providers' narrative notes. These notes vary considerably in terms of completeness, accuracy, and clarity; an observation that highlights the usefulness of sharing these documents with patients. This begets the questions, "Why are these records so varied?" and "What are the impacts of these records on quality of care and patient safety?" This movement has just begun and work is needed in many areas. Another concern is that the use of jargon and abbreviations inhibit the patient from understanding their record. This may result in a large number of questions from patients and may lead to a need for providers to write their narratives differently. Some fear it may require simplifying the record.

Change-of-shift Report at the Patient's Bedside

Change-of-shift report occurs when responsibility and accountability for the care of a patient is handed from one nurse to another. Change-of-shift report has typically taken place in a conference room and may be face-to-face or tape recorded. When this report is given away from the bedside, the opportunity to visualize the patient and include the patient and family in the interchange of information is lost (Tidwell et al., 2011). If the change-of-shift report is conducted at the bedside, it allows the patients and families an opportunity to hear and participate in the exchange of information. There are other benefits to the bedside report, including relationship building between staff members, increased patient satisfaction, a higher quality report, and that the patient becomes an additional resource in diagnosis and treatment (Anderson & Mangino, 2006; Griffin, 2010; Wakefield, Ragan, Brandt, & Tregnago, 2012).

Putting Patient Advocates on the Care Team

In Chapter 6, we reported that nursing care is missed less frequently in countries where it is the custom for family members to be in the hospital with their relatives and friends and participate in their care. In China, if a family member cannot be with the patient, then they hire someone to fill that role. How often have you had a nurse friend say they wouldn't go to the hospital without a friend or family member, preferably a nurse? The idea that patients need an advocate, similar to a doula in labor and delivery, is gaining support. Studies are needed to explore the feasibility of making family members a part of the care team.

Training Programs and Tools

Although the need for patient engagement has become increasingly clear, there are few tools that exist to support true engagement of patients and families in care delivery. However, there are growing numbers of training programs and tools being developed. The Sala Institute for Child and Family Centered Care at NYU Langone Medical Center has developed a training program to encourage and support patient engagement. The AHRQ Patient and Family Engagement module of the Comprehensive Unit-based Safety Program (CUSP) toolkit focuses on making sure patients and their family members understand what is happening during the hospital stay, that they are active participants in the patient's care, and that they are prepared for discharge (Agency for Healthcare Research and Quality, n.d.). The Institute for Patient- and Family-Centered Care has developed resources to assist patients and family members, providers, administrators, educators, researchers, and facility designers with engagement (Institute for Patient- and Family-Centered Care, 2013). The Visiting Nurse Association of America (VNAA) has posted materials on their website that can be used to foster engagement (VNAA, n.d.).

There are also advances in technology that help patients connect with their health care providers and health information. Meaningful-use objectives include engaging consumers, patients, and their families in their healthcare, and a growing number of patients and their families want to be electronically connected to their healthcare providers and information. Many stakeholders feel that the meaningful-use requirements are the foundation of their patient engagement movement. In Stage 1 of meaningful use, several objectives focus on patient engagement, including:

- Providing patients with an electronic copy of their health information, upon request;
- Providing patients with an electronic copy of their discharge instructions, upon request;
- Sending reminders to patients per patient preference for preventive/follow-up care; and
- Providing clinical summaries for patients for each office visit.

In Stage 2 of meaningful use, patient engagement requirements expand. One of the most widely discussed Stage 2 objectives is to provide more than 50% of patients with timely, online access to their health information, and have more than 5% of patients view, download, or transmit their health information to a third party. Additionally, patients must also have the ability to send a secure message through certified EHR technology to the care provider or team, and more than 5% of patients must send a message. Given the industry pushback on these measures in the proposed rule, CMS lowered thresholds in the final Stage 2 rule from 10% to 5%.

Patient Councils and Committee Memberships
A Patient/Family Advisory Council joins patients and families with members of the healthcare team to provide advice on methods of

enhancing the hospital experience. Patients and families are invited to serve on hospital committees to provide the customer viewpoints and ideas on improving quality and safety. They offer a perspective that has largely been ignored in health care. Patients and family members should also be invited to participate in other committees (West & Brown, n.d.).

Mass General launched its first Patient and Family Advisory Council more than 10 years ago to bring together patients, family members, and hospital staff in an ongoing effort to enhance the patient and family care experience (Massachusetts General Hospital, 2014). The Advisory Council at Johns Hopkins has provided input and feedback to the following initiatives: food service, patient portal, patient safety journal, interactive TV, patient ID process, patient satisfaction survey, and the new adult emergency department (Johns Hopkins Medicine, n.d.). The National Institute for Children's Health Quality (NICHQ) has developed guidelines for developing advisory committees in pediatric practices (NICHQ, 2014). At Mayo, One Voice Patient & Family Advisory Council gives voice to patients and their families in the design and operations of cardiovascular clinical services. They also have a newsletter written by and for patients. These are just a few examples.

Having patients and family members participate in advisory committees is beneficial for both patients and organizations. For organizations, it offers a way to receive and respond to consumers, to adopt policies and programs to meet the needs of the patients and families, and to enhance cooperation and partnership among the staff and patients. It can also strengthen the relationship between the organization and the community. For patients and families, this participation can lead to an enhanced understanding of and support for the organization. In addition, community members can gain skills relevant to patient care, such as listening and telling their own stories.

Summary

Patient engagement as a strategy to decease missed nursing care was the subject of this chapter. Positive outcomes and barriers to patient engagement, along with specific strategies to overcome these issues, are described. These include: liberal visitation, interdisciplinary rounds at the patient's bedside, including family members in rounds, providing patients with access to and the ability to write on their own healthcare record, performing the change-of-shift report at the patient's bedside, putting patient advocates on the care team, developing training programs and tools, creating patient councils, and involving patients and families in healthcare organization committee memberships.

References

Agency for Healthcare Research and Quality. (n.d.). The comprehensive unit-based safety program (CUSP) toolkit. Retrieved from http://www.ahrq.gov/professionals/education/curriculum-tools/cusptoolkit/index.html

Agoritsas, T., Bovier, P. A., & Perneger, T. V. (2005). Patient reports of undesirable events during hospitalization. *Journal of General Internal Medicine, 20*(10), 922–928.

Allegranzi, B., Conway, L., Larson, E., & Pittet, D. (2014). Status of the implementation of the World Health Organization multimodal hand hygiene strategy in the United States of America health care facilities. *American Journal of Infection Control, 42*(3), 224–230.

Allegranzi, B., Gayet-Ageron, A., Damani, N., Bengaly, L., McLaws, M. L., Moro, M. L, ... Pittet, D. (2013). Global implementation of WHO's multimodal strategy for improvement of hand hygiene: A quasi-experimental study. *The Lancet Infectious Diseases, 13*(10), 843–851.

Al-Shorbaji, N., & Geissbuhler, A. (2012). Establishing an evidence base for e-health: The proof is in the pudding. Bulletin of the World Health Organization. Retrieved from http://www.scielosp.org/scielo.php?pid=S0042-96862012000500002&script=sci_arttext

Anderson, C. D., & Mangino, R. R. (2006). Nurse shift report: Who says you can't talk in front of the patient? *Nursing Administration Quarterly, 30*(2), 112–122.

Basch, E., Artz, D., Dulko, D., Scher, K., Sabbatini, P., Hensley, ... Schrag, D. (2005). Patient online self-reporting of toxicity symptoms during chemotherapy. *Journal of Clinical Oncology, 23*(15), 3552–3561.

Beckjord, E. B., Finney Rutten, L. J., Squiers, L., Arora, N. K., Volckmann, L., Moser, R. P., & Hesse, B. W. (2007). Use of the internet to communicate with health care providers in the United States: Estimates from the 2003 and 2005 Health Information National Trends Surveys (HINTS). *Journal of Medical Internet Research, 9*(3), e20.

Berwick, D. M., & Kotagal, M. (2004). Restricted visiting hours in ICUs: Time to change. *Journal of the American Medical Association, 292*(6), 736–737.

Carlson, B., Riegel, B., & Thomason, T. (1998). Visitation: Policy versus practice. *Dimensions of Critical Care Nursing, 17*(1), 40–47.

Carman, K. L., Dardess, P., Maurer, M., Sofaer, S., Adams, K., Bechtel, C., & Sweeney, J. (2013). Patient and family engagement: A framework for understanding the elements and developing interventions and policies. *Health Affairs, 32*(2), 223–231.

Cohen, E. (2010). *The empowered patient: How to get the right diagnosis, buy the cheapest drugs, beat your insurance company, and get the best medical care every time.* New York: Ballantine Books.

Charmel, P. A., & Frampton, S. B. (2008). Building the business case for patient-centered care. *Healthcare Financial Management, 62*(3), 80–85.

Chase, D. (2012). Patient engagement is the blockbuster drug of the century. *Forbes: Pharma & Healthcare.* Retrieved from http://www.forbes.com/sites/davechase/2012/09/09/patient-engagement-is-the-blockbuster-drug-of-the-century/

Cypress, B. S. (2012). Family presence on rounds: A systematic review of literature. *Dimensions of Critical Care Nursing, 31*(1), 53–64.

Davidson, J. E., Powers, K., Hedayat, K. H., Tieszen, M., Kon, A. A., Shepard, E., ... Armstrong, D. (2007). Clinical practice guidelines for support of the family in the patient-centered intensive care unit: American College of Critical Care Medicine Task Force 2004-2005. *Critical Care Medicine, 35*(2), 605–622.

Davis, R. E., Jacklin, R., Sevdalis, N., & Vincent, C. A. (2007). Patient involvement in patient safety: What factors influence patient participation and engagement? *Health Expectations, 10*(3), 259–267.

Davis, R. E., Koutantji, M., & Vincent, C. A. (2008). How willing are patients to question healthcare staff on issues related to the quality and safety of their healthcare? *Quality and Safety in Health Care, 17*(2), 90–96.

Duncan, C. (2007). An exploratory study of patient's feelings about asking healthcare professionals to wash their hands. *Journal of Renal Care, 33,* 30–34.

Duncanson, V., & Pearson, L. S. (2005). A study of the factors affecting the likelihood of patients participating in a campaign to improve staff hand hygiene. *British Journal of Infection Control, 6,* 26–30

Entwistle, V. A., & Quick, O. (2006). Trust in the context of patient safety problems. *Journal of Health Organization and Management, 20*(5), 397–416.

Epstein, R. M., & Street, R. L. (2008). *Patient-centered care for the 21st century: Physicians' roles, health systems and patients' preferences.* Philadelphia, PA: American Board of Internal Medicine Foundation.

Erasmus, V., Daha, T. J., Brug, H., Richardus, J. H., Behrendt, M. D., Vos, M. C., & van Beeck, E. F. (2010). Systematic review of studies on compliance with hand hygiene guidelines in hospital care. *Infection Control and Hospital Epidemiology, 31*(3), 283–294.

Frey, B., Ersch, J., Bernet, V., Baenziger, O., Enderli, L., & Doell, C. (in press). Involvement of parents need to get published data in critical incidents in a neonatal-paediatric intensive care unit. *Quality and Safety in Health Care.*

Friedman, S. M., Provan, D., Moore, S., & Hanneman, K. (2008). Errors, near misses and adverse events in the emergency department: What can patients tell us? *Canadian Journal of Emergency Medicine, 10*(5), 421–427.

Gladwin, J. (2007). Giving patients open access to medical records would help nurses improve care. *Nursing Times, 103*(25), 14.

Greenfield, S., Kaplan, S., & Ware, J. E. (1985). Expanding patient involvement in care. Effects on patient outcomes. *Annals of Internal Medicine, 102*(4), 520–528.

Griffin, T. (2010). Bringing change-of-shift report to the bedside: A patient- and family-centered approach. *The Journal of Perinatal & Neonatal Nursing, 24*(4), 348–353.

Hibbard, J. H., Mahoney, E. R., Stock, R., & Tusler, M. (2007). Do increases in patient activation result in improved self-management behaviors? *Health Services Research, 42*(4); 1443–1463.

Hurst, I. (2001). Vigilant watching over: Mothers' actions to safeguard their premature babies in the newborn intensive care nursery. *Journal of Perinatal & Neonatal Nursing, 15*(3), 39–57.

Institute for Patient- and Family-Centered Care. (2013). Tools for change. Retrieved from http://www.ipfcc.org/tools/index.html

Institute of Medicine. (2011). *Patients charting the course: Citizen engagement in the learning health system—Workshop summary.* Washington, DC: National Academies Press.

Johns Hopkins Medicine. (n.d.). Patient and family advisory council. Retrieved from http://www.hopkinsmedicine.org/the_johns_hopkins_hospital/about/patient_family_advisory_council/index.html

Johnstone, M. J., & Kanitsaki, O. (2006). Culture, language, and patient safety: Making the link. *International Journal for Quality in Health Care, 18*(5), 383–388.

Kleiberg, C., Davenport, T., & Freyenberger, B. (2006). Open bedside rounds for families with children in pediatric intensive care units. *American Journal of Critical Care, 15*(5), 492–496.

Kleinpell, R. M. (2008). Visiting hours in the intensive care unit: More evidence that open visitation is beneficial. *Critical Care Medicine, 36*(1), 334–335.

Kuo, G. M., Phillips, R. L., Graham, D., & Hickner, J. M. (2008). Medication errors reported by US family physicians and their office staff. *Quality and Safety in Health Care, 17*(4), 286–290.

Lamba, A. R., Linn, K., & Fletcher, K. E. (2014). Identifying patient safety problems during team rounds: An ethnographic study. *BMJ Quality & Safety, 23*(8), 667–669.

Lehmann, L. S., Brancati, F. L., Chen, M. C., Roter, D., & Dobs, A. S. (1997). The effect of bedside case presentations on patients' perceptions of their medical care. *New England Journal of Medicine, 336*(16), 1150–1155.

Lewis, C., Knopf, D., Chastain-Lorber, K., Ablin, A., Zoger, S., Matthay, K., ... Pantell, R. (1988). Patient, parent, and physician perspectives on pediatric oncology rounds. *The Journal of Pediatrics, 112*(3), 378–384.

Longtin, Y., Sax, H., Leape, L. L., Sheridan, S. E., Donaldson, L., & Pittet, D. (2010). Patient participation: Current knowledge and applicability to patient safety. *Mayo Clinic Proceedings, 85*(1), 53–62.

Lyons, M. (2007). Should patients have a role in patient safety? A safety engineering view. *Quality and Safety in Health Care, 16,* 140–142.

Martin, G. P., & Finn, R. (2011). Patients as team members: opportunities, challenges and paradoxes of including patients in multi-professional healthcare teams. *Sociology of Health & Illness, 33*(7), 1050–1065.

Massachusetts General Hospital. (2014). Patient and family advisory councils. Retrieved from http://www.massgeneral.org/patientadvisorycouncils/

Muething, S. E., Kotagal, U. R., Schoteetker, P. J., Gonzalez del Ray, J., & DeWitt, T. G. (2007). Family-centered bedside rounds: A new approach to patient care and teaching. *Pediatrics, 119*(4), 829–832.

Muller, T. (2003). Typical medication errors in oncology: Analysis and prevention strategies. *Onkologie, 26*(6), 539–544.

National Institute for Children's Health Quality. (2014). *Creating a patient and family advisory council: A toolkit for pediatric patients.* Retrieved from http://www.nichq.org/sitecore/content/medical-home/medical-home/resources/pfac-toolkit

Parnes, B., Fernald, D., Quintela, J., Raya-Guerra, R., Westfall, J., Harris, D., & Pace, W. (2007). Stopping the error cascade: A report on ameliorators from the ASIPS collaborative. *Quality and Safety in Health Care, 16*(1), 12–16.

Perneger, T. (2008). The Council of Europe recommendation Rec(2006)7 on management of patient safety and prevention of adverse events in health care. *International Journal for Quality in Health Care, 20*(5), 305–307.

Rodak, S. (2013). AHA report: Patient engagement is the key to triple aim of health reform. *Becker's Infection Control & Clinical Quality.* Retrieved from http://www.beckershospitalreview.com/quality/aha-report-patient-engagement-is-key-to-triple-aim-of-health-reform.html

Roland, P., Russell, J., Richards, K. C., & Sullivan, S. C. (2001). Visitation in critical care: Processes and outcomes of a performance improvement initiative. *Journal of Nursing Care Quality, 15*(2), 18–26.

Rosen, P., Stenger, E., Bochkoris, M., Hannon, M. J., & Kwoh, C. K. (2009). Family-centered multidisciplinary rounds enhance the team approach in pediatrics. *Pediatrics, 123*(4), e603–e608.

Salas, E., Wilson, K. A., Murphy, C. E., King, H., & Baker, D. (2007). What crew resource management training will not do for patient safety: Unless.... *Journal of Patient Safety, 3*(2), 62–64.

Santiago, C., Lazar, L., Jiang, D., & Burns, K. E. (2014). A survey of the attitudes and perceptions of multidisciplinary team members towards family presence at bedside rounds in the intensive care unit. *Intensive & Critical Care Nursing, 30*(1), 13–21.

Sax, H., Uckay, I., Richet, H., Allegranzi, B., & Pittet, D. (2007). Determinants of good adherence to hand hygiene among healthcare workers who have extensive exposure to hand hygiene campaigns. *Infection Control and Hospital Epidemiology, 28*, 1267–1274.

Schnackenberg, A. K., & Tomlinson, E. C. (2014). Organizational transparency: A new perspective on managing trust in organization-stakeholder relationships. *Journal of Manangement.* Advance online publication. doi:10.1177/0149206314525202

Schulmeister, L. (1999). Chemotherapy medication errors: Descriptions, severity, and contributing factors. *Oncology Nursing Forum, 26*(6), 1033–1042.

Schwappach, D. L. (2008). "Against the silence": Development and first results of a patient survey to assess experiences of safety-related events in hospital. *BMC Health Services Research, 8*, 59.

Schwappach, D. L. (2010). Review: Engaging patients as vigilant partners in safety: A systematic review. *Medical Care Research and Review, 67*(2), 119–148.

Simon, S. K., Phillips, K., Badalamenti, S., Ohlert, J., & Krumberger, J. (1997). Current practices regarding visitation policies in critical care units. *American Journal of Critical Care, 6*(3), 210–217.

Simons, R. J., Baily, R. G., Zelis, R., & Zwillich, C. W. (1989). The physiologic and psychological effects of the bedside presentation. *New England Journal of Medicine, 321*(18), 1273–1275.

Sutton, E., Eborall, H., & Martin, G. (2014). Patient involvement in patient safety: Current experiences, insights from the wider literature, promising opportunities? *Public Management Review.* Advance online publication. doi: 10.1080/14719037.2014.881538

Swift, E. K., Koepke, C. P., Ferrer, J. A., & Miranda, D. (2001). Preventing medical errors: Communicating a role for Medicare beneficiaries. *Health Care Financing Review, 23,* 77–85.

Tang, C. S., Chung, F. F., Lin, M. C., & Wan, G. H. (2009). Impact of patient visiting activities on indoor climate in a medical intensive care unit: A 1-year longitudinal study. *American Journal of Infection Control, 37*(3), 183–188.

Taylor, B. B., Marcantonio, E. R., Pagovich, O., Carbo, A., Bergmann, M., Davis, R. B., ... Weingart, S. N. (2008). Do medical inpatients who report poor service quality experience more adverse events and medical errors? *Medical Care, 46*(2), 224–228.

The Joint Commission. (2008). Speak up initiatives. Retrieved from http://www.jointcommission.org/speakup.aspx

Tidwell, T., Edwards, J., Snider, E., Lindsey, C., Reed, A., Scroggins, I., ... Brigance, J. (2011). A nursing pilot study on bedside reporting to promote best practice and patient/family-centered care. *The Journal of Neuroscience Nursing, 43*(4), e1–e5.

Unruh, K. T., & Pratt, W. (2006). Patients as actors: The patient's role in detecting, preventing, and recovering from medical errors. *International Journal of Medical Informatics, 7*(Suppl. 1), S236–S244.

VNAA. (n.d.). Training programs: Patient education. Retrieved from http://vnaablueprint.org/PatientEngagementTraining.html

Wakefield, D. S., Ragan, R., Brandt, J., & Tregnago, M. (2012). Making the transition to nursing bedside shift reports. *The Joint Commission Journal on Quality and Patient Safety, 38*(6), 243–253.

Wald, J. S., Middleton, B., Bloom, A., Walmsley, D., Gleason, M., Nelson, E., ... Bates, D. W. (2004). A patient-controlled journal for an electronic medical record: Issues and challenges. *Studies in Health Technologies and Informatics, 107*(Pt 2), 1166–1170.

Wanzer, M. B., Booth-Butterfield, M., & Gruber, K. (2004). Perceptions of healthcare providers' communication: Relationships between patient-centered communication and satisfaction. *Health Communication, 16*(3), 363–383.

Wasson, J. H., MacKenzie, T. A., & Hall, M. (2007). Patients use an internet technology to report when things go wrong. *Quality & Safety in Health Care, 16*(3), 213–215.

Weingart, S. N., Cleary, A., Seger, A., Eng, T. K., Saadeh, M., Gross, A., & Shulman, L. N. (2007a). Medication reconciliation in ambulatory oncology. *The Joint Commission Journal on Quality and Patient Safety, 33*(12), 750–757.

Weingart, S. N., Gandhi, T. K., Seger, A. C., Seger, D. L., Borus, J., Burdick, E., ... Bates, D. W. (2005a). Patient-reported medication symptoms in primary care. *Archives of Internal Medicine, 165*(2), 234–240.

Weingart, S. N., Hamrick, H. E., Tutkus, S., Carbo, A., Sands, D. Z., Tess, A., ... Phillips, R. S. (2008). Medication safety messages for patients via the web portal: The MedCheck intervention. *International Journal of Medical Informatics, 77*(3), 161–168.

Weingart, S. N., Pagovich, O., Sands, D. Z., Li, J. M., Aronson, M. D., Davis, R. B., ... Phillips, R. S. (2005b). What can hospitalized patients tell us about adverse events? Learning from patient-reported incidents. *Journal of General Internal Medicine, 20*, 830–836.

Weingart, S. N., Price, J., Duncombe, D., Connor, M., Sommer, K., Conley, K. A., ... Ponte, P. R. (2007b). Patient reported safety and quality of care in outpatient oncology. *The Joint Commission Journal on Quality and Patient Safety, 33*(2), 83–94.

Weingart, S. N., Rind, D., Tofias, Z., & Sands, D. Z. (2006). Who uses the patient internet portal? The PatientSite experience. *Journal of the American Medical Informatics Association, 13*(1), 91–95.

Weingart, S. N., Toth, M., Eneman, J., Aronson, M. D., Sands, D. Z., Ship, A. N., ... Phillips, R. S. (2004). Lessons from a patient partnership intervention to prevent adverse drug events. *International Journal for Quality in Health Care, 16*(6), 499–507.

West, M., & Brown, L. (N d.). *A tool kit for creating a patient and family advisory council.* JBC Healthcare. Retrieved from http://www.theberylinstitute.org/resource/resmgr/webinar_pdf/pfac_toolkit_shared_version.pdf

Wielawski, I. M. (2014). OpenNotes: Putting medical record transparency to the test. In S. L. Isaacs & D. C. Colby (Eds.), *To improve health and health care* (Vol. XVI). San Francisco, CA: Robert Wood Johnson Foundation/Jossey-Bass.

Wilkin, S. (2012). Patient engagement is the holy grail of health care. *KevinMD.com.* Retrieved from http://www.kevinmd.com/blog/2012/01/patient-engagement-holy-grail-health-care.html

World Health Organization. (2005). *The World Alliance for Patient Safety: Global patient safety challenge 2005–2006. Clean care is safer care.* Retrieved from http://www.who.int/patientsafety/events/05/GPSC_Launch_ENGLISH_FINAL.pdf

World Health Organization. (2008). *World Alliance for Patient Safety Forward Programme 2008–2009.* Retrieved from http://www.who.int/patientsafety/information_centre/reports/Alliance_Forward_Programme_2008.pdf

— 16 —

Technology Strategies

by
Ron Piscotty, PhD, RN-BC

The purpose of this chapter is to provide a description of information technologies that could be used to decrease missed nursing care. There has been scant research into how technology can reduce missed nursing care in general, but there are strategies such as reminders and checklists that have been used to remind nurses to provide required nursing care (Chen et al., 2013; Hatler, Hebden, Kaler, & Zack, 2010; Huang et al., 2004). While these reminders have been mainly paper-based, there is a movement in the United States to utilize electronic documentation systems with the elimination of paper systems to improve patient safety and quality (Healthy People 2020, 2015; Institute of Medicine [IOM], 1999, 2001, 2003, 2009).

The technologies explored in this chapter begin with existing technologies frequently found in the acute care setting. Experimental or novel technology that may be used to reduce missed nursing care is also presented.

The technologies reviewed in this chapter often contain, in some part, alarms, alerts, or reminders for the nurse that a care activity has been completed or needs to be completed. Alerts, alarms, and reminders are prevalent in the clinical setting and nurses may be prone to alert or alarm fatigue. Alert or alarm fatigue will be briefly discussed. While the focus of this chapter is on the use of technology to reduce missed nursing care, it is important to note that technology alone will neither solve nor prevent all errors in care. Thus, it is important to discuss the role of technology in quality improvement. This chapter will also present gaps in our current knowledge regarding the interaction between technologies and missed nursing care. Finally, future directions in the use of technology to decrease missed nursing care will be explored.

Why Technology?

It is hypothesized that an electronic system that has nursing reminders should result in decreased missed nursing care. In several studies, discussed in previous chapters, the major reasons for missing nursing care were found to be labor resources, material resources, and communication, in that order. In addition, several other reasons were uncovered and are presented in those chapters. In this chapter, the three major reasons for missing nursing care are examined to determine what technologies might assist to decrease missed nursing care. See Table 16.1 for a summary of technologies to address missed nursing care.

The primary reason for missed nursing care was related to nurse staffing adequacy, specifically labor resources (Gravlin & Bitner, 2010; Kalisch, 2009; Kalisch, Landstrom, & Williams, 2009; Lawless, Wan, & Zeng, 2010). The level and type of nurse staffing predicts the amount of missed nursing care (Kalisch, Tschannen, & Lee, 2011). There are many explanations for why inadequate staff results in more missed care (e.g., no time to provide all the care, teammates unavailable to assist in giving care, etc.). Another reason decreased staffing results in missed nursing care is its potential to increase distractions and interruptions.

Pape (2002) described a distraction as anything that diverts one's attention from achieving a desired goal. As discussed earlier in Chapter 4, the primary impact of distraction is the filling of working memory due to information overload or competing attention (Pape et al., 2005). Pape and colleagues (2005) stated that working memory is where temporary information is stored, and since distractions can impact working memory, they may result in a loss of concentration, leading to missed nursing care. Brixey and colleagues (2007) noted that interruptions in work settings such as aviation, nuclear power plants, and health care could result in catastrophic failures, including loss of life. Interruptions and distractions can have an impact on nurses' working memory. Unless

TABLE 16.1. **Summary of technologies to address missed nursing care.**

Missed nursing care item	Technological solution
Ambulation three times per day or as ordered	Worklist, order list, alert, reminder, mobile tracking devices
Turning patient every two hours	Pressure sensor system, alerts, reminders, worklist, order list
Feeding patient when the food is still warm	Barcode/Radiofrequency identification (RFID) to send alert
Setting up meals for patients who feed themselves	Barcode/Radiofrequency identification (RFID) to send alert, patient initiated requests/reminders
Medications administered within 30 minutes before or after scheduled time	EHR, electronic medication administration record, dashboard, alerts, reminders (particularly for medications that are due at atypical administration times)
Vital signs assessed as ordered	Worklist, order list, electronic flowsheet, alerts, reminders, dashboard, monitors that upload vital signs
Monitoring intake/output	Smart pumps, reminders, worklist, order list
Full documentation of all necessary data	EHR with standardized nursing documentation integrated with smart pumps and monitors
Patient education about illness, tests, and diagnostic studies	EHR, reminders, worklist, order list
Emotional support to patient and/or family	Reminder on worklist for provider to assess for needed support, patient-/family-initiated requests/reminders
Patient bathing/skin care	Reminder, worklist, order list
Mouth care	Reminder, worklist, order list
Hand washing	RFID, hand sanitizer sensors
Patient discharge planning and teaching	Reminder, worklist, order list
Bedside glucose monitoring as ordered	Reminder, worklist, order list, integrated with EHR for automatic documentation
Patient assessments performed each shift	Reminder, worklist, order list, dashboard
Focuses reassessments according to patient condition	EHR reminders based on previous assessments using clinical decision support (CDS), reminder, worklist, order list
IV/Central line site care and assessments according to hospital policy	CDS, worklist, order list, reminders
Response to call light is initiated within 5 minutes	Call-light system can escalate to text pager, smart phone, or personal communication device
PRN medication requests acted on within 15 minutes	Client-initiated request/reminders delivered to nurse, EMAR
Assess effectiveness of medications	Reminder in EHR, worklist, EMAR, order list
Attend interdisciplinary care conferences whenever held	Text messaging, personal communication device
Assist with toileting needs within 5 minutes of request	Text messaging, personal communication device
Skin/Wound care	CDS, worklist, order list, reminder

the nurse is reminded of the original task in some way, a nursing intervention may be missed. Nursing care reminders are an intervention to remind nurses of nursing care missed as a result of frequent interruptions in the clinical setting (Kalisch & Aebersold, 2010).

The second most common reason for missed care is material resources (Gravlin & Bitner, 2010; Kalisch, 2009; Kalisch et al., 2009, 2011). Specifically, missing equipment/supplies, medications, and equipment that is not functioning (Kalisch et al., 2009). In these cases, the nurse must wait for the delivery of the material resources or seek them out in another part of the facility. This is an interruption, which can result in forgetting to complete nursing care. Electronic reminders may be useful in addressing a lack of material resources as the nurse waits for the missing equipment, supplies, or medications to arrive. The reminder may serve as a cue that the activity or intervention needs to be completed.

The third most common reason for missed nursing care is communication and teamwork (Kalisch, 2009; Kalisch et al., 2011). This includes problems such as communication breakdowns and inadequate handoffs, among others. Electronic reminders may improve communication and teamwork and as such decrease the amount of missed nursing care. The reminder may serve to notify the nurse that a particular activity or intervention has not been completed.

Technology Solutions
Electronic Health Record
A common form of technology used within many acute care hospital organizations is the electronic health record or EHR. An EHR is defined as a digital version of the patient's health records (Office of the National Coordinator for Health Information Technology [ONC], n.d.). According to the ONC, EHRs:

- Contain a patient's medical history, diagnoses, medications, treatment plans, immunization dates, allergies, radiology images, and laboratory and test results;
- Allow access to evidence-based tools that providers can use to make decisions about a patient's care; and
- Automate and streamline provider workflow.

The EHR has many functions. The National Research Council (2003) listed eight core functions of the EHR:

1. Collection of health information and data
2. Result management

3. Order management
4. Decision support
5. Electronic communication and connectivity
6. Patient support
7. Administrative processes and reporting
8. Reporting and population health

The implementation of EHRs for all Americans by 2014 was a goal of the Bush Administration (White House, 2004). Under an executive order, ONC was established (White House, 2004). The charge of ONC is to coordinate the implementation of healthcare information technology (HIT) throughout the nation ("About ONC", n.d.). The push for all Americans to have EHRs was also a goal of the American Recovery and Reinvestment Act of 2009 that was signed into law by President Obama. The act allocated nearly 36 billion dollars for the increased implementation of HIT in the country (Healthcare Information Management and Systems Society [HIMSS], 2010). The act requires that eligible professionals and hospitals demonstrate meaningful use of HIT or face financial penalties starting in 2015 ("Are there penalties for providers who don't switch to electronic health records (EHR)?", n.d.).

Within the EHR there are several functions that may help to decrease the amount of missed nursing care. The functions would include CDS systems, nursing documentation, electronic medication administration record (EMAR), barcode medication administration (BCMA), order lists, worklists or queues, and dashboards.

Clinical decision support systems

Clinical decision support (CDS) systems are a form of technology used within the electronic health record and are also available as standalone systems. These systems typically utilize reminders, prompts, and/or alerts to decrease missed nursing care. These reminders, prompts, or alerts are based on algorithms that analyze data that is entered into the electronic health record. When certain data is entered, an alert, alarm, or reminder is triggered. The alert can be delivered to the nurse in a variety of ways using technology. The most common is an alert or reminder in the EHR, but the alert or reminders can also be sent to pagers and smart phones via text messaging. The alerts or reminders are often integrated into other applications of the EHR such as nursing documentation, EMAR, BCMA, and dashboards, discussed in the following paragraphs.

Structured nursing documentation in EHR
The EHR typically includes structured nursing documentation. The documentation by the nurse in the EHR is usually standardized. A benefit of structured nursing documentation is a more complete record (Li & Korniewicz, 2013). One of the commonly missed nursing care activities is incomplete documentation; structured nursing documentation in the EHR may improve documentation completion. The structured documentation in EHRs requires the nurse to document key components of the patients' current condition. Standardized drop-down lists allow all nurses to document using the same terminology. Also, based on the nurses' documentation, additional fields may become available for the nurse to document. For example, if a nurse is documenting a pain assessment and indicates that the patient is in pain, a complete pain assessment would need to be completed. Additionally, within the EHR there are required sections of documentation that must be addressed before the nurse can move on to the next section of documentation. The EHR also allows for the longitudinal documentation of patient education (Hebda & Czar, 2013). Documentation prompts built into the EHR may decrease missed patient education. Also, having a longitudinal patient education record reduces redundancy and unnecessary effort by nurses.

Electronic medication administration record, barcoding, and automated dispensing cabinets
Although dose omissions that are considered adverse drug events are rare (Coleman, McDowell, & Ferner, 2012), the electronic medication administration record (EMAR) contained within the EHR may help reduce the number of missed or delayed medications. The EMAR contains both a complete list of medications that the patient has been prescribed via computerized provider order entry (CPOE) during their visit, as well as a means for documenting and viewing the administration of medications. The EMAR can be sorted into various displays that list only currently active medication orders, discontinued medication orders, or all medication orders since admission. The EMAR may also contain visual or textual cues that may alert the nurse that a medication is due or past due (Coleman et al., 2012). The EMAR may interact with other applications in the EHR such as worklists and dashboards (discussed below) to display medications due or past due. The EMAR may also prevent errors of commission as the EMAR readily displays drug-to-drug interactions, duplicate drug orders, contraindicated drugs, and allergy warnings (Coleman et al., 2012).

Barcoding is another form of technology that is becoming the norm in the acute care setting. It is typically used with the electronic medication administration record found within the EHR and is called barcode medication administration or BCMA. Barcode medication administration is defined as the use of a barcode scanner to document the administration of prescribed medications. Functions of BCMA are to ensure that the five "rights" of medication administration are completed, including the right person, drug, dose, route, and time. The basic steps in administering medication with BCMA require the nurse to scan the patient's identification band with a barcode reader and then the medication (Voshell, Piscotty, Lawrence, & Targoz, 2013). The person, drug, dose, route, and time must match what is listed in the EHR or an alert will be displayed that the nurse must then address (Voshell et al., 2013). An example of how BCMA can prevent missed nursing care is that some medications may require multiple pills. The dosage of a drug may be 800 mg but only comes in a 400 mg form. If only one pill is administered, the patient would have an omission of care, as they did not receive the proper dosage of medication. BCMA prevents this by notifying the nurse that the proper dosage has not been scanned. BCMA may also improve surveillance and decrease errors of commission as part of a closed-loop medication administration system. The system easily identifies drug-to-drug interactions, contraindicated drugs, wrong drug or dose, or wrong patient, which are then communicated to the nurse via the EHR.

Automated dispensing cabinets are common in the acute care setting. The cabinets contain and dispense patient medications and often are located in a secure centralized location on the nursing unit. The cabinets can be freestanding or they may be interfaced with a pharmacy management system and/or the EHR. One example of these cabinets is the Pyxis MedStation. The Pyxis MedStation contains patient medications that have been ordered by a prescriber. The station requires the nurse enter a username and passcode (Hammer, 2009) or may contain biometric identification such as fingerprint scanning to access the medications. The nurse then selects the patient from a screen. Once the patient is selected, a medication profile is populated to show which medications have been ordered for the patient. The nurse can then select the medication that they plan to administer from the cabinet. The availability of such a dispensing cabinet may have a significant impact on missed nursing care. If present, the nurse can readily access patient medications from the dispensing cabinet and will not need to wait for the pharmacy to deliver the medication (Stachowiak, 2013). Also, due to the integration with the EHR and pharmacy management system, the time to first dose may be improved due to improved notification and communications between prescribers, nurses, and pharmacists.

Stachowiak (2013) also notes that there are issues with automated dispensing cabinets that may disrupt nursing workflow. She notes that recommendations on the proper administration of medication require the nurse to access the cabinet, administer the medication to the patient, and then document the medication. The nurse would then go back to the cabinet and repeat the process for the remaining patients. Stachowiak (2013) estimated that this process takes a minimum of 15 minutes to complete per patient. Therefore, if a nurse has several patients, medications may not be administered on time, resulting in an omission of timely care. Stachowiak (2013) recommends that the workflow be changed to reflect the actual practice of nursing. An example would be to store medications in the patient rooms or offer a mobile dispensing cabinet.

Order list

The order list within the EHR provides a list of all patient care orders entered for a particular hospital visit. The order list thus may serve as a reminder to provide prescribed care and may aide in the reduction of missed nursing care. The list includes orders for medications, laboratory tests, radiological exams, ancillary services, and nursing care activities, among others. The order list is generated primarily from the computerized provider order entry (CPOE) but can be populated through documentation via the CDS. The order list, like the EMAR, can be customized to view all orders, active orders, or discontinued orders, among others. As with orders written on paper, the nurse is responsible for viewing the electronic order list to review entered orders to ensure they are appropriate and carried out in a timely manner. The order list also displays alerts or warnings related to medication prescribing and duplicate orders.

Worklists/queues and dashboards

Worklists/queues and dashboards are functions within the EHR that provide textual and visual indicators of required nursing activities that need to be completed. A worklist or queue is an electronic list that contains patient demographic information and all care orders (Lykowski & Mahoney, 2004). The worklist or queue provides textual indicators of required nursing activities that need to be completed.

Typically, it is a list of nursing care activities that have been ordered for each patient, each shift. When the nurse documents that the activity has been completed, it automatically falls off the list.

Dashboards are another form of technology in the EHR that provide more visual cues and summaries of patient status and care activities that need to be completed. Dashboards are digital visual displays of pertinent clinical and/or administrative data and information (Wells, 2009). Figure 16.1 is an example of a clinical dashboard developed for nursing staff in a Singapore Hospital. The visual displays can include different colors (such as red, yellow, and green) to indicate priority, icons to indicate an activity, or text messages. The number of new orders for patients, medications due, and patient length of stay can also be included in dashboard displays. The dashboard can be located within the EHR where the individual nurse views the information or it may be located on the nursing unit on large digital displays that can be seen by nursing staff or other healthcare providers. The dashboard is typically integrated with clinical systems such as the EHR (Tan, Hii, Chan, Sardul, & Mah, 2013; Wells, 2009). The data from the clinical system is then processed and displayed on the dashboard for users to view (Tan et al., 2013; Wells, 2009).

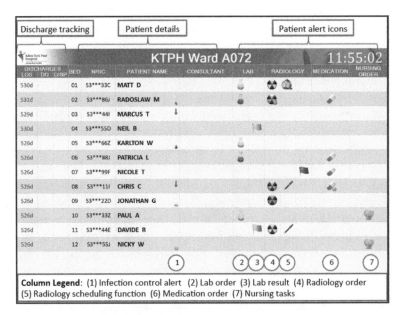

FIGURE 16.1. **Screenshot of the dashboard on a touch screen computer.**
Reproduced with permission from: Tan, Y., Hii, J., Chan, K., Sardual, R., & Mah, B. (2013).
An electronic dashboard to improve nursing care. Studies in Health Technology and
Informatics, 192, *109–194.*

Tan and colleagues (2013) conducted a survey study to examine nurses' perceptions regarding a clinical dashboard implemented in a Singapore Hospital. The dashboard, named "Andon System," was implemented in five wards and in the radiology department. The purpose of the dashboard was to alert nurses to STAT orders, abnormal results, and infection control alerts. The final sample included 106 nurses. The authors reported that 86% of the nurses reported using the dashboard each shift. The mean satisfaction score of the dashboard use was 3.6 out of 5 on a Likert-type scale with 1 = strongly disagree and 5 = strongly agree. The authors concluded that a well-designed clinical dashboard might result in improved quality of nursing care (Tan et al., 2013).

Coleman, Hodson, Brooks, and Rosser (2013) conducted a retrospective time-series analysis to determine if there were changes in overdue medication doses after implementing several interventions to address the problem. The intervention occurred over a 4-year period and included the implementation of a clinical dashboard indicating overdue or omitted doses and subsequent visual cues located in the EHR for doses of overdue medications (Coleman et al., 2013). With regard to the clinical dashboard, there was a significant reduction in the number of overdue medications, but unfortunately, this was not the case with the visual indicators (Coleman et al., 2013). The authors conclude that a clinical dashboard can decrease the amount of overdue or omitted medications (Coleman et al., 2013).

Electronic Reminders

Electronic nursing care reminders are a specific form of clinical decision support that was examined by Piscotty and Kalisch (2014) and Piscotty, Kalisch, Gracey-Thomas, and Yarandi (2015b) to determine if reminder usage was related to missed nursing care. In the descriptive studies, 165 and 124 nurses were surveyed regarding their nursing care reminder usage and missed nursing care (Piscotty & Kalisch, 2014; Piscotty et al., 2015b). A significant negative relationship was found between reminders and missed nursing care, indicating that nurses who reported using reminders more frequently described missing less nursing care (Piscotty & Kalisch, 2014; Piscotty et al., 2015b). Piscotty, Kalisch, and Gracey-Thomas (2015a) also examined the relationship between electronic reminders, the perceived impact of technology on practice, and their relationship to missed nursing care. It was discovered that nurses that rated technology as more supportive of their practice missed less care. This indicates that reminder usage combined with a positive perception of the use of HIT on practice results in a greater decrease in missed nursing care (Piscotty et al., 2015a).

Social Media

Social media use in the healthcare setting is increasing. Social media could be used to decrease missed nursing care by creating an online community for nurses on a nursing unit or hospital. The purpose of the group could be to post information regarding rates of missed nursing care, current strategies to reduce missed nursing care, and feedback from nurses and administrators. The main concern with creating such a group may be the fact that undesirable information regarding the amount of missed nursing care may be made public. The best option available would be to use a commercial social networking site such as Facebook and create a private group that cannot be accessed by the public. Only those invited by the group's leader could access and contribute to the site. Another option that is becoming more commonly available is internal Facebook-like pages that are hosted on an organization's intranet. The internal intranet option is not made available to the public and can only be viewed within the organization.

Individual Communication Devices

Phones, pagers, and other communication devices can be used to deliver reminders or alerts to nurses. The information is usually delivered in the form of a text message. The nurse can then view the message and act upon it. The information delivered by these devices can aid in reminding the nurse that a patient needs required care or has missed care that needs to be delivered, and aid in surveillance of abnormal vital signs and cardiac arrhythmias.

A form of this type of technology is the Vocera Communication Badge, which is an individual communication device that the nurse wears throughout the shift (Figure 16.2). Urgent alarms or information in the nurse's current location are communicated via the device. The nurse can follow up on the alarm by calling a physician, nurse practitioner, or other staff to investigate the urgent situation using the device. The individual communication devices could be used to decrease missed nursing care by integrating them with nurse call systems (discussed below), EHRs, and other technology systems ("Healthcare", n.d.). An example of use might be that a patient has requested pain medication by using the nurse call system. The nurse can then be notified via the personal communicator that the patient is

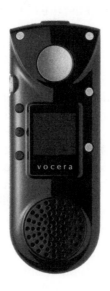

FIGURE 16.2. **Vocera Communication Badge.**
Reproduced with permission from Vocera Communications, Inc.

in need of medication. The nurse can then ensure that the medication is administered in a timely manner.

Nurse Call Systems

Nurse call systems have been found in acute care settings for many decades. These typically consist of a system that allows the patient to notify a central station that they require some type of assistance. Early systems included lighted indicators outside patient rooms to indicate to the nursing staff that a patient required assistance. Additionally, nurse call systems contained two-way communication between the patient's room and the nurses' station. An employee could connect directly to the patient room and inquire about the request. The staff member could then notify the appropriate individual to address the situation. New technology within nurse call systems allows a more dynamic communication system. Patients can be directly connected to their nurse. Also, the new systems are able to prioritize requests from patients (Blandford, Heindel, & McLaughlin, 2013). The systems also contain tracking software that can record how quickly a call is answered.

An example of the nurse call system is the Hill-Rom Nurse Communication System. Hammer (2009) describes that the nurse wears a badge locator. The nurse can then be located in either the central station or in each patient's room. The nurse can also communicate with the central station or another room. Hammer states that during focused interviews, the technology was viewed as potentially valuable, but not frequently put into use. Hammer concludes that the system needs to be used more frequently by nurses to be deemed effective.

Smart Pumps and Monitors

Smart pumps are intravenous pumps that have enhanced computerized technology to improve safety and quality of intravenous infusions (Harding, 2013; Jahansouz, Rafie, Chu, Lamott, & Atayee, 2013). Smart pumps may help to ensure accurate intake monitoring. Smart pumps may also directly interface with the EHR, and the appropriate volume for the infusions can then be automatically entered into the EHR and verified by the nurse. This would result in improved accuracy of intake of intravenous fluids and medications. Smart pumps also provide alerts regarding safe medication infusion. These alerts can aid in proper surveillance of the medication administration. An example might be that a medication must be infused over a certain period of time. The smart pump has a drug database or library that contains this information (Harding, 2013; Jahansouz et al., 2013). When the nurse scans the medication, the pump will notify the nurse if the rate of administration is within the normal parameters for that medication (Harding, 2013; Jahansouz et al., 2013).

Biomedical monitors such as vital sign machines and telemetry monitors are also a technology that could possibly decrease the amount of missed nursing care. Smart monitors often interface with the EHR. Data from these machines can be automatically uploaded into the EHR and verified for accuracy. This improves the accuracy and rate of documentation of these physiologic measures. Additionally, monitors often have built-in alarms. These alarms can be adjusted to individual patients. These alarms can alert the nurse of decreased or increased heart rate, apnea, or abnormal vital signs.

Mobile Technology

Mobile technology is being introduced in the acute care setting as it allows the nurse to conduct more aspects of care at the bedside. Reminders and alerts can be delivered to varying mobile devices. Popular mobile devices include smartphones and tablets. Increasingly, EHR vendors are developing applications that can be downloaded on a mobile technology device that allows access to patient records and even allows documentation of care via the EHR. Next generation mobile technology such as Google Glass, smart watches, and smart clothing are currently being developed and tested in the acute care setting.

Google Glass, for example, allows for information to be displayed in a non-distracting way via a small screen attached to the device. The Google Glass looks like, and is worn like, a traditional pair of glasses (Muensterer, Lacher, Zoeller, Bronstein, & Kubler, 2014). The Glass contains a central processing unit, touchpad, display screen, high-definition camera, microphone, bone-conduction transducer, and wireless connectivity (Muensterer et al., 2014). The screen provides a heads-up display of pertinent information to the wearer. This could be used to bring pertinent information regarding patient care or patient requests to the nurse. Glass also allows communication via voice command that would allow nurses to interact with other nurses or staff members. A demonstration of the Google Glass can be viewed at the following website: http://www.healthcare.philips.com/main/about/future-of-healthcare/.

The Google Glass is currently being piloted in the Emergency Department of Beth Israel Deaconess Medical Center (BIDMC) with physicians ("Emergency providers see big potential for Google Glass", 2014). The physicians are using the device to interact with the EHR to view patient information on the device as well as to page others for assistance ("Emergency providers see big potential for Google Glass", 2014).

Muensterer and colleagues (2014) conducted an exploratory study to determine the usefulness, advantages, and disadvantages of the Google Glass in a pediatric surgical practice. The Glass was found to be useful for photo and video documentation, making phone calls, and looking up billing codes and information on the Internet (Muensterer et al., 2014). Advantages were ease of use and comfort, while disadvantages were poor battery life, data security, and call quality (Muensterer et al., 2014). The authors conclude that while the Google Glass has useful features and is easy to use, it would need improved hardware reliability and data security features, and applications specific to the provider's workflow in order to be effective (Muensterer et al., 2014).

Another group of new devices on the market are smart watches. Like the Google Glass, smart watches contain a small screen that provides pertinent information to the wearer. The current versions of these watches have been developed to be an extension of smartphones. The smart watches can communicate with the smart phone, displaying text messages as well as making voice calls. Nurses can wear the smart watches and important patient information can be delivered to the device.

Smart clothing has been in development for many years. Smart clothing can contain communication devices, tracking devices such as radio frequency identification (RFID), or other type of sensors. The smart clothing could also be developed for both patients and nurses. An example might be the incorporation of a communication device and RFID that can be accessed by the nurse or others to communicate and track movements. Smart clothing technology may also be used to monitor physiologic measures of the patient such as heart rate, respirations, and cardiac rhythms. Abnormal or critical readings can then be communicated to the nurse to take action.

Technology has been designed to track and document patient activity, such as ambulation, using sensors and RFID. One company that has developed this technology is Tractivity. Tractivity has developed a wearable sensor and a corresponding tracking and reporting system (J. Watson, personal communication, April 29, 2014). Additionally, there is an array of activity-tracking sensors available on the market that monitor activity and could be used to track patient mobility. Activity-tracking devices come in the form of wearable watches or sensors that can be attached to clothing or the body. The devices include such brands as the Fit Bit, Nike FuelBand, and Jawbone UP. The devices can be used to monitor patient steps, stairs climbed, calories burned, and sleep patterns.

Biomedical Sensors
A variety of biomedical sensors exist to measure things such as pressure. Pressure sensors could be used with software to develop a patient turning system to decrease the incidence of pressure ulcers. An example of this is the MAP System developed by Wellsense ("Mattress sensing MAP System prevents pressure ulcers," 2013), in which the pressure sensors are able to determine the patient's last turn position and forecast the next position. The information is displayed in the patient's room at the bedside or to a device such as Google Glass to notify nursing staff that the patient needs to be turned ("Mattress sensing MAP System prevents pressure ulcers," 2013). Additionally, CDS could be deployed within the system to send alerts and reminders if it has been a significant time since the patient has been turned.

Currently, there are technologies available that can track hand hygiene in the acute care setting, two of which can determine the amount of cleanser and number of times the dispenser was accessed. The information can then be interpreted for trends in increased or decreased usage of cleanser (Sodre da Costa et al., 2013). A positive trend may or may not necessarily be a clear indication of improved hand hygiene as other factors such as an increase in patient census may cause an increase in use.

Combinations of technologies that incorporate sensors and RFID can track not only if the cleanser system was accessed, but also the employee that accessed it and their location at the time. The Hill-Rom Hand Hygiene Compliance Solution is one example (http://www.hill-rom.com/usa/Products/Category/Clinical-Workflow-Solutions/Hill-Rom-Hand-Hygiene-Compliance-Solution1). The sensor is typically attached to a cleanser dispenser, and can detect when the alcohol cleanser is used (Edmond et al., 2010). There are also devices that contain an RFID that can determine who is using the hand cleanser (Marra & Edmond, 2014). Employees each wear a badge that interacts with the RFID system, which then identifies who is using the cleanser device. The information can then be sent wirelessly to a display in the patient room that indicates if the employee has washed their hands and then serves as a visual reminder to the employee that hand hygiene has not been completed (Marra & Edmond, 2014). The information collected by the system can also be analyzed to determine employee compliance with hand hygiene.

Patient-centered Technology
Patient-initiated reminders or requests are another form of technology that could possibly be used to decrease missed nursing care. The technology puts the patient in charge of reporting certain aspects of health status including such things as pain levels or requests for medication. An example of this would be for a patient to document via a graphical user interface on their bedside display their pain score and desire for pain medications. This information would then be forwarded to the nurse via the EHR or other mobile technology such as a text pager or smart phone.

Another form of patient-centered technology is electronic or digital patient whiteboards. Many organizations currently utilize non-digital (traditional) whiteboards in patients' rooms to post information such as the date, name of nurse, name of provider, discharge date, and daily patient goals, all of which must be updated on a daily basis by using a dry-erase marker. Digital whiteboards, however, can be displayed on screens in the patient room, located on a wall within view of the patient or accessed via the patient's television monitor. One example that is currently available is The Interactive Patient Whiteboard by Getwellnetwork (http://www.getwellnetwork.com/solutions/tools/interactive-patient-whiteboard). The digital whiteboards can be updated via information interfaced with the EHR or changed at a central station each shift. As noted in Chapter 8 of this book, patients are able to recognize aspects of missed nursing care; therefore, including information that patients can report as missed on the digital whiteboard may decrease the amount of missed nursing care.

Technology and Quality Improvement

Implementing technology alone will not decrease errors. Technology must be implemented in organizations that have a culture with a focus on safety and redesigning workflow to improve quality of care (Brokel & Harrison, 2009; Byrne, 2013). Many issues arise with the adoption of technology in the healthcare setting. One is that the technology must either fit within the current workflow of the organization or the workflow needs to be redesigned in order to incorporate the technology into the future structure of the organization (Piscotty & Tzeng, 2011). Introducing technology with disregard to existing workflow can result in unintended consequences of technology implementation (Aarts, Ash, & Berg, 2007; Ash, 2007; Harrison, Koppel, & Bar-Lev, 2007). Although these consequences can be positive, many that have been identified have been negative and have likewise negatively impacted patient safety and quality of care.

Alert or Alarm Fatigue

Many of the technologies discussed in this chapter provide alerts, alarms, or reminders to nurses, but one of the negative effects of excessive or irrelevant alerts is something called alert or alarm fatigue. Alert or alarm fatigue can lead to providers ignoring all alerts, thus potentially missing one that could have prevented serious harm to a patient. The ability to customize these alarms has been limited by vendors and organizations in order to reduce liability (Kesselheim, Cresswell, Phansalkar, Bates, & Sheikh, 2011). Kesselheim and colleagues (2011) suggest through their analysis that modifications can be made to alerts and alarms that reduce or mitigate risk of litigation to these parties and actually decrease the burden on providers and limit related fatigue. The Joint Commission (2013) has also made alarm system safety one of the National Patient

Safety Goals. The national safety goals are to heighten organizational awareness of the risks associated with alarms and develop measures to mitigate those risks (TJC, 2013).

Gaps in Knowledge

The main gap in knowledge regarding technology and missed nursing care is that the efficacy of these technologies in reducing missed nursing care has not been established. A consequence of this lack of established efficacy is that it is not known which technologies successfully address specific aspects of missed nursing care and result in an improvement. Additional gaps relate to the lack of interoperability among technologies and to the lack of integration of new healthcare technologies with existing ones, such as the EHR. *Interoperability* refers to disparate technology systems that can work together and exchange data and information in a meaningful manner. A lack of *integration* leaves technology in silos and pertinent patient information is not shared among systems. A final gap is that many aspects of nursing care are not documented in either the paper record or the electronic record. One reason for this may be inconsistency of nursing documentation in using standardized nursing languages.

Future Directions and Research

As technology improvements and advancements continue, they will be implemented in the clinical setting at a rapid pace. Extensive research will be needed to determine the impact of these technologies on nursing practice, quality of care, and safety. Interoperability of HIT is a national priority, and as such, future technologies must be able to interact with each other to provide a seamless operating experience for the user. The national trend in consumer electronics is the movement from large, stationary computing devices to smaller mobile ones. This trend is also quickly becoming more common in the clinical setting. Many HIT vendors are heeding this trend by tying mobile applications that can be used on smart phones and tablets to their main product (e.g., EHRs). Nursing researchers need to start examining the impact that these novel devices can have on improving patient care by reducing the amount of missed nursing care. Without this research, nursing will continue to lag behind other healthcare professions that are already quickly embracing and experimenting with these devices in their practice settings.

References

Aarts, J., Ash, J., & Berg, M. (2007). Extending the understanding of computerized physician order entry: Implications for professional collaboration, workflow and quality of care. *International Journal of Medical Informatics, 76*(1), S4–S13.

About ONC. (n.d.). *HealthIT.gov:Newsroom.* Retrieved from http://www.healthit.gov/newsroom/about-onc

Are there penalties for providers who don't switch to electronic health records (EHR)? (n.d.). Retrieved from http://www.healthit.gov/providers-professionals/faqs/are-there-penalties-providers-who-don%E2%80%99t-switch-electronic-health-record

Ash, J. (2007). The extent and importance of unintended consequences related to computerized provider order entry. *Journal of the American Medical Informatics Association, 14*(4), 415–423.

Blandford, A., Heindel, J., & McLaughlin, M. (2013). New technology: A centralized nurse call system. *Nursing2013, 43*(3), 18–20.

Brixey, J., Robinson, D., Johnson, C., Johnson, T., Turely, J., & Zhang, J. (2007). A concept analysis of the phenomenon interruption. *Advances in Nursing Science, 30*(1), E26–E42.

Brokel, J., & Harrison, M. (2009). Redesigning care processes using an electronic health record: A system's experience. *The Joint Commission Journal on Quality and Patient Safety, 35*(2), 82–92.

Byrne, M. (2013). Redesign of electronic health records for perianesthesia nursing. *Journal of PeriAnesthesia Nursing, 28*(3), 163–168.

Chen, Y., Chi, M., Chen, Y., Chan, Y., Chou, S., & Wang, F. (2013). Using a criteria-based reminder to reduce use of indwelling urinary catheters and decrease urinary tract infections. *American Journal of Critical Care, 22*(2), 105–114.

Coleman, J., Hodson, J., Brooks, H., & Rosser, D. (2013). Missed medication doses in hospitalised patients: A descriptive account of quality improvement measure and time series analysis. *International Journal for Quality in Health Care, 25*(5), 564–572.

Coleman, J., McDowell, S., & Ferner, R. (2012). Dose omissions in hospitalized patients in a UK hospital: An analysis of the relative contribution of adverse drug reactions. (8), 677–683.

Edmond, M., Goodell, A., Zuelzer, W., Sanogo, K., Elam, K., & Bearman, G. (2010). Successful use of alcohol sensor technology to monitor and report hand hygiene compliance. *Journal of Hospital Infection, 76*(2010), 354–372.

Emergency providers see big potential for Google Glass. (2014). *ED Management.* Available from http://go.galegroup.com/ps/i.do?id=GALE%7CA364819131&v=2.1&u=lom_waynesu&it=r&p=AONE&sw=w&asid=e2b696455e8e840527da1557efc2ad32

Gravlin, G., & Bittner, N. (2010). Nurses' and nursing assistants' reports of missed care and delegation. *The Journal of Nursing Administration, 40*(7–8), 329–335.

Hammer, S. (2009). *The role of physical design and informal communication and learning in reducing stress and gaining competency among new nurse graduates* (Unpublished master's thesis). Cornell University, Ithica, NY.

Harding, A. (2013). Intravenous smart pumps. *Journal of Infusion Nursing, 36*(3), 191–194.

Harrison, M., Koppel, R., & Bar-Lev, S. (2007). Unintended consequences of information technologies in health care: An interactive sociotechnical analysis. *Journal of the American Medical Informatics Association, 14*(5), 542–549.

Hatler, C., Hebden, J., Kaler, W., & Zack, J. (2010). Walk the walk to reduce catheter-related bloodstream infections: Using evidenced-based practices, nurses can help prevent deadly infections linked to central venous catheters. *American Nurse Today, 5*(1), 26–30.

Healthcare. (n.d.). Retrieved from http://www.vocera.com/industry-solution/healthcare

Healthcare Information and Management Systems Society. (2010). *HIMSS health information exchange: ARRA HITECH FAQs related to HIE.* Retrieved from: http://www.himss.org/files/HIMSSorg/content/files/12_04_09_ARRAHITECHHIE_FactSheet.pdf

Healthy People 2020. (2015). Health communication and health information technology. Retrieved from http://www.healthypeople.gov/2020/topics-objectives/topic/health-communication-and-health-information-technology

Hebda, T., & Czar, P. (2013). *Handbook of informatics for nurses and healthcare professionals* (5th ed.). Upper Saddle River, NJ: Pearson Education Inc.

Huang, W., Wann, S., Lin, S., Kunin, C., Kung, M., Lin, C., ... Lin, T. (2004). Catheter-associated urinary tract infections in intensive care units can be reduced by prompting physicians to remove unnecessary catheters. *Infection Control and Hospital Epidemiology, 25*(11), 974–978.

Jahansouz, F., Rafie, S., Chu, F., Lamott, J., & Atayee, R. (2013). Impact of smart infusion pump implementation on intravenous patient-controlled analgesia medication errors. *California Journal of Health-System Pharmacy, 25*(5) 145–150.

The Joint Commission. (2013). Alarm system safety. R^3 *Report,* Issue 5. Retrieved from http://www.jointcommission.org/assets/1/18/R3_Report_Issue_5_12_2_13_Final.pdf

Institute of Medicine. (1999). *To err is human: Building a safer health system.* Washington, DC: National Academies Press.

Institute of Medicine. (2001). *Crossing the quality chasm: A new health system for the 21st Century.* Washington, DC: National Academies Press.

Institute of Medicine. (2003). *Keeping patients safe: Transforming the work environment of nurses.* Washington, DC: National Academies Press.

Institute of Medicine. (2009). *Interactive list of comparative effectiveness research (CER) areas.* Washington, DC: National Academies Press. Retrieved from http://www.iom.edu/en/Reports/2009/ComparativeEffectivenessResearchPriorities.aspx

Kalisch, B. (2009). Nurse and nurse assistant perceptions of missed nursing care: what does it tell us about teamwork? *The Journal of Nursing Administration, 39*(11), 485–493

Kalisch, B., & Aebersold, M. (2010). Interruptions and multitasking in nursing care. *The Joint Commission Journal of Quality and Patient Safety, 36*(3), 126–132.

Kalisch, B., Landstrom, G., & Williams, R. (2009). Missed nursing care: errors of omission. *Nursing Outlook, 57*(1), 3–9.

Kalisch, B., Tschannen, D., & Lee, K. (2011). Do staffing levels predict missed nursing care? *International Journal for Quality in Health Care, 23*(3), 302–308.

Kesselheim, A., Cresswell, K., Phansalkar, S., Bates, D., & Sheikh, A. (2011). Clinical decision support systems could be modified to reduce 'alert fatigue' while still minimizing the risk of litigation. *Health Affairs, 30*(12), 2310–2317.

Lawless, J., Wan, L., & Zeng, I. (2010). Patient care 'rationed' as nurses struggle under heavy workloads—survey. *Nursing New Zealand, 16*(7), 16–18.

Li, D., & Korniewicz, D. (2013). Determination of the effectiveness of electronic health records to document pressure ulcers. *Medical-Surgical Nursing, 22*(1), 17–25.

Lykowski, G., & Mahoney, D. (2004). Computerized provider order entry improves workflow and outcomes. *Nursing Management, 35*(2), 40G–40H.

Marra, A., & Edmond, M. (2014). New technologies to monitor healthcare worker hand hygiene. *Clinical Microbiology and Infection, 20*, 29–33.

Mattress sensing MAP System prevents pressure ulcers. (2013). *MedGadget.* Retrieved from http://www.medgadget.com/2013/07/mattress-sensing-map-system-prevents-pressure-ulcers.html

Muensterer, O., Lacher, M., Zoeller, C., Bronstein, M., & Kubler, J. (2014). Google Glass in pediatric surgery: An exploratory study. *International Journal of Surgery, 12*(2014), 281–289.

National Research Council. (2003). *Key capabilities of an electronic health record system: Letter report.* Washington, DC: The National Academies Press.

Office of the National Coordinator for Health Information Technology. (n.d.). *What is an electronic health record (EHR)?* Retrieved from http://www.healthit.gov/providers-professionals/faqs/what-electronic-health-record-ehr

Pape, T. (2002). *The effect of nurses' use of a focused protocol to reduce distractions during medication administration* (Unpublished Doctoral dissertation). Texas Woman's University, Houston, TX.

Pape, T., Guerra, D., Muzquiz, M., Bryant, J., Ingram, M., Schranner, B., … Welker, J. (2005). Innovative approaches to reducing nurses' distractions during medication administration. *Journal of Continuing Education in Nursing, 36*(3), 108–116.

Piscotty, R., & Kalisch, B. (2014). The relationship between electronic nursing care reminders and missed nursing care. *Computers, Informatics, Nursing, 32*(10), 475–481.

Piscotty, R., Kalisch, B., & Gracey-Thomas, A. (2015a). Impact of healthcare information technology on nursing practice. *Journal of Nursing Scholarship, 47*(4), 287–293.

Piscotty, R., Kalisch, B., Gracey-Thomas, A., & Yarandi, H. (2015b). Electronic nursing care reminders: Implications for nurse leaders. *Journal of Nursing Administration, 45*(5), 239-242.

Piscotty, R., & Tzeng, H. (2011). Exploring the clinical information system implementation readiness activities to support nursing in hospital settings. *Computers, Informatics, Nursing, 29*(11), 648-565.

Sodre da Costa, L., Neves, V., Marra, A., Sampaio Camargo, T., Fatima dos Santos Cardoso, M., da Silva Victor, E., ... Edmond, M. (2013). Measuring hand hygiene compliance in a hematology-oncology unit: A comparative study of methodologies. *American Journal of Infection Control, 41*(2013), 997-1000.

Stachowiak, M. (2013). Automated dispensing cabinets: Curse or cure? *American Journal of Nursing, 113*(5), 11.

Tan, Y., Hii, J., Chan, K., Sardual, R., & Mah, B. (2013). An electronic dashboard to improve nursing care. *Studies in Health Technology and Informatics, 192*, 109-194.

Voshell, B., Piscotty, R., Lawrence, J., & Targosz, M. (2013). Barcode medication administration work-arounds: A systematic review and implications for nurse executives. *Journal of Nursing Administration, 43*(10), 530-535.

Wells, B. (2009). Developing clinical dashboards. *Computerworld, 43*(19), 28-31.

White House. (2004). Transforming health care: The President's health information technology plan. Retrieved from http://georgewbush-whitehouse. archives.gov/infocus/technology/economic_policy200404/chap3.html

Index